Fine Needle Aspiration
for the Clinician

Fine Needle Aspiration for the Clinician

Joseph A. Linsk, M.D.

Chief, Department of Hematology, Oncology
Associate Pathologist
Atlantic City Medical Center
Atlantic City, New Jersey
Associate Professor of Medicine
Hahnemann Medical School
Philadelphia, Pennsylvania

Sixten Franzen, M.D.

Director, Division of Cytology
Department of Tumor Pathology
Karolinska Hospital
Stockholm, Sweden

J. B. Lippincott Company

Philadelphia

London Mexico City New York
St. Louis São Paulo Sydney

Acquisitions Editor: Lisa A. Biello
Sponsoring Editor: Delois Patterson
Manuscript Editor: Virginia M. Barishek
Indexer: Angela Holt
Design Director: Tracy Baldwin
Designer/Coordinator: Charles W. Field
Production Supervisor: Kathleen Dunn
Production Coordinator: George V. Gordon
Compositor: Ruttle, Shaw & Wetherill, Inc.
Printer/Binder: The Murray Printing Company

6 5 4 3 2 1

Library of Congress Cataloging-in-Publication Data

Linsk, Joseph A.
    Fine needle aspiration for the clinician.

    Includes bibliographies and index.
    1. Biopsy, Needle. 2. Cancer—Diagnosis.
3. Diagnosis, Cytologic. I. Franzen, Sixten.
II. Title. [DNLM: 1. Biopsy, Needle. WB 379 L759f]
RC270.3.N44L56 1986   616.07'58   85-16051
ISBN 0-397-50678-3

The authors and publisher have exerted every effort to ensure that drug selection and
dosage set forth in this text are in accord with current recommendations and practice at
the time of publication. However, in view of ongoing research, changes in government
regulations, and the constant flow of information relating to drug therapy and drug
reactions, the reader is urged to check the package insert for each drug for any change
in indications and dosage and for added warnings and precautions. This is particularly
important when the recommended agent is a new or infrequently employed drug.

Preface

This book is an outgrowth of many years' experience in clinical medicine, particularly clinical oncology, during which the technique of fine needle aspiration has been applied diligently. From its inception, aspiration cytology has been the province of cytologists and cytopathologists without whom the securing of diagnostic material would have been an empty exercise. Out of this experience a number of books on cytopathology have been written, beginning with the pioneer work of J. Zajicek and including our previous own text on the subject.

To date no book has been written for the clinican. As a result there is a lack of interest, or more specifically, a lack of knowledge of fine needle aspiration as a clinical diagnostic tool. Clinicians reflexly reach for diagnostic help from radiography and laboratory. For nonpalpable or obscure disorders, imaging techniques are often necessary. However, for many clinical disorders the "target" is immediately evident or is discovered easily by the clinician relying on his physical senses. It is our perception that the basic exercise of medicine, namely defining the disease process, has been blunted by reliance on technology. Our experience as clinicians and cytologists has shown us that the application of this method, among its other salutary effects, heightens the clinical senses, resulting in quicker discovery of disease and quicker solutions of problems.

This book is concerned with a broad area of clinical medicine—namely, neoplastic and allied diseases—that in multiple guises, confronts the practicing physician daily.

The clinician does not have to become a cytologist to use fine needle aspiration any more than he must become a radiologist to order a CT scan.

If he will recognize the potential value of fine needle aspiration, learn where to apply it (just as he knows when to order an x-ray), and then with rapidly learned dexterity, do the aspiration, both he and the patient will be benefitted greatly. Cytologists and pathologists are standing by to rapidly interpret slides that are submitted.

This text will stress economy—of time, space, technology, patient anxiety, and money. It will to some extent offer a solution to part of the spiraling complexity and cost of modern medicine.

Joseph A. Linsk, M.D.
Sixten Franzen, M.D.

Contents

10. The Skeleton   282

11. Central Nervous System Lesions   299

Appendix: Case Panorama   308

Index   333

Acronyms

ABC   Aspiration biopsy cytology
NHL   Non-Hodgkin's lymphoma
L–H   Lymphocytic–histiocytic
FNA   Fine needle aspiration
CT   Computed tomography
IVP   Intravenous pyelogram

Introduction

Clinical medicine has played the role of reluctant lover to fine needle aspiration for several decades. Workers in the field of fine needle aspiration are beginning to sense a consummation of the marriage. The whole thrust of diagnostic medicine since the perfection of the physical examination has been toward acquiring data through clinical observations, morphology, measurements, and imaging techniques. In the past decade, high technology—which is delicate, complex, and expensive—has proliferated riotously to the same end: the acquisition of data to help reveal the diagnosis and prepare for the treatment. The application of this enormous outpouring of scientific effort to clinical problem solving[4] may have produced the negative effect of dulling the clinical sensibilities of practicing physicians. Reaching for the CT scan has become almost a reflex action. Many physicians working in hospitals are acutely aware that this kind of reflex unfortunately has replaced basic examination, including the laying on of hands.

This has compounded the difficulties of introducing fine needle aspiration into clinical diagnostic medicine. It is a clinical technique that requires a return to basics, including anatomy, both topographic and relational, histopathology and the basis of disease, and physical diagnosis. For nonpalpable pathologic disorders of the head, chest, and abdomen, the application of imaging techniques is necessary.

Perhaps one of the most gratifying and intellectually stimulating aspects of aspiration cytology, as Nils Söderström* emphasized, is the moment of surprise or gratification when the unexpected or anticipated smear appears on the microscope. Fitting it into the clinical pattern—the diagnostic formulary of the clinician and the dynamic pathology of the disease process—quickens and enriches the pleasure of clinical oncology and clinical medicine in general.

Finding cells that are out of place triggers a series of clinical questions:

What is the primary source?
By which route did the cells arrive at the target area?
Do they change the stage of the tumor?
Do they render the patient incurable?
What is the differential diagnosis of cells not clearly identified?
Do the cells arise from a current or previously existing known primary,
   or could they denote a second primary?

There is no more essential act than the direct examination of the cellular pathology since, to paraphrase Sutton's Law, "That's where the

* Personal communication.

disease is!'' Also of critical importance to the clinician is the axiom that an accurate rapid diagnosis increases the patient's confidence and strongly supports compliance to proposed therapy.

What Is Fine Needle Aspiration Cytology?

Fine needle aspiration cytology is a diagnostic tool that was introduced into clinical practice in 1930.[20] Although it has become widely accepted in the past two decades, it is still little known to the vast number of practicing clinicians for several reasons. With the exception of the Karolinska Institute in Stockholm where some lectures about fine needle aspiration cytology are given each year to medical students,* it has not to our knowledge been introduced formally into medical school curricula. With rare exceptions,† none of the approved pathology training programs in the United States has incorporated any formal teaching. None of the approved United States medical residency training programs is introducing trainees to the method. As a result, apart from a general awareness, practicing clinicians lack knowledge of the method and certainly are not using it.

Aspiration cytology is a diagnostic biopsy method in which cells and tissue fluid are extracted from a tumor or a nodule using a syringe and a fine needle. Using the fine needle (22 gauge to 25 gauge) virtually assures an atraumatic procedure that is acceptable to the patient. The extracted material is smeared skillfully on a microscope slide (see Technique), and is either air dried or fixed. Then it can be stained rapidly, and diagnosis may be rendered promptly. The material aspirated consists of single cells and cell clusters, and the yield may number in the thousands. When an epithelial tumor is the target, the entire smear most often will consist of tumor cells, generally intact. Contrast this to exfoliative cytology in which the cells are either shed or scraped from the lesion, and often few cancer cells are intermixed with many benign epithelial or stromal cells and inflammatory, degenerated cells and cell debris. Such smears require somewhat laborious screening by trained technologists and then review by a pathologist. On the other hand, the diagnosis of an aspiration smear very often can be made at a glance or after a brief perusal by an experienced cytopathologist.

The cell clusters obtained on aspiration may present structural formations such as alveolar groups, cell balls, monolayers, and papillary projections, which allow tumor typing in many cases.[16] In effect, the material is a microbiopsy with a high level of correlation with histopathology.[8,29]

The technique outlined below allows the clinician to extend the examination into the palpable and nonpalpable lesion producing part or all of the syndrome for which the patient has sought help. It allows the

---

* Personal communication, T. Löwhagen.
† Personal communication, D. Rosenthal.

clinician to complete the examination at one patient encounter without the necessity of postponement, return visit, referral to a remote specialist, and scheduling operating room time, all of which frustrate the patient and heighten his anxiety.[9]

The Evolution of Fine Needle Aspiration Cytology

The discipline of fine needle aspiration cytology has had a curious evolution. For much of the past 50 years, the major innovations and the seminal publications have appeared through the interest and effort of clinicians.[10,17,26,29] The enthusiasm and energy brought to this method is well known to all physicians who practice this clinical science. A simple, fast, and accurate method that is unencumbered by major preparations, hospital reservations, medico-legal complications (for the most part), technological complexities, and a large staff has and should have great appeal to the individual physician who must deal daily with complicated and frustrating problems.

In spite of its attractiveness, the general clinician has not shown a major interest in using aspiration cytology. This is due in part to his dependence on cytopathologic diagnosis that has not always been encouraged by pathologists (see below). However, most clinicians have had no exposure or training and have adhered tenaciously to traditional diagnostic methods (shown later in Fig. 1-1).

THE ROLE OF THE PATHOLOGIST

Those pathologists who are interested in morphology gradually have converted themselves into part-time clinicians to gather the material* because clinicians in their institutions have not taken the initiative.

Such pathologists, and many others who have established symbiotic relationships with clinicians, have been responsible for the vast outpouring of papers on the subject in the past 20 years. Almost without exception, these papers present the cytopathology of all varieties of palpable and nonpalpable lesions. The technique of puncture is explained briefly, and clinical correlation is scarcely mentioned. With few exceptions, pathologists who make major contributions to clinical diagnoses and understanding of the disease process do not think clinically. They are not trained in history taking or physical examination. They are as uncomfortable in the clinical arena as the clinician is behind the microscope.

The interpretation of microscope slides is nevertheless crucial to the process of aspiration biopsy. It requires study and experience, and at this time suffers from the failure of the educational discipline of pathology to incorporate formal programs into the curriculum. Therefore, the average pathologist must depend on clinicians for material, and must rely on in-

---

* Personal communications, S. Dahlgren and W.J. Frable.

dependent study and sporadic tutorials for information. Nevertheless, pathologists are expressing great interest, and in many and possibly all pathology departments diagnoses are being rendered on few or many slides during the course of one year.

With a few noteworthy exceptions, at present the clinical aspects of a patient (including history, physical findings, and integration of laboratory and imaging procedures) are separated from the interpretation of microscopic preparations. This dichotomy has been a major disadvantage in developing the method for general use.

A few physicians and pathologists have acquired the knowledge and experience to carry out the aspirations expertly and to read their own smears. This produces optimum diagnostic results. Worldwide, such hybrids are few, and recruiting these individuals into all central, regional, community, and private hospitals is highly unlikely.

For the most part, particularly in community and regional hospitals where most patients are seen, material is submitted sporadically to pathologists, many of whom try to respond with prompt diagnoses but often with trepidation. This is compounded by the extraordinarily poor material they are often called upon to interpret. The material may be sparse, intermixed with blood and fluid, traumatized, and contaminated. Its quality reflects the clinician's lack of interest in this diagnostic process. This is analogous to the cervical Pap smears received by pathologists from presumably trained and interested gynecologists, which range from excellent to unreadable.

THE ROLE OF THE CLINICIAN

As clinicians who have acquired some expertise in microscopy, we are alert to the potential value of fine needle aspiration cytology to clinical diagnosis and management. It is, in fact, a clinical tool that is available to the practicing or institutional physician and allows him to maintain more detailed control of his patient's progress. This hands-on technique cements the doctor–patient relationship.

Fine needle aspiration cytology in our practice immediately follows the fundamental history and physical examination in which a target lesion such as enlarged lymph node, thyroid nodule, breast mass, or abdominal, pelvic, or rectal lesion has been revealed. In most instances, it precedes x-ray, scans, special chemical analyses, and consultation with subspecialists. This is illustrated in the series of diagnostic schemata in which the traditional series of examinations and studies are intercepted by fine needle aspiration, which will yield a definitive diagnosis promptly in most cases (Fig. 1-1).

Before reviewing the utility of fine needle aspiration to the various medical and surgical subdivisions, several general responsibilities of the clinician should be stressed.

(Text continues on p. 7.)

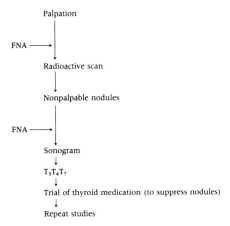

Comment: FNA combined with clinical judgment sharply reduces diagnostic testing,
A   time, and cost.

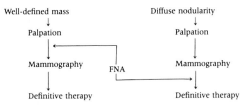

Comment: Well-defined palpable masses should be aspirated for diagnosis and bilateral
mammography carried out to detect other nonpalpable disease.
        Nodular breasts without a dominant lump should have mammography first, which
B   may direct FNA or require a stereotactic approach.

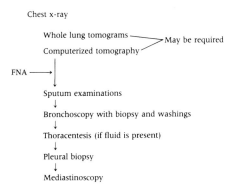

Comment: FNA may eliminate prolonged hospitalization in addition to reducing the
C   morbidity and cost of multiple procedures (see Case 5-2).

FIGURE 1-1: Fine needle aspiration and the diagnostic profile. (A) Thyroid nodules, enlargements, and tumors. (B) Breast tumors. (C) Lung and mediastinal tumors. (D) Abdominal masses. (E) Renal masses. (F) Prostatic nodules or masses. (G) Enlarged cervical nodes. (H) Bone lesions. (I) Miscellaneous targets. (*Figure continues on pp. 6 and 7.*)

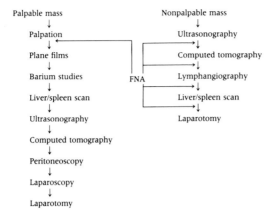

Comment: FNA is carried out at once on palpable lesions and may eliminate a large number of studies, as well as forestall surgery.

FNA may be introduced after any of the visualizing procedures, and it may eliminate further study.

D

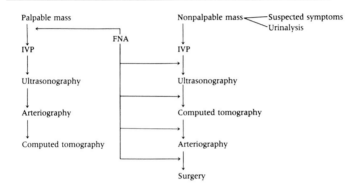

Comment: Palpable renal mass should be diagnosed immediately with FNA, eliminating imaging procedures. Puncture of nonpalpable mass requires imaging procedures (Case 1-1).

E

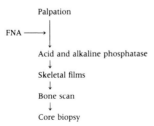

Comment: Prompt establishment of the diagnosis by FNA eliminates core biopsy. Other ancillary studies are related to staging, but are sometimes done before the diagnosis of prostatic carcinoma is established in an effort to obtain indirect evidence. Computed tomography and lymphangiography may be used for staging, after primary diagnosis is established, and may provide further targets for FNA.

F

Figure 1-1 *(continued)*

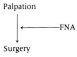

Palpation

↓ ←————FNA

Surgery

Surgical violation of the neck for diagnosis of metastatic disease is contraindicated.

Comment: FNA cytology will yield the following diagnoses and prompt the accompanying studies:
　If squamous: Detailed head and neck examination
　If nonsquamous: Judicious search for primary below the clavicle
　If lymphoid: Mixed, well differentiated
　　　　　　　　Search for focal infection
　　　　　　　　Viral studies
　　　　　　　　In children—observe for several weeks
　　　　　　　　Biopsy if no regression or diagnosis
　　　　　　Monomorphic and/or poorly differentiated
　　　　　　　　Bone marrow
　　　　　　　　Chest x-ray
G　　　　　　　Surgical biopsy

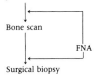

X-ray alteration with or without pain, tenderness, swelling

Bone scan

FNA

Surgical biopsy

Comment: Open bone biopsies are rarely necessary if FNA can be carried out. X-ray
H　control may not be necessary if there is point tenderness, swelling, or palpable defect.

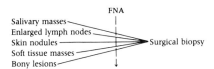

FNA

Salivary masses
Enlarged lymph nodes
Skin nodules ————————→ Surgical biopsy
Soft tissue masses
Bony lesions

Comment: Surgical biopsy should always be preceded by FNA to guide the surgical
I　approach and more often to forestall it. Sialograms can usually be eliminated.

FIGURE 1-1 *(continued)*

1. The patient usually welcomes a brief and reassuring discussion outlining the purpose and goals of the procedure. Hazards should be mentioned and in some cases should be stressed at this point, depending on the particular anatomic structure to be penetrated (such as lung or abdominal viscera). It is useful and accurate to point out to the hesitant patient that the alternative to a puncture may be a surgical procedure, often with general anesthesia. It has not been our habit to obtain signed consent for fine needle aspiration or for bone marrow puncture. As a practical matter, is saves time and discussion and avoids raising unnecessary questions. This approach results from the confidence gained in performing well over one hundred thousand punctures with vanishingly rare complications or difficulties. However, informed consent is entirely the prerogative of the private or institutional physician carrying out the procedure, and its necessity varies considerably with the anatomic structure.

2. The clinician should not begin aspirating without instruction. The procedure is deceptively simple. Initial aspirations may miss the target. Even if they are on target, adequate material may not be obtained. If material is obtained, it may be prepared and smeared ineptly, rendering a proper microscopic reading difficult or impossible. Frustration and disenchantment will occur rapidly, and the method will be rejected as worthless. During a recent attempt to introduce fine needle aspiration into a large oncology department in a medical school, the staff pleaded lack of personnel and lack of time. Eventually, an initial puncture of an abdominal mass was performed as the first attempt in the department. No significant material was obtained and the entire method was dropped.

3. Physicians who consciously or unconsciously delete unsatisfactory surgical or other subspecialist adjuvant colleagues, laboratories, and radiology services from their diagnostic and therapeutic support system should not settle for imperfect procedures and results in this critical diagnostic method. Therefore, they must address themselves diligently to perfecting their technique. With fine needle aspiration, the clinician is carrying out a procedure as important and intrinsic as the basic physical examination. Diligent palpation of the breast or auscultation of the heart is not more crucial than extracting diagnostic material with a fine needle. The care exercised should be the same.

Therefore, attention must be addressed to obtaining an adequate sample even after instruction has been received. With experience, the extraction of significant material can be identified on the unstained smear. For example, aspiration of a firm neck mass that yields only goblets of translucent fat on the smear obviously has missed the target. With the ease of repeat aspiration, perseverance until a proper specimen is obtained becomes essential. The technique of smearing is considered the most critical step in achieving a satisfactory result (see below). After instruction and experience, good results usually are obtained.

One of the pitfalls of the method is the clinician's bland self-assurance that his smears are quite satisfactory, and that diagnostic difficulties are entirely the pathologist's. By reviewing an execrable smear with a referring clinician, we were able to bring about a change in his technique.

4. Awareness of the place of fine needle aspiration biopsy in clinical medicine is very important to the clinician. No physician can do everything. His critical faculties require that he know when to call a surgeon, what kind of surgeon, and which surgeon. He also must know when to request imaging procedures. The wide and immediate availability of such complex and expensive diagnostic measures test to the highest degree the discriminative function of the physician.[4] Therefore, he must be more than cursorily familiar with tomographic studies, bone scans, lung scans, hidascans, mugascans, and so forth. If not, the provider simply will serve up whatever is requested, however absurd it is. The same rules apply to use of the laboratory where the clinician has a potpourri of studies to choose from.

It is apparent that many clinicians will not find the procedural aspects of fine needle aspiration congenial and will elect not to do the procedures. It is precisely this group who should be knowledgeable about the place of fine needle aspiration in the diagnostic workup and who should have a readily accessible referral station that will carry out the procedure and promptly report results. Attention to the nine diagnostic schemata illustrated in Figure 1-1 will help divert the flow of diagnostic procedures into efficient channels.

Integrating the Method into Clinical Practice

It is our perception that fine needle aspiration is primarily a flexible clinical tool available to physicians rather than a laboratory or pathology procedure. How it is used depends on the focus of the clinician. This book is divided into detailed discussions of regional lesions and the clinical and procedural approach to them. However, an overview of the individual clinician's role in applying the method should be useful. It is apparent that there is considerable overlap among some areas of clinical interest. An example is head and neck tumors, which potentially are the responsibility of general surgeons, otorhinolaryngologists, plastic surgeons, and head and neck surgeons. The following discussions are limited to one specialist or another.

Fine Needle Aspiration and the Physical Examination

In 1976, an interesting study by C. Everett Koop entitled *Visible and Palpable Lesions in Children* was published.[13] It presented a series of patients whose cases dramatically illustrated the importance of basic physical examination. Laboratory and imaging studies were not used.

Fine needle aspiration is an extension of the physical examination. Having defined the lesion physically (or by imaging techniques) the diagnosis can be rendered directly and immediately by the puncture technique.

Conversely, continued application of the puncture technique improves skills in physical diagnosis. Alertness in observation and heightened tactile sensibilities are salutary by-products. As the following chapters illustrate, techniques of palpation and the ability to focus attention become important attributes of the perceptive clinician. It has been our experience that clinicians who actively refer patients for aspiration acquire increased sensitivity to lesions they previously either would have not noticed or would have ignored. Patients referred for aspiration of 5-mm palpable masses in the thyroid or breast, which turn out to be papillary carcinoma of the thyroid or minimal carcinoma of the breast, are not rare.

The possibility of atraumatic diagnosis of a lesion so small that the clinician might feel absurd to refer for surgical excision provides an improved sense of security for those knowledgeable in the method.

THE ROLE OF THE PRIMARY PHYSICIAN

In traditional medicine, the first doctor encountered by the patient is the primary physician. The patient may have a localized disorder, or the physician may discover it in the course of his examination. Areas of interest that call for consideration of fine needle aspiration are varieties of skin nodules, sebaceous cysts, enlarged cervical lymph nodes (particularly in children), varieties of goiter, cystic or nodular breasts, hepatomegaly, and enlarged inguinal nodes.

The details of managing specific regional lesions are in the following chapters. Of general importance to the primary physician, however, is the ready availability of fine needle aspiration for referral and prompt communication of results.

Some primary physicians in our experience have embraced the method and submit slides for diagnosis.

THE ROLE OF THE ONCOLOGIST

Medical oncology is one of the most rapidly expanding divisions of medical practice. Research in and application of chemotherapy appears to dominate the literature. Metastatic disease is the major application of therapy, and primary tumors are still the province of surgeons and radiotherapists. As a result, medical oncologists often fail to see initial lesions that are referred from primary care physicians directly to surgeons or radiotherapists. This is unfortunate, since the oncologist is by definition trained in all aspects of neoplastic disease and is in the best position to plan and direct the course of treatment of the patient. Also, because he is a trained internist, the oncologist can take a holistic view of the patient, including cardiopulmonary, renal, hepatic, cerebral, and psychological aspects.

Acquiring the knowledge and skill of aspiration biopsy is a singular asset to the medical oncologist. It places him in a position not only to evaluate the patient, but in many cases to render a rapid outpatient diagnosis. The availability of these skills in regional centers will prompt the primary physician to refer the patient rapidly for initial diagnosis to the oncologist. Without question, the patient with neoplastic disease is best served by early review of his problem with an oncologist rather than a late consultation after a plan of therapy and numerous procedures are already in place.

Experience has shown that reporting on aspiration biopsy at staff meetings and clinical conferences is a valuable educational aid and will alert the staff to early oncologic referral.

From a practical standpoint, an even more valuable use of aspiration biopsy is the follow up of previously treated patients. The earliest detection of skin nodules and lymph nodes may be followed promptly by aspiration, rapid diagnosis, and rapid treatment. Enlarged livers with questionable scans, positive but not definitive bone scans, a solitary pulmonary nodule in a patient with prior extrathoracic carcinoma, postirradiation induration, and other examples considered in this book are all clinical problems distinctly in the province of the medical oncologist. There is no better method of evaluation than aspiration biopsy.

Failure to incorporate this method into major oncologic clinics is a curious omission in this modern era.

THE ROLE OF THE RADIOTHERAPIST

Follow up is an extremely important function of the radiotherapist. Detailed examination of the tumor site and regional nodes yields a harvest of local indurations, nodules, masses, and nodal enlargements. Experience has shown that the most inconspicuous asymmetry may yield cancer cells. Without the needle aspiration technique, a choice must be made between further follow up after an appropriate interval or referral for surgical biopsy, both of which may be inconvenient for the patient. This is due to the fact that radiotherapy units, apart from large urban centers, are regionalized. Therefore, the patient may have to travel considerable distance, particularly in less populated countries and areas.

Personal experience has shown also that adding needle aspiration to the diagnostic method provides the radiotherapist with significant personal assurance that he has carefully performed his follow up function.

THE ROLE OF THE RADIOLOGIST

The clinical radiologist (intervention radiology) has been responsible for initiating the present widening interest in fine needle aspiration. As a result, the more difficult, hazardous, and complex procedures were used much more commonly than the simple aspiration of palpable surface lesions. Nevertheless, the increasing presentation of cytologic material to pathology departments stimulated and, in fact, mandated an interest in and perfection of morphologic diagnosis of the material. This led to requests from pathology departments for other types of material and the general interest was aroused.

The radiologist aids and directs punctures of the brain, base of the skull, thyroid, skeleton, lungs, mediastinum, liver, pancreas, retroperitoneum, and pelvis. He also performs many of the punctures, particularly of the lungs, pancreas, and retroperitoneum. It is important that all clinicians recognize the availability and value of these procedures when planning the diagnostic work-up of many of these patients.

THE ROLE OF THE GENERAL SURGEON

Common clinical problems referred for surgical evaluation are scalp masses, salivary gland and thyroid masses, lateral neck masses, enlarged nodes in all regions, breast masses, abdominal and rectal masses, and soft tissue swellings. The patient may or may not have undergone considerable diagnostic study before the referral. The surgeon has the option at point of referral, depending on prior studies, to schedule the patient for an incisional or excisional procedure.

Preoperative diagnosis has been in our experience an extremely valuable aid to the surgeon in planning the procedure. Knowing the nature of the mass beforehand—that a salivary mass is a mixed tumor, a thryoid nodule is a papillary carcinoma, a neck mass is a squamous metastasis, a breast mass is fat necrosis, and a muscle mass is a sarcoma—is an important asset for the surgeon.

Many other examples will be cited in the chapters to follow, but the general clinical principle of obtaining maximum information before major invasion of the patient is completely applicable. Awareness of the potential of fine needle aspiration encourages the surgeon to obtain the information either by carrying out the aspiration or by referring the patient.

Peroperative fine needle aspiration[16] is also a useful tool for the surgeon in the diagnosis of pancreatic and retroperitoneal tumors when excisional biopsy might be hazardous.[15,19]

THE ROLE OF THE UROLOGIST

Facility with fine needle aspiration will allow the urologist to diagnose renal tumors preoperatively. Fortified with cell type and differentiation, he may opt for preoperative radiation of a Wilms' tumor or hypernephroma. He also will spare unexpectedly nonmalignant lesions as illustrated in the following case.

Case 1-1

The patient was a 50-year-old woman with mild persistent leukocytosis. During the workup, urinalysis revealed microscopic hematuria. IVP followed and was interpreted as showing a possible renal lesion. She was referred to a large university medical center for angiography (this was before the era of CT scans). An avascular mass was identified and surgery was recommended. A left nephrectomy was performed. Bisection of the resected specimen revealed a prominent mass of pelvic fat (called a lipoma). No other tumor was found.

However compelling the radiographic picture, there is no loss in obtaining preoperative cytologic confirmation.

Transrectal aspiration of the prostate is an enormous clinical aid to the urologist in planning therapy or follow up. This is discussed in Chapter 7.

There has been great reluctance to puncture the testicle. One major use of fine needle aspiration has been in fertility studies, as described in Chapter 3. A more important use is for the early diagnosis of tumors when they appear as questionable lesions. The clinician in his wisdom may elect to observe them rather than do a biopsy. Patient compliance is always an unknown factor, and allowing a patient with a potential tumor to slip away without diagnosis may be a lethal hesitation.

Our experience confirms the high diagnostic utility of testicular puncture without evidence of deleterious effects.

THE ROLE OF THE PULMONARY PHYSICIAN
AND THE THORACIC SURGEON

Recognizing that pulmonary lesions discovered on chest films can be reached safely and that a biopsy can be done with the fine needle has altered and reversed many of the traditional diagnostic methods in chest disease (see Fig. 1-1C). Although sputum examination is noninvasive, can be done for the ambulatory patient, and has a fairly high diagnostic yield,[2] it must be remembered that reported studies originated in major centers with highly specialized personnel. The overall yield from sputum examinations in the community or regional hospital is considerably lower. In addition, with the exception of small cell anaplastic carcinoma, definitive cancer therapy may not be undertaken on the basis of sputum diagnosis without confirmation.[2] Beyond sputum examination, fine needle aspiration has rapidly become the most direct, timesaving, and definitive method of diagnosis in many (if not most) cases. The diagnosis of cancer on fine needle aspiration of a pulmonary mass is definitive, and cancer therapy can follow without histology. The role of bronchoscopy and other techniques is considered in Chapter 5.

Experience has shown that the reordering of the traditional approach takes place quickly when the radiologist and chest physician collaborate to secure cytologic specimens. Initially, only large and obviously inoperable tumors are punctured to provide a morphologic diagnosis for radiotherapy. Subsequently, smaller peripheral lesions are punctured. They are noteworthy for not yielding sputum, and they are beyond the reach of bronchoscopy. Finally, smaller central lesions have been aspirated. For the primary clinician, awareness of the possible uses of aspiration enables him to make the appropriate referral.

THE ROLE OF THE OTORHINOLARYNGOLOGIST

Although most ear, nose, and throat lesions are exposed and are easily available for surgical biopsy, fine needle aspiration adds a valuable tool. Patients are generally encountered in office practice and consultation. Visualization of a lesion of the palate, pharynx, tonsil, tongue, or oral mucosa may be followed promptly by local spray anesthesia and rapid extraction of diagnostic material, which allows treatment planning. Not all suspicious lesions are cancer, as illustrated later in Case 1-2 in which a typical ''cancer'' turned out to be an inflammatory lesion. Fine needle aspiration will spare the patient surgical biopsy in uncomfortable and tender sites.

Salivary gland masses often present puzzling problems that are dealt with by sialograms and surgical extirpation or biopsy. Fine needle aspiration should be a useful tool for the otorhinolaryngologist, who is frequently the primary physician or the first point of reference.

Submandibular glands, which are often the site of chronic inflammation, may be easily confused with enlarged lymph nodes. The question is settled by fine needle aspiration.

Finally, postsurgical follow up of intraoral lesions is aided by the availability of puncture of suspicious areas of induration.

THE ROLE OF THE NEUROSURGEON

Puncture of the brain is rapidly becoming a valuable adjuvant method in neurosurgery. Deep-seated and more superficial lesions can be reached, and accurate cytologic diagnosis can be rendered both about the presence of tumor and tumor type (see Chap. 11). The calvarium may be entered through small holes. Techniques are discussed in Chapter 11.

Illustrative examples of the utility of this method are presented in the Appendix (see Cases A-3, A-4, and A-6).

What Is the Place of Fine Needle Aspiration in Clinical Medicine?

Having reviewed the potential for applying fine needle aspiration by individual groups of physicians, it is important to take an overview of clinical medicine, and find out precisely why and where this clinical tool should enter firmly into diagnostic conditioning.

Clinical medicine seeks to prevent, detect, diagnose, and manage human disorders. Initial evaluation continues to be the history and physical examination, although all practicing physicians become aware that, as their training period fades, this performance becomes less complete. To some extent this may be due to greater experience and an ability to focus on the clinical problem and ignore apparently uninvolved systems. But to a larger extent, the physician comes to rely on laboratory imaging and other technical procedures to screen the patient for disease.

Medical training dictates the requisition of routine studies. Formerly, complete blood count, urinalysis, and VDRL were done. However, now VDRL has been deleted, and a chemistry profile of up to 26 studies, which might routinely include thyroid, iron, and triglyceride values, has been added. Use of the clinical laboratory is clearly one of the pillars of clinical practice taught in medical school, stressed in residency training, and incorporated reflexively into post-training practice.

Chest x-ray became a routine order in most hospitals in the 1950s with other films, such as barium enema, ordered as indicated. All physicians are aware of the intensification of use and the proliferation of types of imaging procedures since then. In many centers, the ease of ordering a CT scan regardless of its cost has increased the volume of use to the point that they are just short of routine. Without questioning the need for all these studies, there seems little question that they have become an important part of the physician's thinking and planning when dealing with a clinical problem.

The same observations can be made about adjuvant studies in cardiology. They have progressed far beyond the routine electrocardiogram to include echocardiograms, myocardial scans, and even coronary visualization.

Exfoliative cytology began fitfully in the 1940s. Now it is a major tool of practicing physicians, particularly for studies of the genital and pulmonary tracts. Few doctors fail to recognize the importance of the Pap test, and if they forget, their patients will remind them. The place of and need for outpatient pulmonary and urinary cytology may not be as well entrenched as it should be in some arenas.

We may summarize the physician's thinking when confronting a clinical problem. He will listen quietly to the patient's complaint and ask a few pertinent questions. He then examines the affected area if it is localized, and may cursorily examine a few other areas, and probably will record the blood pressure. At this point, the whole world of technology is open to him, and he may order from a large array of diagnostic aids or possibly refer the patient to a subspecialist. In reviewing more sophisticated case studies and reports (for example, cases in the *New England Journal of Medicine,* or entire seminars devoted to one disease process), the systematic analysis of the patient's problems proceeds as outlined above.

With a few exceptions worldwide, the technique of fine needle aspiration has not been incorporated into the thinking of the average clinician. Faced with a clinical problem, the diagnosis of which might be correctly surmised but not definitively established by his initial encounter, he will seek aid in ancillary, usually indirect or tangential procedures and studies. Examples of this are the subject of the following chapters, and include enlarged nodes; salivary and thyroid swelling; intraoral masses; breast disorders; pulmonary lesions; hepatosplenomegaly; abdominal and pelvic masses; anal, vulvar, rectal, and testicular abnormalities; and soft tissue and bony lesions.

It is not necessary for the private and institutional practicing physician to have an x-ray unit in his office to know when to order appropriate films. And although laboratory tests are essential, he cannot run his own sophisticated laboratory. Similarly, it is not necessary to become skilled in the techniques of fine needle aspiration and certainly not in cytologic interpretation, even though these skills are useful. However, it is essential to know the potential yield of fine needle aspiration, how it will aid and more often specifically make the diagnosis, and when and where to apply it. Such knowledge should be as much a part of the clinician's thinking as the knowledge that tells him to order a venogram, a creatinine level, or an echocardiogram.

It is precisely the position occupied by fine needle aspiration in the diagnostic plan that forms the substance of the following chapters. Reaching beyond that to the technical aspects and to cytologic interpretation is, for the clinician, a further but secondary step. If the clinician requests fine needle aspiration to help to diagnose, pathologists, cytologists, radiologists, oncologists, and other clinicians ultimately will be available to answer the request. The precise entrance of fine needle aspiration into the diagnostic schemata is outlined in Figure 1-1.

The Generic "Tumor"

The referral of patients for oncologic opinion or fine needle aspiration with a designated diagnosis is not uncommon. The request will often state, "Please evaluate cervical or axillary nodes, salivary tumor, breast tumor, gynecomastia, liver mass, enlarged spleen," and so forth. Listed in Table 1-1 are clinical look-alikes that highlight the importance of considering palpable and visualized clinical masses as generic "tumors."

The clinician is faced with a mass that requires a diagnosis. Some tumors, if large and fungating or massively infiltrating, are clinically unequivocal malignancy, but the nature of most masses can only be surmised. Most seasoned clinicians have experienced surprise findings revealed after possible unnecessary surgery or after unintended neglect of a malignant neoplasm. In addition, the attempt to separate tumors clinically into primary and metastatic categories frequently will meet with failure.

It is useful to think of "tumors" regionally rather than in terms of organ site. Although most tumors appearing in the lungs, breast, thyroid, and so forth probably arise in those organs, thinking of tumors as generic rather than type-specific will enable the physician to maintain a more imaginative concept of the possible diagnoses.

The Technique

Although there are numerous published techniques for fine needle aspiration, all suitable for the individual clinician or aspirator, the following method has been used with success continuously for 30 years. It is simple, usually yields satisfactory smears, is easily adaptable to most targets, and requires minimal preparation and few instruments.

Two important considerations are identifying the target and analyzing the angle of puncture most likely to extract useful material. Skirting a lesion, miscalculating depth, or penetrating to a necrotic center all may result in absent, insufficient, or unsatisfactory cellular content.

The basic tools required are a 10- or 20-cc plastic syringe, a 22-gauge needle, 2.54 cm or 3.8 cm (1 in or 1.5 in) long, two microscope slides with frosted ends, and an alcohol pad. After a time, a one-handed syringe with a glass barrel (the Franzen syringe) was added. A more recent addition was the one-handed synringe holder into which the plastic syringe could be

TABLE 1-1: **Clinical Look-Alikes**

Clinical Diagnosis	Cytologic Diagnosis
Sebaceous cyst	Subcutaneous metastasis
Tumor of salivary gland	Sialadenitis
Enlarged cervical node	Salivary gland
	Branchial cleft cyst
	Cervical rib
	Carotid body tumor
Metastatic node	Inflammatory node
Carcinoma of the thyroid	Subacute thyroiditis
Enlarged axillary nodes	Axillary breast lobule
	Carcinoma of axillary tail of breast
Breast carcinoma	Fat necrosis
	Hematoma
	Granular cell myoblastoma
	Senile duct ectasia
	Cyst
Lung abscess	Cavitating carcinoma
Tuberculosis cavity	Lung abscess
Liver neoplasm	Distended gallbladder
	Postnecrotic cirrhosis
	Liver cyst
Splenomegaly	Renal tumor
	Lymphomatous nodes
	Retroperitoneal sarcoma
	Left lobe of liver
	Carcinoma of splenic flexure
Pelvic metastasis	Fibroid uterus
	Ovarian mass
Presacral metastasis	Chordoma
Hemorrhoid	Basaloid carcinoma
Primary rectal carcinoma (anterior wall)	Prostate carcinoma
Lipoma or fibroma of soft tissue	Sarcoma

fitted snugly. The latter has become part of the standard procedure in our clinics. Finally, the Franzen needle guide, which is used for transrectal and transvaginal punctures, was added, with a 22-cm, 22-gauge needle. These tools are illustrated in Figures 1-2, 1-3, and 1-4.

THE PUNCTURE

Palpable lesions may be punctured according to the following steps. Techniques for puncturing nonpalpable lesions are described in later chapters.

1. The target is transfixed with one hand.
2. The one-handed syringe holder with syringe and needle is poised over the target.
3. The needle is passed into the mass after prior indication to the patient (Fig. 1-5).

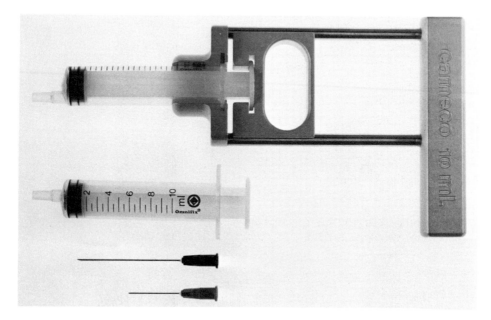

FIGURE 1-2: These are the basic tools for fine needle aspiration. Needles may vary in size from 1 cm to 20 cm. Syringes and holders also vary in size.

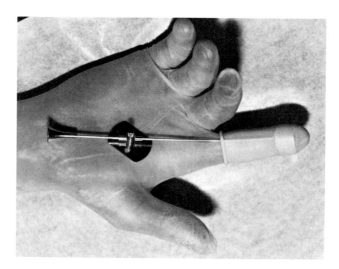

FIGURE 1-3: The needle guide is affixed to the index finger with a finger cot.

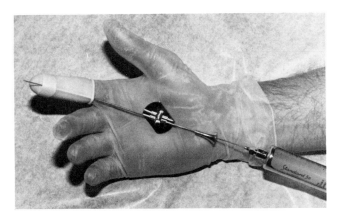

FIGURE 1-4: The needle point may extend as much as 3 cm beyond the guide ring. The finger should palpate above the target.

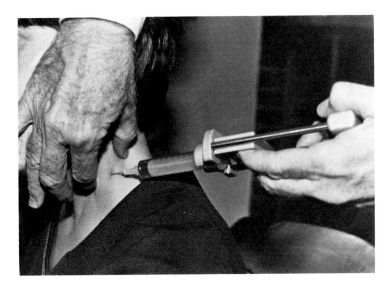

FIGURE 1-5: The mass is transfixed and the needle is inserted briskly.

4. A full 10 cc of suction is applied.
5. The needle tip is oscillated within the target briefly, in one channel, maintaining suction (Fig. 1-6).
6. Suction is released and the needle is withdrawn.
7. The needle is separated and air is drawn into the syringe (Fig. 1-7).

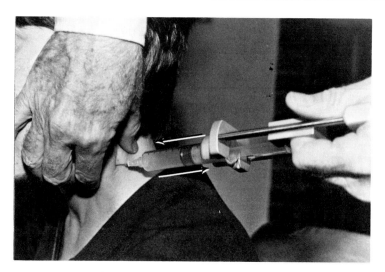

FIGURE 1-6: With suction applied, the syringe and needle are oscillated (*arrows*) in one channel.

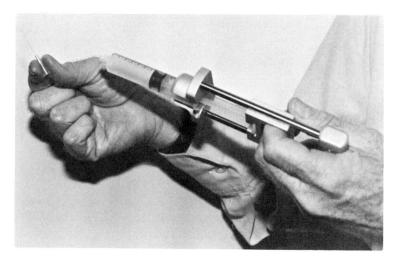

FIGURE 1-7: The needle is separated and air is drawn into the syringe.

8. The needle is reattached and the material that is contained entirely within the needle barrel is expelled onto a glass slide (Fig. 1-8). The material will be liquid, semisolid, or gelatinous (Fig. 1-9).

THE SMEAR

The extracted material now on the glass slide is smeared according to the following steps.

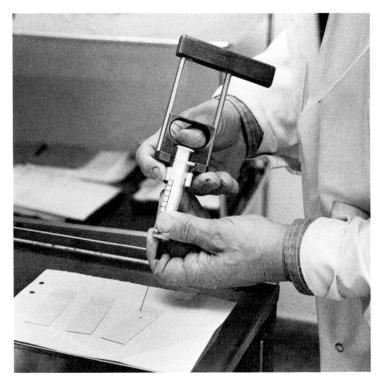

FIGURE 1-8: The needle is reattached, and the material within the needle barrel is expelled onto a glass slide.

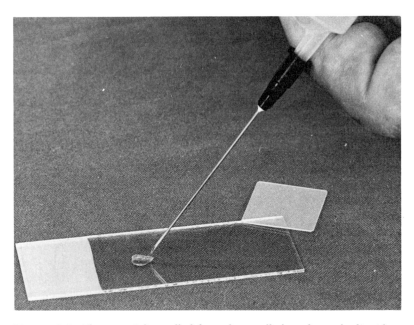

FIGURE 1-9: The material expelled from the needle barrel may be liquid or gelatinous.

1. The material is pressed down gently and drawn out to a feathered edge. A second slide or Bürker cover slip may be used (Fig. 1-10). Larger particles left behind are drawn out further.
2. If the material is more liquid, it is pulled in the same fashion as a blood smear. Before completing the feathering process, the particles are lined up across the slide. At that point, the slide or cover slip is raised and turned, and the spreading is completed by pressing the particles out as described in Step 1. The smear will have a thin and a thick part (Fig. 1-11). Varieties of smears are illustrated in Figure 1-12.
3. The smear is either air dried, sprayed, or dropped into fixative.

THE STAIN

Details of rapid staining methods have been presented in several publications.[8,12,21–23] The following techniques also may be considered.

1. At the Karolinska Institute, May–Grünwald–Giemsa stain has been used satisfactorily for 30 years to stain air-dried material.
2. Both Wright's stain and Diff-Quik* are alternative Romanowsky's stains.
3. Hematoxylin also has been used successfully for air-dried material.
4. Fixed slides are stained by the routine Papanicolaou's method.
5. A rapid Papanicolaou's method also has been used.

COMMENT ON THE TECHNIQUE

A great deal of practice is necessary to assure adequate sampling and good smearing. Fresh tissue samples are recommended for practice. Samples of liver and kidney tissue have been used successfully for demonstration at tutorials. The degree of success or failure in technique can be determined only by looking at the stained material microscopically or enlisting a pathologist to review the slides.

Starting out immediately puncturing patients may provide early success but more often will result in poor smears and frustrating results. Where a cyst is evacuated, a droplet of the material can be expressed in a slide and smeared. If any particles are floating, they should be separated out by decanting the fluid and then smearing the particles. This also applies to bloody material. Decanting the blood promptly to visualize the particles is important to avoid clotting. Depending on the source, the fluid can be centrifuged and the sediment thus obtained can be smeared.

The basic technique applies whether the target is palpable or nonpalpable. Nonpalpable targets (intracranial, intrathoracic, and retroperitoneal) are discussed in the following chapters. However, after penetrating the mass the procedure is the same.

*Harleco, Gibbstown, NJ.

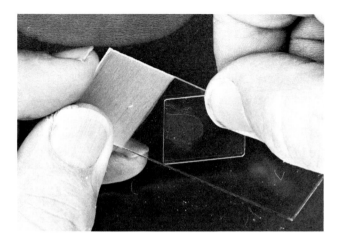

FIGURE 1-10: Smears are made with either a Bürker cover-slip or a second slide.

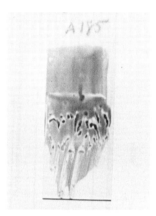

FIGURE 1-11: A two-phase smear. Smears must be made so that lesional material is spread broadly.

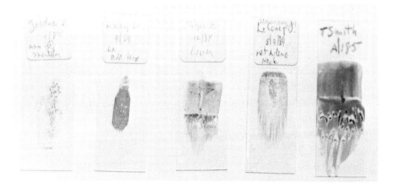

FIGURE 1-12: Five slides illustrate an assortment of smears.

Cytologic Pitfalls

The frequency of misinterpreting smears progressively gives way as experience is gained. The following sources of error vary widely in their likelihood of occurrence. Only an ongoing experience will allow the interpreter of slides to appreciate the possibilities for error.

1. Fragments of striated muscle stain royal blue with Romanowsky's and orange with Papanicolaou's. They may be confused with keratinization seen in squamous aspirates.
2. Chronic sialadenitis presenting clinically as a hard mass may yield sheets of ductal cells that will simulate a tumor.
3. Atypical epithelial cells associated with Hashimoto's thyroiditis may be read as suspicious for neoplasm.
4. Follicular smears from the thyroid cannot be categorized as malignant or benign, and this should be avoided.[18]
5. Highly reactive lymph nodes may yield increased numbers of atypical histiocytes. The risk of overdiagnosing lymphoma is reduced by the requirement to confirm with histology, but care and clinical judgment are necessary to determine when and if surgical biopsy should be done.
6. Breast inflammation may yield large numbers of histiocytes on smear, simulating a tumor.
7. Marked epithelial cellularity with atypia in breast aspiration may simulate carcinoma. It is important to examine individual cells and search for stripped nuclei.[16]
8. In pulmonary aspirates, atypical histiocytic proliferation can simulate a tumor.
9. A mixture of mucin and atypical cells (bronchial mucin with metaplastic bronchial epithelium) may simulate a mucinous carcinoma in pulmonary aspirates.
10. Clear cell lung tumors may simulate metastatic hypernephroma.
11. Clear cell thyroid and pelvic tumors also may be confused with metastatic hypernephroma.
12. Renal puncture may yield histiocytic proliferations from perinephric inflammation, simulating hypernephroma.
13. Atypical glandular and ductal proliferation associated with pancreatitis may simulate a tumor.
14. Masses of aggregated hepatocytes with poor cellular definition may be misinterpreted as tumor groups.
15. Intraluminal intestinal mucin may suggest mucinous adenocarcinoma on smear.
16. Metastatic pigmented melanoma to the liver may simulate hepatoma with bile.
17. Granulomatous prostatitis may be mistaken for tumor.
18. High lateral transrectal puncture of the prostate may yield atypical

large cells, which are normal for seminal vescicles but may be mistaken for prostatic carcinoma.

19. Plump histiocytes with large nucleoli seen in nodular fasciitis may be mistaken for sarcoma.

Errors in cytologic judgment, particularly false-positive diagnoses, are infrequent and decrease progressively with experience. It should be kept in mind that in the presence of a suspicious clinical picture, a positive cytologic diagnosis rendered by an experienced cytologist should not be discarded because of negative histology without further study (see Case 4-7).[27,29]

Clinical Pitfalls

If initial experience with the method is successful, enthusiasm increases and expectations rise. The results should be reviewed regularly in a sober manner to avoid unnecessary punctures and particularly to avoid over-reading slides. All statements about the low percentage of false-positive and false-negative diagnoses refer to work done by experienced cytopathologists and clinicians. The failure of critical self-evaluation, then, is the first and most important pitfall.

A high percentage of false-negative diagnoses results from the aspiration technique, not the microscopy. Of course, failure to reach the target will produce slides negative for tumor. Unsatisfactory smears are unreadable and produce unsatisfactory reports. In the larger sense, a high percentage of false-negative diagnoses because of poor technique reduces confidence in the method, and therefore is a major pitfall.

For the clinician, it is important to remember that a benign aspiration diagnosis in the presence of a clinically suspicious lesion must be dealt with by careful follow up or surgical biopsy. The failure to recognize that the clinical picture overrides negative cytology is a serious pitfall.

The following case illustrates the importance of clinical follow up and the exercise of caution.

Case 1-2

The patient was a 72-year-old retired physician with long-standing chronic lymphocytic leukemia for which he had studiously avoided medical counsel. He finally presented himself for evaluation of a firm ulcerated lesion at the right lateral border of his tongue.

On examination, he had generalized lymphadenopathy, splenomegaly palpable at 5 cm, atrial fibrillation with mild congestive failure, and marked stasis dermatitis of his legs with two plus edema. The tongue lesion was clinically a carcinoma.

Laboratory studies disclosed the following values: hemoglobin, 9.8 g/dL; white count, 98,000/mm^3, with 99% lymphocytes and numerous smudge cells; and platelets, 106,000/mm^3. On protein electrophoresis there was marked reduction of gammaglobulin.

At a joint conference with the radiotherapy department, the radiotherapist agreed to treat the patient based on a confirming cytologic diagnosis of carcinoma. It was felt that the patient's immune and physical status were so poor that a wedge biopsy should be avoided. In addition, the patient declined wedge biopsy.

Fine needle aspiration was performed. The needle entered through intact mucosa and was angled to the center of the mass. Aspiration yielded an inflammatory exudate. The patient was instructed to rinse with warm saline and take penicillin.

When he returned for a repeat aspiration in 4 days, the lesion had shrunk markedly. Ultimately, it regressed completely.

COMMENT In this case, uniform clinical judgment that the lesion was a carcinoma was wrong. The initial aspiration was considered to be a false-negative diagnosis, but clinical follow up confirmed that the lesion was indeed inflammatory.

Hazards

The fine needle is by definition 22 gauge (0.7 mm inner diameter) or smaller. The fineness is limited only by the flexibility of the needle barrel. An extremely flexible needle barrel may make penetration of the skin and guidance to deeper targets difficult. Tissue trauma produced by this instrument has been minimal based on years of practical experience. In our experience, fine needle aspiration effects on histologic diagnosis have been without significance.

Nevertheless, the following traumatic effects must be considered: bleeding and hematomas; infection; seeding of the needle pathway and tumor dissemination; pneumothorax; release of malignant cyst contents into the peritoneal cavity; bile peritonitis; and arterial hemorrhage and thrombosis.

BLEEDING AND HEMATOMAS

Proper technique requires that pressure be applied to all superficial puncture sites. Breast and thyroid punctures in particular may produce significant hematomas, and a large ecchymosis may occur in the breast if careful pressure is not applied. Surgeons occasionally will express annoyance at the presence of a breast hematoma, but hematomas have not compromised surgical technique. Small targets such as nodules or nodes may be obscured by hematomas produced by the initial puncture. It may be necessary to wait for resorption of the blood.

Hemoptysis can be caused by puncture, bleeding, and communication with a bronchus. It is sometimes alarming, but invariably it is self-limited.

Bleeding from a splenic puncture has occurred once in our experience. The patient required transfusions on the following day, but no surgery. Hepatic or retroperitoneal bleeding has not been seen in our experience or reported.

An adrenal hemorrhage can be a potential hazard. Hematuria after renal puncture occurs but is without clinical significance. On the other hand, fairly brisk urethral bleeding has occurred after prostatic puncture. It suggests the presence of large veins, information that is important in the event of possible prostatic surgery.

INFECTION

Infection following fine needle aspiration is rare. We have not seen it after any puncture of palpable masses. Infection after transcranial, transthoracic, and transabdominal punctures is also unknown in our experience. This includes punctures of abscesses and acute inflammation (Case A-13), although in the clinical context, antibiotics would be administered. Transabdominal puncture of the retroperitoneum may pass through the colon. We have seen colon organisms intermixed with cells in cytologic smears.[16] In spite of this, infections have not been reported.

Transrectal puncture of the prostate may result in serious bacteremias and septicemias.[5,6] However, it is a rare event, and can be avoided if no attempt is made to puncture prostates suspected of acute prostatitis. Theoretically, similar results may occur after transrectal or transvaginal puncture of pelvic masses, but this has not been reported.

SEEDING OF THE NEEDLE PATHWAY AND TUMOR DISSEMINATION

The development of a tumor nodule at the site of puncture is an extremely rare event in our experience. Ascitic tumors subject to paracentesis may seed and a tumor nodule will appear at the puncture site. This, of course, is not a fine needle aspiration. A rare subcutaneous nodule has appeared in our experience following lung puncture for bronchogenic carcinoma. The literature contains similar reports.[7,25] Other reports of implantation tumor have occurred with a large-bore needle.[28] One reason for the absence of reports following aspiration of common targets such as breast, lymph nodes, and thyroid is that therapy promptly follows with extirpation or ablation of the tumor. In effect, implantation tumor does not pose a hazard that should inhibit fine needle aspiration in the appropriate clinical context.

Tumor dissemination is a concern whenever a tumor is disturbed. Concern has extended to fine needle puncture. Several studies that firmly dispel this concern have been published.[1,24]

PNEUMOTHORAX

Transthoracic puncture produces pneumothorax in a high percentage of cases. Most are clinically not significant. The incidence depends on the frequency of follow up films. Films taken immediately after puncture may demonstrate a 10% to 20% pneumothorax. Patients should be observed for several hours, since the air leak may persist and compromise vital capacity. However, outpatient puncture is perfectly feasible.[14]

The rapid development of a large pneumothorax (tension pneumothorax) may require the rapid application of a chest tube with attached Heimlich valve or with underwater drainage. Practically, the latter can be achieved by the rapid insertion of a readily available plastic intravenous catheter with attached tubing and underwater insertion.

Since many patients with lung tumors also have chronic obstructive pulmonary disease, the problem of pneumothorax is compounded. Older patients with large, asymptomatic radiographic tumors that are not resectable for medical reasons, should not be punctured.

Pneumothorax may occur inadvertently when puncture of a rib, intercostal tumor, or small lesion at the edge of a breast is attempted and the needle slips through the ribs.

RELEASE OF MALIGNANT CYST CONTENTS
INTO THE PERITONEAL CAVITY

Inadvertent rupture of an ovarian cystadenocarcinoma is a surgical hazard leading to intraperitoneal tumor dissemination. Puncture of a malignant intraperitoneal cyst theoretically presents the same hazard and has been listed as a contraindication.[3,11] At present, there is no data to confirm or deny the possibility, but such a precaution seems reasonable. This interdiction may be modified under appropriate clinical circumstances, as illustrated in the following case.

Case 1-3

The patient was a 74-year-old woman with congestive heart failure and the residual effects of a stroke. Surgery with anesthesia was not deemed medically feasible. A mass could be palpated in the abdomen. Pelvic examination revealed that the mass apparently rose out of the pelvis. The dome of the mass extended 3 cm above the umbilicus. A CT scan demonstrated a biphasic mass. Ultrasonography demonstrated that the left side of the mass contained fluid. Radiographically, the differential diagnoses included fibroid uterus, sarcoma with degeneration and liquefaction, and cystic ovarian mass.

Fine needle aspiration of the right side of the mass yielded with great difficulty a few apparently benign spindle cells characteristic of leiomyoma. Fine needle aspiration of the left side yielded 10 cc of dark, turbid fluid containing old blood and clusters of enlarged carcinoma cells. Without defining the cancer further, the patient was treated supportively.

BILE PERITONITIS

We have seen one patient with obstructive jaundice in whom puncture of the liver resulted in an acute episode of upper abdominal pain with rebound suggesting bile irritation. The patient recovered with supportive care. Obstructive jaundice may be a relative contraindication, although the liver is regularly punctured in obstructive jaundice with intervention radiologic procedures.

ARTERIAL HEMORRHAGE AND THROMBOSIS

Puncture of a major artery, including the aorta, has been done inadvertently in our experience with no evidence of hemorrhage. During one attempt to aspirate a mediastinal mass under fluoroscopy, the needle could be felt entering the aortic arch with a crunching sensation that suggested an inelastic sclerotic wall. Although this was attended by some anxiety, there were no untoward effects.

Puncture of a carotid body tumor at the bifurcation of the carotid artery is probably contraindicated because of one reported instance of carotid artery thrombosis and stroke. Many carotid body tumors have been punctured, and cytologic diagnoses rendered. Where a neck mass cannot be identified by angiography, careful aspiration may be considered.

Dealing with Patient Reactions to the Diagnosis of Cancer

The direct and immediate diagnosis of cancer is a frequent occurrence in fine needle aspiration of palpable and nonpalpable lesions. The aspirating physician (who may also be a cytopathologist) may not be the primary physician. However, there is no question that he has established contact and some degree of relationship with the patient in the brief encounter consisting of the pre-puncture discussion and the procedure.

Some physicians consider their role purely technical: obtain the specimen; make the diagnosis; and write the report. This is probably not a totally satisfactory sequence. Experience has shown that pre-puncture discussion relaxes the patient and improves the ease of obtaining the specimen. Increased patient acceptance also will permit repeat punctures as indicated.

Clinical contact with the patient, particularly the laying on of hands, increases patient expectations. All pathologists, radiologists, and clinicians who use the method may anticipate questions from the patient. The patient is often aware, or he may be told, that staining and diagnosis may be carried out at once. A selected but increasing number of physicians have the facility of aspirating, quickly staining, and immediately reviewing the smear. This has the advantage of allowing a repeat puncture during the same patient visit if the target has not been reached or if the material is scant. Many patients may have travelled some distance, sometimes reluctantly, and a technical failure may result in noncompliance with a follow up appointment. Therefore, a number of physicians will be aware of the diagnosis during the initial patient visit, and then will be faced with the frequent, though not inevitable, question: "What do I have?" or "Is it cancer?" Referring clinicians receiving immediate diagnostic data also will be faced with the similar problem of responding to a patient's emotionally charged question. Although most clinicians have developed through experience a *modus vivendi* in dealing with the announcement of cancer, the rather abrupt revelation of cancer yielded by fine needle aspiration, often in the face of an innocuous lesion, may require adjustments in the conduct of practice.

The aspirating physician necessarily must be guided by the advice and consent of the referring physician where this is proffered. Families also may insist that the patient be spared the diagnosis of cancer and such a constraint must be dealt with on an individual basis.

Our experience has shown us that in the absence of prior restraint, direct answers should be given to the queries about cancer. Smears negative for cancer should be reported freely to the patient. Negative smears invariably please the patient, but the necessity of continuing to deal with a palpable or radiographically demonstrated lesion on a clinical basis must be stressed. It may require surgical biopsy or continued follow up until the lesion is resolved or its significance understood. A cardinal error is dismissal without follow up or recommendation of such.

With positive smears, the answer is "Yes, the smear is malignant."

"Does that mean I have cancer?"

"Yes, it is a cancer, but fortunately it appears to be an early case so we may have very good curative treatment."

The point of this hypothetical exchange is that the patient always must be left with a positive feeling. A positive response can be made in almost all cases without violating the prognostic facts.

When the aspirating physician elects not to respond to the question, he then may indicate that the smears require more study (which they may), and that he will phone the report to the referring physician. The referring physician then will be faced with the same problem of communication. Where possible, discussion with the patient should not take place on the telephone.

In the interest of minimizing patient and family anxiety, we have found that this positive approach is the most effective.

Conclusion

Fine needle aspiration is an important skill for clinicians of all specialties, but particularly for those who are more likely to see the patient during his initial encounter. It is a skill that should be incorporated into medical school and residency training programs. Failure to present it during basic medical training is responsible in part for its sluggish acceptance in clinical practice.

Physicians who do the puncture and read the slides receive a unique intellectual gratification. For other physicians, knowledge of when to request puncture immeasurably improves clinical efficiency. Experience has shown that awareness of the puncture method results in the elimination of many more complex, expensive, and time-consuming studies.

The clinician is best served by understanding the importance and problems of cytologic interpretation, and he is encouraged to maintain a cooperative relationship with the cytopathologist. Failure to submit carefully prepared smears is a major pitfall that will be recognized by the cytopathologist. It is important for the clinician to respond positively to critical evaluation of smears.

Limitations of the method must be kept clearly in mind.[3,11] Just as the cytopathologist must be cautioned to acquire expertise before assuming responsibility for diagnoses that might result in major therapy, similarly the clinician will find that considerable practice after appropriate instruction ultimately will yield the best results. Major causes of failure are the inability to reach the target, extract cells after reaching it, or smear them properly. This may occur even with large, easily palpable masses and can lead to early discouragement. Remember that a negative yield does not exclude cancer!

Poor results also occur when physicians with serious intent are overconfident in a deceptively simple technique. They also may occur when the technique is performed too casually. Even a simple technique requires a measure of attention and practice.

For those physicians who can correlate their findings on physical examination with the information yielded by aspiration and finally with end-results data, a singular enhancement of their knowledge and pleasure in medical practice will take place.

The chapters that follow contain numerous cross-references. Even though regions and organs are highlighted, clinical cases and illustrations relating to other regions are included in various chapters. This will stress the interrelatedness of the entire clinical spectrum. It also will challenge the imagination of the clinician and help break down fixed ideas that so often impede the search for a final diagnosis.

REFERENCES

1. Berg JW, Robbins GF: A late look at the safety of aspiration cytology. Cancer 15:826, 1962
2. Caya JG, Wollenberg NJ, Clowry LJ: The significance of "positive" respiratory cytology. Determinations in a series of 327 patients. Am J Clin Pathol 82:155, 1984
3. Christopherson WW: Cytologic detection and diagnosis of cancer: Its contributions and limitations. Cancer 51:1201, 1983
4. Cutler P: Problem Solving in Clinical Medicine: From Data to Diagnosis. Baltimore, Williams & Wilkins, 1979

5. Edson RS, Van Scoy RE, Leary FJ: Gram-negative bacteremia after trans-rectal needle biopsy of the prostate. Mayo Clin Proc 55:489, 1980
6. Esposti PL, Elman A, Worlen H: Complications of transrectal aspiration biopsy of the prostate. Scand J Urol Nephrol 9:208, 1975
7. Ferrucci JT Jr: Malignant seeding of the tract after thin-needle aspiration biopsy. Radiology 130:345, 1979
8. Frable WJ: Thin Needle Aspiration Biopsy. Philadelphia, WB Saunders, 1983
9. Frank SE: Lessons. JAMA 252:2014, 1984
10. Franzen S, Giertz G, Zajicek J: Cytologic diagnosis of prostatic tumors by transrectal aspiration biopsy: A preliminary report. Br J Urol 32:193, 1960
11. Hajdu SI, Melamed M: Limitations of aspiration cytology in the diagnosis of primary neoplasms. Acta Cytol 28:337, 1984
12. Hammar SP, Bartha M, Riecks L et al: Technical aspects of thin-needle aspiration biopsy. Lab Med 11:227, 1982
13. Koop CE: Visible and Palpable Lesions in Children. New York, Grune & Stratton, 1976
14. Lalli AF, McCormick LJ, Zelch M et al: Aspiration biopsies of chest lesions. Radiology 127:35, 1978
15. Lightwood R, Reber HA, Way LW: The risk and accuracy of pancreatic biopsy. Am J Surg 132:189, 1976
16. Linsk JA, Franzen S: Clinical Aspiration Cytology. Philadelphia, JB Lippin-cott, 1983
17. Lopes-Cardoza P: Atlas of Clinical Cytology. Hertogenbosch, Harga, 1976
18. Löwhagen T, Linsk JA: Aspiration cytology of the thyroid gland. In Linsk JA, Franzen S (eds): Clinical Aspiration Cytology, pp 61–83. Philadelphia, JB Lippincott, 1983
19. Lund F: Carcinoma of the pancreas. Acta Chir Scand 135:515, 1969
20. Martin HE, Ellis EB: Biopsy by needle puncture and aspiration. Ann Surg 92:169, 1930
21. Meyers DS, Yokota SB, Teplitz RL: Letter to the editor. Acta Cytol 27:81, 1984
22. Pak HY, Yokota SB, Teplitz RL et al: Rapid staining technique employed in fine needle aspiration of the lung. Acta Cytol 25:178, 1981
23. Pak HY, Yokota SB, Teplitz RL: Letter to the editor. Acta Cytol 27:81, 1984
24. Schreeb T, Von Amer O, Skovsted G: Renal adenocarcinoma. Is there a risk of spreading tumor cells in diagnostic puncture? Scand J Urol Nephrol 1:270, 1967
25. Sinner WN, Zajicek J: Implantation metastases after percutaneous trans-thoracic needle aspiration biopsy. Acta Radiol [Diagn] (Stockh) 17:473, 1976
26. Söderström N: Fine Needle Aspiration Biopsy. Stockholm, Almqvist & Wilksell, 1966
27. Tao L-C, Weisberg G, Ritcey EL et al: False "false-positive" results in diagnostic cytology. Acta Cytol 28:450, 1984
28. Wolinsky H, Lischner MW: Needle track implantation of tumor after per-cutaneous lung biopsy. Ann Intern Med 71:359, 1969
29. Zajicek J: Aspiration Biopsy Cytology I and II. Basel, S Karger, 1973, 1979

The Head and Neck Region (Excluding the Thyroid and CNS)

2

The head and neck region provides a variety of targets for fine needle aspiration. They arise from structures within the region and engrafted onto the region by a metastatic or inflammatory process. The application of fine needle aspiration to the diagnosis of several targets in this area has received considerable attention in published reports.[21,22,42,63,71]

Primary and Secondary Lesions

Lesions in the head and neck suitable for fine needle biopsy fall into three groups: (1) primary pathologic processes (Table 2-1); (2) secondary pathologic processes (Table 2-2); and (3) multicentric disorders with target areas in the region.

Clinical identification of a lesion may be quite accurate, and treatment may be rendered on clinical grounds. An aphthous ulcer of the tongue is an example. On the other hand, an indurated ulcerated lesion of the tongue may be deceptive (see Case 1-2). Similarly, most nodular masses in the neck may be identified clinically as enlarged lymph nodes, but submaxillary and submandibular salivary gland enlargements, carotid body tumors, neural tumors (Case A-9), and others may be present unexpectedly.

Diseases initiated in the head and neck area may remain localized (*e.g.,* mixed tumor of the parotid), or they may metastasize (*e.g.,* nasopharyngeal carcinoma) and become part of a larger or systemic syndrome. On the other hand, an unknown primary arising below the clavicles not infrequently will make itself known by an enlargement in the neck[70] (see Cases 2-9 and 2-10).

Finally, known multicentric disorders such as infectious mononucleosis, sarcoidosis, non-Hodgkin's lymphoma, and Kaposi's sarcoma may display prominent targets in the head and neck region. Such lesions require careful history and physical examination and possibly laboratory studies such as a heterophil titer to understand the process.

Therefore, it must be recognized that many if not all palpable or visualized lesions must be considered evidence of an unknown disease process until the tissue is sampled and examined. Clinical examination alone can suggest the disease process but cannot yield a definitive diagnosis that will allow therapy. Some dermatologic lesions, such as a typical seborrheic

TABLE 2-1: Primary Lesions of the Head and Neck

Inflammatory	Neoplastic	Undefined
Sebaceous cyst	Squamous carcinoma of skin	Branchial cysts
Nodular fasciitis	Basal cell carcinoma	Eosinophilic granuloma (local-
Sarcoid	Sweat gland tumors[43]	ized)*
Tuberculosis	Lipoma	
Actinomycosis[53]	Orbital lymphoma	
Pyogenic le-	Intraorbital tumors	
sions	Primary nodal and extranodal	
	lymphomas	
	Kaposi's sarcoma[27]	
	Hodgkin's and non-Hodgkin's	
	lymphomas (stage I)	
	Calcifying epithelioma of Mal-	
	herbe	
	Tumors of tongue, tonsil, pal-	
	ate, mucosa, salivary gland,	
	carotid body, lacrimal gland,	
	glomus jugulare, skull†	
	Pituitary tumor‡	

* See also Case 10-5.

† Osteogenic sarcoma in Paget's disease, chordoma, meningioma (with skull erosion), and plasmacytoma (solitary).

‡ Chromophobe and eosinophilic adenomas, craniopharyngioma, and suprasellar
germinoma.[34]

keratosis, have highly diagnostic appearances, but they are exceptions and
treatment is not usually contemplated. Basal cell carcinomas, particularly
in the paranasal and periorbital regions, are highly characteristic, but biopsy
is always required before surgery. Surgical, usually punch, biopsy is carried
out, and fine needle aspiration is not a primary diagnostic measure. However, the fine needle is extremely useful in defining the edges of the tumor
before plastic surgery. Characteristic plugs of small basal cells are extracted
easily[42] (Fig. 2-1).

Examination of the head and neck should be preceded by questions to
elicit the location of a lesion previously discovered by the patient and
considered insignificant.

Regions of the Head and Neck

The Scalp

Inspection and palpation of the bald scalp and palpation of the hair-covered
scalp are important parts of a general physical examination and are discussed further in Chapter 9. The most common significant lesion of the
bald scalp is actinic keratosis with its predisposition to squamous carcinoma.

TABLE 2-2: Secondary Lesions of the Head and Neck

Metastatic scalp nodules
  Melanoma
  Breast
  Bronchogenic
  Gastrointestinal
  Thyroid
  Renal
Metastatic lymph nodes
  Same
Lytic skull lesions
  Multiple myeloma
  Metastatic carcinoma
  Eosinophilic granuloma*
Inflammatory lesions†
  Non-neoplastic lymphadenopathy
  Infectious mononucleosis
  Toxoplasmosis
  Cat-scratch disease
  Tuberculosis
  Sarcoid
Hodgkin's and non-Hodgkin's lymphomas (stages II to
    IV)

* Multiple sites; see Case A-3 in Appendix.
† See Chapter 8.

These lesions rarely escape diagnosis on examination by an experienced observer. More subtle, however, is the development of occipital and posterior cervical nodes, which may appear before, during, or after treatment of the primary scalp lesion. Development of posterior cervical nodes several years after treatment of a squamous carcinoma of the scalp was reported in a patient with chronic lymphocytic leukemia with adenopathy, which initially misled the physician.[42]

It is useful to question patients about lesions they might have noted in their hair-covered scalp. Melanoma may be undetected before metastasis. A patient with metastasis to the parotid nodes from a previously unnoted scalp melanoma has been reported.[42]

Probably the most common scalp "tumor" is the sebaceous or epidermoid cyst. The diagnosis is clinically confirmed by the presence of a punctate, plugged orifice from which oily, granular material can be expressed. However, many of these cysts have no orifice. They may be covered by hair. Palpation is not conclusive. Patients may say that they have had the cyst for years. Clinical judgment must be exercised, but the ease of fine needle aspiration would encourage biopsy to rule out a metastatic tumor nodule (see Chap. 9) and squamous carcinoma developing in a cyst. The latter is rare.[68] Clinical problems that arise are illustrated in Case 2-1.

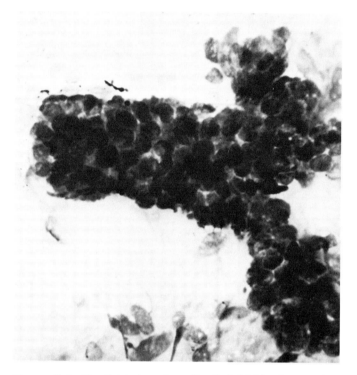

FIGURE 2-1: The tight plug of small cells is highly characteristic of basal cell carcinoma.

Case 2-1

The patient was a 58-year-old man complaining of weakness and fever. On examination of the scalp, two nodules measuring up to 2 cm were palpated. One was of recent origin. Pallor and grade II systolic murmur at the aorta were noted. Results of abdominal examination were negative. Hemoglobin level was 9 g/dL, and erythrocyte sedimentation rate (Wintrob) was 32. Two to four red blood cells were present on microscopic examination of the urine. Fine needle aspiration of the older nodule yielded sour-smelling, gritty squames characteristic of epidermoid cyst. Fine needle aspiration of the recent nodule yielded cytologic smears consistent with hypernephroma.[42] An IVP confirmed the primary origin.

Sweat gland tumors must be included in the differential diagnosis of skin lesions of the scalp, face, and neck.[38,43] They are primarily dermal lesions, and therefore may be distinguished from metastatic nodules, which are often but not always in the subcutaneous compartment. Dermal lesions move *with* the skin, but the skin is moved *over* a metastatic nodule. Although the cytology of these lesions has not been reported in detail, they may be distinguished from squamous carcinoma and, for the most part, from basal cell carcinomas. Malignant varieties are rare.[38]

Lesions of the skull including the calvarium and skull base are considered in Chapter 10.

The Orbit

The orbit is the site of several lesions that can be diagnosed by fine needle aspiration. They are orbital lymphoma; intraorbital tumors; recurrent post-exenteration orbital tumors; and lacrimal gland tumors and granulomas.

ORBITAL LYMPHOMA

Of 60 carefully studied cases originally diagnosed as orbital lymphoma, 20 were defined as benign on historic and histologic review.[39] The most significant aspect of the study from the standpoint of clinical fine needle aspiration was that 54 of the 60 lesions were palpable. In addition, 20 produced proptosis. The lesions were usually freely moveable. As with all lymphomas, their textures were varied, and included firm, rubbery, fleshy, and soft.

Sixteen of the 40 histologically confirmed malignant lymphomas were part of a generalized lymphomatous disorder.[39] Extraction of a lymphoid smear with monomorphic or immature characteristics in the clinical setting of generalized lymphoma should be decisive in the diagnosis of orbital lymphoma (see Case 9-4).

Lymphoid smears in the absence of known extraorbital lymphoma should be examined critically. All clinical data should be submitted to the pathologist. It is useful to know that virtually all orbital lymphomas occur in the sixth and seventh decades.[39] Histologically, benign diagnoses include inflammatory pseudo-tumor, reactive lymphoid hyperplasia, and atypical lymphoid hyperplasia. For the present, cytologic criteria separating benign from malignant orbital lymphoma should parallel the findings previously described for nodal lymphoma.[37]

INTRAORBITAL TUMORS

Intraorbital lesions can be reached with the help of computed tomography. This is illustrated in Case A-5 in which aspiration produced surprise findings (see Appendix). Recurrent post-exenteration orbital tumors are diagnosed easily by fine needle aspiration, and a patient with recurrence of adenoid cystic carcinoma of the lacrimal gland was reported.[42]

LACRIMAL GLANDS

Bilateral enlargement of the lacrimal glands is usually part of a recognized syndrome, such as sarcoidosis. This can be easily confirmed with fine needle aspiration. Aspiration is also an excellent technique for diagnosing a unilateral lacrimal enlargement.

Intra-Oral Tumors

Intra-oral examination requires that the patient be in a relaxed position, either supine or braced in an ear, nose, and throat (ENT) seat. Adequate light from a head lamp or reflector is essential. Inspection and palpation are necessary for adequate examination. The importance of palpation cannot be overemphasized. It often will detect lesions that are missed easily during inspection, and that may be missed when a tongue depressor is relied upon for visualization. Topical anesthetic spray is useful in some patients and is required in most patients prior to aspiration. Both hands are needed to expose, palpate, and aspirate with the one-handed syringe (Fig. 2-2). Before aspiration, the lesion is palpated to assess its texture and limits. This is carried out with the index finger covered by a finger cot or plastic gloves.

The dominant lesion of the tongue and intra-oral mucosa is squamous carcinoma. Biopsy is usually surgical. However, fine needle aspiration of an indurated lesion is easy to accomplish. It is particularly useful to diagnose a primary lesion when metastatic nodes already have been identified. Fungating tumors (Fig. 2-3) will often fail to yield diagnostic histology because of a shallow biopsy, but deeper fine needle aspiration will produce diagnostic smears. Using the fine needle method will also spare a patient the further morbidity of removing a deep wedge of tissue from such a lesion. Figure 2-3 is an example of a tumor that is clinically and unequivocally cancer, but for which the radiotherapist or oncologist requires morphologic

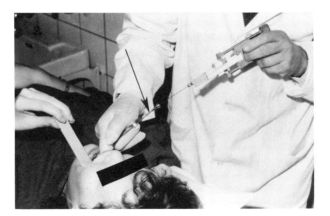

FIGURE 2-2: With the palpating finger on or above the target, the long needle is inserted through the needle guide (*arrow*). This patient was 18 years old and had an adenoid cystic carcinoma.

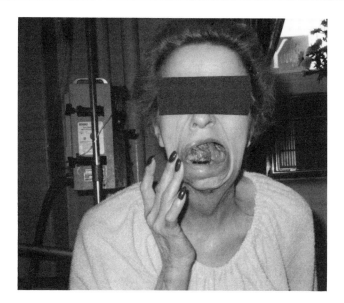

FIGURE 2-3: This patient had a fungating carcinoma of the tongue. On surgical biopsy, only necrosis was obtained. Squamous carcinoma was diagnosed by fine needle aspiration.

confirmation. Granular cell myoblastoma and neural tumors (neurilemomas, schwannomas) have fairly characteristic cytologic pictures that will allow preoperative diagnosis (Case A-9).

The enlarged tonsil should be palpated and inspected (Fig. 2-4). Squamous carcinoma is firm and lymphoma is rubbery. Fine needle aspiration will easily yield smears diagnostic of squamous carcinoma. The tonsil base forms part of Waldeyer's ring, which includes the pharynx, nasopharynx, and base of the tongue. Hyperplastic or frankly tumorous lymphoid tissues are suitable targets for fine needle aspiration. The faucial tonsil is the most frequent site of extranodal non-Hodgkin's lymphoma in the head and neck.[5] Most lymphomas in this region are nodular, poorly differentiated lymphocytic or histiocytic.[5,55] Smears consist of clusters and sheets of enlarged, poorly differentiated lymphoid cells. The distinction between nodular and diffuse histologies cannot be made by smears. Surgical biopsy is necessary. Gastrointestinal lymphoma was noted in 17.6% of Waldeyer's ring lymphomas.[3,55] Gastrointestinal (GI) studies should be performed when lymphoma is diagnosed in the region of Waldeyer's ring.

An enlarged tonsil yielding well-differentiated lymphocytes ordinarily cannot be defined as lymphoma by cytologic smear. Surgical biopsy is necessary to establish a diagnosis after suitable treatment and observation to allow regression, similar to the procedure for enlarged cervical nodes (see Chap. 8).

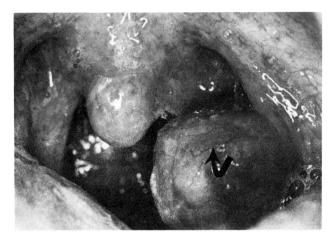

FIGURE 2-4: The enlarged tonsil (*curved arrow*) is a fairly easy target to aspirate after it is sprayed with local anesthesia.

Aspiration may yield surprise findings, as illustrated in the following case.

Case 2-2

The patient was an 80-year-old man who was brought from some distance to the clinic for evaluation of a firm left cervical node, fixed and measuring 1.5 cm. Clinically, it appeared to be a typical metastatic squamous carcinoma. Intra-oral examination revealed an obvious enlarged left tonsil that also was somewhat firm to palpation. Fine needle aspiration of both sites yielded sheets of moderately differentiated plasma cells. Sternal puncture was carried out at the same visit, and it established a diagnosis of myeloma with extramedullary extension. Further studies were obtained, and the patient was referred back with an outline of therapy to his primary physician.

The head and neck region is the most common site for extramedullary plasmacytoma.[16]

The soft palate is a site of salivary gland tumors in addition to squamous carcinoma. Mixed tumors,[42] muco-epidermoid tumors, and acinic cell tumors have been observed. Fine needle aspiration yields diagnostic smears. Preoperative identification of tumor type guides surgery.

Squamous carcinoma of the base of the tongue may be an inapparent primary in the presence of identified metastatic cervical nodes. At the initial screening by a clinician, before detailed head and neck examination with direct and indirect laryngoscopy, palpation after anesthetic spray will detect induration and nodularity. Utilizing the prostate needle guide and long needle (see Fig. 2-2) indurated areas in all parts of the oral cavity can be aspirated and diagnosis of squamous or other carcinoma documented. The poor cure rate summarized from the literature and reported in a new series by Rollo and co-workers[58] undoubtedly results in part from late diagnosis. Incorporating palpation of the tongue base into regular examination of all patients who have even minimal symptoms will improve the results by establishing early diagnosis.

Clinical awareness of intra-oral lesions is often delayed because of the patient's failure to notice an enlarging or ulcerating tumor. Enlarged tonsils or uvula, and a bulging posterior pharyngeal wall may not be detected by the patient during an early stage. Indurated and ulcerated malignant lesions of the tongue, lips, and gums often are recognized as inflammatory. Tumor may be found inadvertently during examination for a more common disorder such as pharyngitis. Intraoral melanoma is an example.[9]

Finally, lesions may be elicited during a complete search for a primary tumor or during a primary physical examination.

Facial Lesions

Primary basal cell carcinomas, as noted above, infrequently become targets for fine needle aspiration. Diagnosis of recurrence and determination of the extent of a tumor will be made by extracting basal cells through a needle as small as 25 gauge (see Figs. 9-10, 9-11). An invasive basal cell carcinoma may tunnel through the subcutaneous tissue without surface evidence, and the aspirating needle must be placed judiciously.[32] Post-radiation recurrence may be difficult to detect clinically because of the radiation-associated induration. Sampling of the suspicious area will be necessary.

Maxillary sinus tumors may erode bone and bulge the cheek, presenting a suitable target for fine needle aspiration. Surgical biopsy of such a tumor is difficult. This is, of course, a late manifestation of antral carcinoma, but because about 80% of paranasal sinus cancers arise in this compartment,[12] such cases do appear in the clinic sometimes after prolonged treatment for "sinusitis." Crusted squamous lesions of the lip and nasal vestibule should be aspirated promptly with a fine needle, or scraped, and smeared. Aspiration should be performed tangentially to extract cells from the base of the lesion. The alternative to prompt biopsy too often is observation, local applications, patient noncompliance, and ominous delay. A cytologic diagnosis of cancer will initiate therapy quickly. Surgical biopsy, sometimes punch biopsy, is necessary if cytologic preparations are nondiagnostic, and to determine extent of infiltration. Case A-1 illustrates the usefulness of fine needle aspiration in difficult and selected sites (see Appendix).

Sebaceous cysts, sweat gland tumors, nodular melanomas, and cutaneous lymphoid aggregates (see below) and lymphomas are all palpable lesions that may be sampled and diagnosed to allow surgical planning.

Lymphoid nodules may appear randomly in the subcutaneous fat. They produce a small bulge that can be punctured. The yield in three patients has been small, well-differentiated lymphocytes. None of the three has developed a lymphoproliferative disorder in 3 to 5 years. Twelve cases were studied, of which one involved the nose and three the conjunctiva.[20] Six of the twelve patients developed malignant lymphoma. Immunocytochemical studies revealing monoclonality may predict a malignant course. Subcutaneous skin nodules are not uncommon in the course of a known lymphoma. Identification by fine needle aspiration may allow treatment with radiation using a small portal, particularly in facial deposits, as Case 2-3 illustrates.

Case 2-3

The patient was a 55-year-old woman who presented with a stage I chronic lymphocytic leukemia. After 1 year, a hemolytic anemia supervened, and she was treated with chlorambucil (Leukeran) and steroids, with improvement. The disease then assumed the aspect of non-Hodgkin's lymphoma with no further evidence of leukemia. Nodes fluctuated in size for several years in different regions. At 5 years, a 0.5-cm nodule was palpated in the fleshy portion of the anterior chin. It was aspirated and treated with radiation using a small portal. Two additional lymphoid infiltrates appeared in the cheek and forehead. Both were identified and treated. The disease progressed over a 12-year period, and the patient died.

Primary cutaneous lymphoma is discussed in Chapter 9.

Finally, patients who present with ostensibly benign lesions may plan to have plastic surgery (Fig. 2-5). Such lesions should be sampled preoperatively, so that after a meticulous plastic procedure it is not discovered that the diagnosis was amelanotic melanoma, leiomyosarcoma, and so forth, necessitating further surgery.

Salivary Glands

Preoperative diagnosis of salivary gland masses is a valuable clinical aid.[6,47,51] Smears obtained by fine needle aspiration will separate lesions immediately into operative and nonoperative cases. Lesions in which excisional therapy is optional (o), unnecessary (u), or contraindicated (c) are listed below:

Acute sialadenitis	(u)
Chronic sialadenitis	(o)
Intraglandular lymphadenitis	(u)

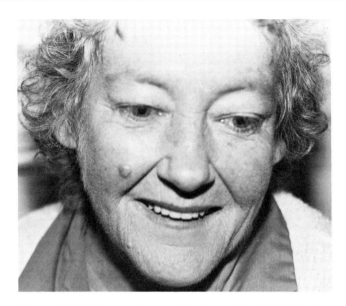

FIGURE 2-5: The nonpigmented lesion on the right side of this patient's face had enlarged recently. A nodular amelanotic melanoma cannot be excluded clinically. Preoperative fine needle aspiration is indicated.

Metabolic disorders	(u)
Benign cystic lesion (Fig. 2-10)[24]	
(see later sections branchial cysts)	(o)
Lymphoepithelial lesion[7]	(o)
Sarcoid (Heerfordt's disease)	(u)
Lipoma[35]	(o)
Primary lymphoma: Hodgkin's disease	
and non-Hodgkin's type	(o)
Extranodal extension of lymphoma:	
Hodgkin's and non-Hodgkin's	(u)
Metastatic and undifferentiated carcinoma	(c)

Smears consisting of intact and degenerated granulocytes, sometimes with the appearance in the syringe of thin pus, are diagnostic of acute suppurative sialadenitis. The gland is enlarged and usually tender. Overlying skin may be reddened.

Chronic sialadenitis presents problems both clinically and cytologically. It is one source of false-positive evaluation. There may be a firm mass that will not regress. In our experience, however, excision has been carried out only when the cytologic diagnosis was false-positive or suspicious, an infrequent occurrence.

Intraglandular lymphadenitis is diagnosed when the mass yields polymorphous lymphoid smears. Inflammation is confirmed in the presence of regional infection, suspected cat scratch, and fairly prompt regression. Tuberculous parotid lymphadenopathy has been reported with error in diagnosis in many with the usual diagnostic measures.[54] Aspiration of granular necrotic material may yield fairly diagnostic smears. Some of the material should be stained for acid fast bacillus (AFB) and cultured. Clinical evaluation and clinical suspicion are important.

The cause of soft bilateral enlargement of the parotid glands usually can be recognized from the clinical context. The glands may be infiltrated with fat in chronic alcoholism with cirrhosis. Benign enlargement has been reported in bulimia (compulsive overeating and vomiting).[41] Patients with dehydration, terminal illness, and diabetes occasionally have glandular enlargement. Fine needle aspiration will yield cytologically normal glandular fragments.

Cysts that yield squamous smears (characteristic of branchial cysts) or clear fluid, with collapse and no residual, can be observed. Where there is suspicion of tumor, however, excision must be considered (see below). Unexpected benign lesions may be present.

Benign lymphoepithelial lesions (Mikulicz's disease,[66] Godwin's disease,[25] Sjögren's disease[64]) may yield a reasonably characteristic cytologic picture. Sjögren's (sicca) syndrome with involvement of the lacrimal glands, conjunctiva, intraoral and nasal mucosa, and polyarthritis will confirm the diagnosis.

Sarcoidosis (Heerfordt's disease, uveoparotid fever) is diagnosed readily on examination of smears by an experienced observer. There is often bilateral involvement of the parotid gland. This is seen most commonly in black female patients in the second and third decades of life. Lacrimal glands may be involved, simulating Sjögren's syndrome. However, the cytology is distinctive.

Facial nerve paralysis in the presence of parotid masses or infiltrations is a pitfall in diagnosis. Severe nonspecific chronic inflammation can produce a desmoplastic reaction with compromise of the facial nerve.[42] Similarly, sarcoidosis of the parotid gland may result in facial nerve paralysis.[26] Both of these inflammatory lesions may be confused with invasive carcinoma, which produces similar paralysis.[65]

Lipoma is an uncommon tumor.[35] However, when a satisfactory cytologic diagnosis is made, particularly in an older patient, it may be left *in situ.*

Hodgkin's and non-Hodgkin's lymphoma may involve intraglandular lymph nodes as part of regional or generalized nodal disease. In that context, cytologic diagnosis is straightforward and surgery is unnecessary.

Primary extranodal salivary gland lymphoma has been reported in detail by Hyman and Wolff.[31] They encountered only one case of Hodgkin's disease in a group of 33 patients with lymphomas. All pathologic types of non-Hodgkin's lymphoma were described, and origin in intraglandular lymph nodes was definite in six cases and likely in a number of others. In four cases, contiguous lymphoepithelial lesions were evident.

From the standpoint of fine needle aspiration, extraction of lymphoid smears characteristic of lymphoma[37] would permit nonsurgical treatment (radiation and chemotherapy) in elderly patients or in other patients with medical disorders that increase surgical risk. Whether potentially surgical lesions will be treated nonsurgically based on cytologic diagnosis will depend on the physician's confidence in the diagnosis and results of future studies.

METASTATIC AND UNDIFFERENTIATED CARCINOMA

Patients with poorly differentiated or undifferentiated carcinomas that are clinically invading the surrounding tissues are probably poor surgical subjects and would be better served by radiation and chemotherapy. Perceptions of operability vary from surgeon to surgeon. Fine needle aspiration can establish the fact of high grade malignancy.

Metastasis to the parotid is illustrated in the following case.

Case 2-4

The patient was a 64-year-old black woman referred for aspiration of a mass in the right parotid gland. The gland appeared to be densely infiltrated, and was fixed to the surrounding tissue with some skin puckering. The central elevated portion was aspirated. The smears had none of the characteristic cytologic patterns of the variety of primary salivary gland tumors that have been described.[42] Therefore, the mass was considered to be a primary undifferentiated carcinoma. In spite of radiotherapy, the disease progressed rapidly. At autopsy, a moderate-sized, poorly differentiated ductal carcinoma was found within the fatty tissue on one pendulous breast. The pathology was the same as that in the mestastasis.

COMMENT Spread to the scalp occurred from this metastatic mass. Discontinuous invasion of the scalp by breast carcinoma is discussed in Chapter 9.

OPERATIVE LESIONS SPECIFICALLY IDENTIFIED
BY FINE NEEDLE ASPIRATION

Salivary gland tumors that present palpable targets for fine needle aspiration include those of the three largest paired glands: the parotid, submaxillary, and sublingual. Mucus and serous glands lie submucosally throughout the oral cavity, palate (hard and soft), and parts of the pharynx. Any of these surfaces may be a site of tumor formation that can become a target for fine needle aspiration.[13,52] The cytologic yield from these tumors is the same as that from the three major paired groups, and in most cases it will identify the following tumor types:

Benign
    Mixed tumor (pleomorphic adenoma)
    Warthin's tumor (papillary cystadenoma lymphomatosum)
    Oncocytoma

Malignant
    Malignant mixed
    Adenoid cystic
    Acinic cell
    Mucoepidermoid
    Adenopapillary
    Squamous

For the clinician, oncologist, and surgeon, information resulting from fine needle aspiration is critical to management. Separation of benign and malignant tumors allows surgical planning and provides important data for both the patient and the surgeon. The importance of cooperation between clinician and pathologist cannot be overstated. Familiarity with cytologic as well as clinical principles is quite useful if not mandatory.

SPECIFIC PRIMARY CELL TYPES

The diagnosis of Warthin's tumor should alert the clinician to the possibility of bilaterality. Malignant tumors have been seen,[42] but they are distinctly rare. Excision can be limited with little fear of recurrence. Pleomorphic adenoma (mixed tumor) tends to recur, and ultimately may transform to a malignant lesion. So-called benign mixed tumors also can metastasize.[42] Smears may be extremely cellular with little or no stroma. This is a pitfall in cytologic diagnosis. Diagnosis is aided by the physical examination and history. Recurrence or neglect leading to a massive lobulated tumor present for years is highly characteristic. Most surgical procedures, meticulously done, will require only removal of the superficial lobe without damage to the seventh nerve.

Oncocytomas are benign, although cytologically benign cases with invasion have been seen.[15] The tumor is encapsulated. Therefore, ablation is necessary but radical surgery is not.

Survival rates of patients with the main malignant tumor types are illustrated in Figure 2-6.

Fine needle aspiration may be used to separate mucoepidermoid and adenoid cystic tumors into types with better and worse prognosis. The more malignant tumors produce early fixation, dimpling, and ulceration of the skin. The less malignant mucoepidermoid tumors raise this type as a group into a better prognostic category (see Fig. 2-6). Adenoid cystic carcinoma has been divided into solid (better prognosis) and trabecular or cribiform

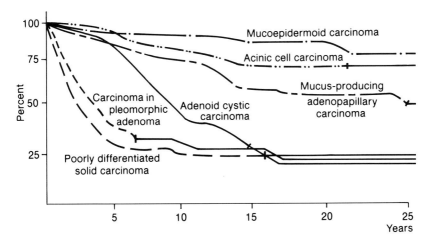

FIGURE 2-6: Carcinoma of the parotid gland. Survival rate in the main carcinoma types. Full line denotes fewer than 10 observations. (Adapted from Blanck C: Carcinoma of the Parotid Gland. Master's thesis, Acta Universitatis Upsaliensis, Uppsala, 1974.)

(poorer prognosis) types.[17,52] These types can be appreciated cytologically[42] and an approach to surgical planning can be considered. Because of their location in the head and neck region, the extent of a local procedure with its consequent disfigurement is an important issue, as is the question of radical neck dissection in the absence of palpable nodes. The recurrence of adenoid cystic carcinoma may be insidious. A high index of suspicion coupled with frequent fine needle aspiration of even slightly indurated areas will disclose early recurrence.

In general, cytologic criteria will guide therapy in the other malignant tumor types. As with other cancers, the initial procedure often determines the future of the patient. Some tumors, such as acinic cell carcinoma (identified by fine needle aspiration), enlarge in a painless slow-growing fashion, yet may have infiltrating borders. Knowing the tumor types preoperatively, particularly when dealing with rare or infrequent lesions, allows time for research and preparation. Outside of the few specialized centers worldwide, surgeons and oncologists cannot accumulate large personal experience with individual tumor types, and preoperative diagnosis will afford them time to review the subject before the crucial initial procedure.

PITFALLS IN DIAGNOSIS

The clinician, whether he performs the aspiration and refers slides for diagnosis, or simply refers the patient, must utilize all determined clinical data in the final analysis of the cytologic report. All cystic lesions must be evaluated with follow-up aspiration of residual induration. Branchial cysts and Warthin's tumors will yield fairly characteristic smears. Unexplained, poorly cellular cystic fluids, though they may result from simple retention cysts, must be suspicious for mucoepidermoid carcinoma.

Chronic inflammatory reactions may produce a clinical picture simulating malignancy, including seventh nerve paralysis (see above). Similarly, glandular destruction may leave hyperplastic ducts with atypical epithelium and form a delineated tumor mass that can be read as neoplasm on fine needle aspiration—a false-positive result.

Cytologic reports that fail to identify tumor type require further clinical evaluation of the patient. Also, tumors may vary considerably in size, and nodules as small as 1 cm may yield a variety of salivary tumor types, including lethal carcinomas.

Diagnostic problems are illustrated in Case 2-5.

Case 2-5

A healthy 21-year-old man was referred for fine needle aspiration of a left preauricular nodule measuring 1 cm by 1.5 cm. The nodule had been noted 2 months earlier; however, on further questioning, it was determined that it may have been enlarging for 1 year. His family doctor, suspecting an infection, referred the patient to a specialist in infectious diseases. He then was referred to an otolaryngologist, who ordered a sialogram. Findings were normal. The family doctor then sent the patient to an oral surgeon, who referred the patient for fine needle aspiration.

Aspiration yielded typical smears of benign mixed tumor 1 month after the patient had visited his family physician.

COMMENT It is very apparent that the direct route to diagnosis in this patient was fine needle aspiration.

CAROTID BODY TUMORS
PARAGANGLIOMAS

The cytology of carotid body tumors has been defined and reported elsewhere.[19,42] Experience has shown that the morphology is consistently diagnostic.

Carotid body tumor was the admitting diagnosis in only 8 of 43 patients with the tumor. Other diagnoses considered were tuberculosis, lymphadenitis, branchiogenic cyst, benign salivary gland enlargement, schwannoma, malignant lymphoma, carcinoma of thyroid and larynx, and metastatic carcinoma.[40]

Carotid body tumors appear in the region of the carotid bifurcation. They often have a history of growth over a period of months to years. The slow growth and absence of symptoms may result in neglect and late

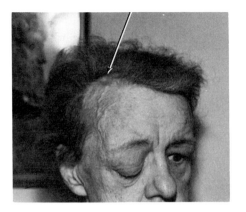

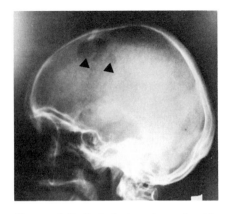

FIGURE 2-7: This patient has a metastatic paraganglioma. The depression in the scalp (*arrow*) is the site of the lytic lesion in the calvarium (see Fig. 2-8). Ptosis and proptosis of the right eye are present.

FIGURE 2-8: Lytic lesions (*arrowheads*) in the calvarium are evident.

presentation of the tumor for diagnosis. The tumor is deep beneath the sternocleidomastoid, and may be tender to palpation. It can be moved horizontally but not vertically. It is more common in hypoxic environments[62] and is associated with chronic diseases causing hypoxia.[49] It may be familial, and there is an increased incidence of bilateral occurrence.[28,61]

Malignancy occurred in 5 of 69 patients with paragangliomas of the head and neck.[40] This was discussed further by Robertson and Cooney.[57] A metastatic ganglioma is illustrated in Case 2-6, which follows.

Case 2-6

The patient was a 63-year-old woman who had a rubbery mass near her right parotid gland. Fine needle aspiration yielded smears that were read by an expert cytopathologist as consistent with paraganglioma. Subsequent surgical biopsy confirmed the diagnosis.

The tumor was deemed nonresectable and the patient received radiation. Retrobulbar invasion occurred 6 months later, with proptosis of her eye (Fig. 2-7). Examination at this time revealed a soft swelling with a central depression in the right anterior scalp (*arrow*). Lytic lesions were present in the calvarium at the same site (Fig. 2-8). The scalp/skull lesion was aspirated easily. Aspiration confirmed the diagnosis of metastatic paraganglioma.

Treatment with streptozotocin produced significant tumor regression.

Figure 2-9 shows a 24-year-old man with a walnut-sized tumor in the right side of his neck. The aspirated material was mixed with blood. Cytologic findings were typical for paraganglioma (carotid body tumor; see Fig. 2-9) and were confirmed on histologic section.

Cytologically, metastatic follicular carcinoma of the thyroid must be considered because of the occasional glandular appearance. Spindle cells that may be reported should not be confused with spindle cell melanoma, medullary carcinoma of the thyroid, neurofibroma, and spindle cell metastatic renal carcinoma.

The tumors are quite vascular and have a characteristic vascular pattern on angiography. This diagnostic procedure is considered safer than fine needle aspiration because of the rare possibility of thrombosis of the carotid artery or hemorrhage. However, needle aspiration was performed in one series of 15 cases and in another series of 13 cases without serious mishap.[19,40]

Paragangliomas are less likely to produce palpable tumor for direct puncture in other locations. In the series of Lack and co-workers, in addition to 44 carotid body tumors, there were 13 vagal body tumors, 8 jugulo-tympanic tumors, 3 nasal tumors, and one in either the orbit, larynx, or aortic arch region.[40]

BRANCHIAL CLEFT CYSTS

The branchial cleft cyst, which usually appears between the ages of 10 and 30,[11,30] is a common target for fine needle aspiration. Zajicek selected 100 cases from the archives at Radiumhemmet and presented the cytology, which is fairly characteristic.[70] Detailed studies of 468 cases at the Armed Forces Institute of Pathology have established that these structures arise as

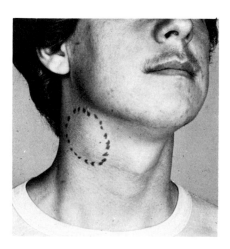 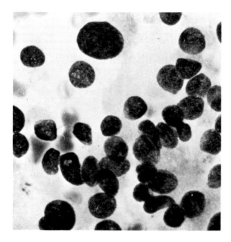

FIGURE 2-9: (*Left*) This patient's neck mass was a generic tumor until it was identified by fine needle aspiration as a paraganglioma. (*Right*) Aspiration cytology showed typical microscopic findings of paraganglioma.

epithelial cysts within lymph nodes rather than from embryonic remnants of branchial cleft epithelium.[10] This explains their presence in sites extrinsic to the topographic region of the sternocleidomastoid muscle.[42] They are found within the parotid gland,[30] the angle of the mandible, the submandibular area, the preauricular area, posterior to the sternocleidomastoid, and the posterior angle of the neck.[10]

The cyst may be a firm, rubbery mass simulating a lymphoid tumor or even metastatic carcinoma. The extraction of fluid, which enters the syringe freely and rapidly, is often a surprise. The fluid is usually a turbid yellowish-gray. Careful palpation and repeat aspiration of residual induration should be performed.

Fourteen branchial cysts in the parotid gland have been collected by Hoffman.[30] Aspiration of fluid may easily lead to a false diagnosis of Warthin's tumor (see below). In the differential diagnosis of branchial cysts in the parotid gland, Hoffman included lymphadenitis, hygroma, lipoma, lymphoma, parotid tumor, and sialadenitis.

In Figure 2-10, we see a patient with a doughy mass of the left parotid gland, which had been present for 6 months. Fine needle aspiration yielded smears consisting of inspissated squames. The cytologic diagnosis rendered was epidermoid cyst, left parotid. This cyst may have been of branchial origin.

CARCINOMA IN BRANCHIAL CLEFT CYST AND
METASTASIS WITH INAPPARENT PRIMARY

The existence of carcinoma arising in a branchial cleft cyst has been questioned by Willis,[68] although he reported one acceptable case. Martin and co-workers proposed four criteria for the diagnosis of primary carcinoma of a branchial cleft cyst.[46] There was only one absolute criterion, namely, histologic demonstration of a cancer developing in the wall of an epithelial-lined cyst in the lateral neck. Bernstein and co-workers presented a case with an acceptable criterion, but stressed that all proposed cases should be supported by a thorough search for an occult primary and that follow-up searches should be maintained after obliteration of the primary lesion.[8]

Fine needle aspiration of a branchial cyst with carcinoma in the wall would yield turbid, possibly hemorrhagic, fluid containing benign squamous cells and clusters of malignant cells. As with all malignant cysts and body fluids, failure to find malignant cells does not exclude cancer. Careful palpation to detect residual induration is essential after evacuation.

Cystic squamous carcinoma is well known, particularly in bronchogenic cancers. Cystic breakdown of metastatic squamous carcinoma in lateral neck nodes may produce fluid by necrosis and suppuration, and may simulate malignancy in a branchial cyst. The fluid yield may be similar, although the likelihood of positive cytology is greater.

Squamous carcinoma metastatic to lateral neck nodes is readily identified by fine needle aspiration (see below). In several series, 8% to 15%

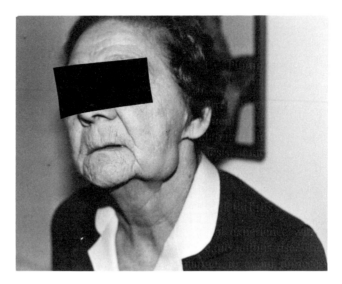

FIGURE 2-10: The mass in this patient's left parotid gland had a doughy consistency and yielded sheets of squames on fine needle aspiration.

of cases failed to reveal a primary source on initial examination,[14,23,33] and in 69% of one group (123 cases), the patients either survived or died without the primary source being found.[4] Obliteration of a malignant branchial cyst by extension of the tumor would make distinction from metastatic carcinoma with an unknown primary impossible.

The Enlarged Lymph Node

Lymph nodes in the head, neck and all regions of the body are deemed "enlarged" depending on the diligence of the examination and the clinical perception of "abnormal." For example, patients are not infrequently referred for fine needle aspiration of nodes that either were not palpated by the aspirating physician or were not considered clinically significant. Normal, noninvolved lymph nodes vary in size from several millimeters (for example, detected in pathologic examination of excised axillary contents), up to a flattened nodule 1 cm in length that might appear in the supraclavicular region (an area not usually subject to antigenic stimulation). On the other hand, small nodes appearing in unexpected regions may be pathologic, as illustrated in Cases 2-7 and 2-8.

Case 2-7

The patient was a 36-year-old physical education instructor with a heightened concern for his physical status. He had palpated a node in the left posterior cervical triangle. On examination, the node was measured 4 mm in greatest dimension. It was firm, and no scalp inflammation could be detected. The node was aspirated with a 25-gauge needle, and yielded a monomorphic smear composed of well-differentiated lymphocytes. On surgical biopsy, the histologic diagnosis was well-differentiated, diffuse non-Hodgkin's lymphoma. The patient was observed without therapy. At age 48 years, he was asymptomatic and had generalized lymphadenopathy with nodes up to 2 cm in greatest dimension.

Diagnosis and management of lymphomatous nodes is discussed in Chapter 8. Clinically enlarged (pathologic) nodes are divided into distinct groups by the findings on fine needle aspiration. Lymphoid smears are yielded by inflammatory, reactive, or lymphomatous nodes (see Chap. 8). The cytologic findings may be quite diagnostic, as illustrated in Case 2-8.

Case 2-8

The patient was an asymptomatic 75-year-old woman who requested examination of a node she had detected in her left posterior cervical triangle. She thought it had appeared suddenly, but agreed that it might have evolved slowly and that she may have just noticed it. There was no significant medical history, and there were no prior surgical procedures. On examination, scalp, orapharynx, nasal passages, external node-bearing regions, and abdomen were normal. The node was solitary, firm, and mobile and measured 1 cm. Her family physician had dismissed it to be rechecked in several months.

Fine needle aspiration yielded an abundantly cellular smear. It was lymphoid on low-power microscopy with no evidence of extraneous epithelial or metastatic cells. On closer examination, the smear was mixed with numerous eosinophils, frequent neutrophils, and a variety of lymphoid cells, including small lymphocytes, numerous transformed cells, and atypical poorly differentiated lymphoid cells with enlarged and multiple nucleoli. On careful examination, rare but convincing Sternberg–Reed cells were seen (Fig. 2-11). Hodgkin's disease was confirmed by biopsy and surgical pathology.

COMMENT The atypical location of the node prompted aspiration.

Detailed discussion of metastatic lymph nodes is presented in Chapter 8. For the clinician, aspiration of cervical nodes is an adjuvant technique that is preceded by careful history, regional and general examination, and formulation of a clinical diagnosis. It has been well established that in 50% of metastatic cervical nodes, the primary source is below the clavicle.[18] This

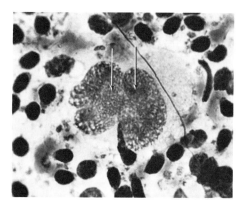

Figure 2-11: Aspirate of lymph node shows Sternberg–Reed cell with giant nucleoli (*arrows*).

is based on a review of 1101 patients with cytologically verified carcinomatous metastasis in cervical lymph nodes. Patients in this review were unselected, recruited from the population of Stockholm and environs. It is clear that the percentages would vary if patients were recruited from the selected population of a head and neck oncology unit or hospital.

For the primary clinician faced with suspicious neck nodes in the adult, examination of the breasts, abdomen, pelvis, and prostate together with chest x-ray is as important as intra-oral examination. Clinical information obtained in such examination will help guide the cytopathologist.

History and physical examinations of the aforementioned regions and the head and neck should be followed immediately by fine needle aspiration. Indirect studies including x-rays, scans, and laboratory determinations produce a low diagnostic yield in comparison with direct sampling of the node. In addition, they are costly and time consuming, and can branch into endless diversionary studies. Cytologically identifiable primary carcinomas are presented in Table 2-3.

Squamous Carcinoma: Geography and Primary Site

For some lesions, location of the metastatic node can be correlated with the primary site with modest success. However, it must be kept in mind that the logical regional spread of carcinoma is regularly altered by prior surgery, including lymphadenectomy, and by radiation, which obliterates lymphatic pathways.[56]

Clinical evaluation of submental nodes gives a low diagnostic yield. Even in the presence of a known squamous carcinoma of the lip, a significant percentage of enlarged submental nodes are reported to be inflammatory. Squamous carcinoma in submental nodes requires careful exami-

TABLE 2-3: Cytologically Identifiable
Primary Carcinomas

THYROID CARCINOMA	LUNG CARCINOMA
Follicular	Oat cell (small)
Papillary	KIDNEY CARCINOMA
Medullary	Hypernephroma
SALIVARY GLAND CARCINOMA	GASTROINTESTINAL CANCER
Adenoid cystic	Signet ring
Adenopapillary	Carcinoid
BREAST CARCINOMA	TESTIS (OVARY)
Apocrine	Seminoma
Magenta bodies	MELANOMA

nation of the lower lip, lower gingiva, floor of the mouth, and buccal mucosa. Particularly in this area, where a small primary could have been surgically removed, it is important to question the patient about prior lesions. A significant number of patients with oral cancers are recruited from noncompliant smokers and drinkers who may fail to volunteer such information.

Nasopharyngeal carcinoma is the major site of occult carcinoma in the head and neck region. As many as 90% of patients with nasopharyngeal carcinoma may present with clinically positive nodes,[48] and more than 50% of these patients had bilateral nodes. Diligent palpation of the angle of the jaw will reveal an enlarged jugulodigastric node, which is a major clinical clue to the diagnosis of nasopharyngeal carcinoma. Where this finding accompanies cranial nerve symptoms, it may explain a puzzling syndrome caused by local invasion of nasopharyngeal carcinoma. Enlarged nodes in the occipital region and posterior triangle are most often due to spread from a scalp lesion. However, nasopharyngeal carcinoma may also be the primary site. Nasopharyngeal carcinoma varies histologically from low grade squamous lesions to poorly differentiated types with characteristics of small or larger cell anaplastic tumors. Many cases are of the poorly differentiated type, and therefore tend to metastasize freely to all areas of the neck and remotely.

Enlarged cervical nodes also may be the presenting sign of small unobtrusive carcinomas of the tongue. They may have a small ulcerating surface while invading deeply, or may even present as a submucosal nodule found only by palpation. Such lesions can be aspirated with a 25-gauge needle immediately after identifying the squamous nature of the metastatic node.

The other primary sites in head and neck (larynx, hypopharynx, base of tongue, nasal cavity, and paranasal sinuses) usually will produce local symptoms before or coincident with the discovery of metastatic nodes.[59,60] The lateral and anterior triangles of the neck are the usual sites of metastasis.

Recurrent disease targets for fine needle aspiration in the head and neck are postoperative and post-irradiation nodes, nodules, scars, and in-filtrations. Fine needle aspiration can be a useful part of the routine post-treatment examination. Finding the earliest recurrence requires careful fin-gertip palpation of the incision and treated area. Post-irradiation induration should be punctured freely on minimal suspicion rather than observed. Dependence on surgical biopsy of this region will delay diagnosis because of concern about negative yield and poor healing. Neither of these consid-erations play a role in aspiration biopsy. Well over 50% of the post-treat-ment smears that we have received for diagnosis (usually from radiotherapy departments) are negative, indicating that aspiration biopsy is used freely. Nevertheless, a significant number of early recurrences are found by this method. Intra-oral palpation also is a useful adjunct to inspection in the follow-up examination. Submucosal nodes and nodules indicating metas-tasis and recurrence will be detected.[48]

Fistulas that fail to heal and local infiltration of tracheostomy sites and laryngostomas are important targets for fine needle aspiration. It will ob-viate wedge biopsy, and can be done early.

Finding squamous cells that range from well to poorly differentiated (best studied by staining with Papanicolaou's stain) in lymph node aspirates is virtually pathognomonic of metastatic squamous carcinoma. Nonsqua-mous cytologic findings that may be identified by an experienced cytologist are listed in Table 2-4. Other metastases not originating in the head and neck are discussed in Chapter 8.

The Unidentified Neck Mass

All experienced clinicians can reasonably separate neck masses into broad categories by careful history and palpation. Lymph nodes, cysts, thyroid enlargements, phlegmonous inflammations, and possibly less common dis-orders such as sarcomas can be sorted out. It is demonstrated repeatedly in this book that no matter how compelling the clinical picture, a morphologic diagnosis (cytology or histology) usually is necessary before undertaking any major therapy. However, lesser therapy—including obser-vation alone, symptomatic treatment (such as moist compresses), or even antibiotic therapy—certainly may be pursued, often successfully, on the basis of clinical perception alone without any biopsy procedure. Careful explanation to the patient or the patient's family of the importance of follow up to be sure that regression occurs is, of course, essential. The following cases illustrate diagnostic measures taken in identifying a neck mass.

Case 2-9

A 68-year-old woman was referred to the oncology clinic because of an enlarging mass in her left anterior neck (Fig. 2-12). The referring physician had made a clinical diagnosis of thyroid tumor of undeter-

TABLE 2-4: Differential Diagnosis of Cervical Nodes*

Adults	Children

BENIGN LYMPHORETICULAR DISORDERS

Adults	Children
Lymphadenitis	Lymphadenitis
Acute	Acute
Chronic	Chronic
Toxoplasmosis	Toxoplasmosis
Infectious mononucleosis	Infectious mononucleosis
Actinomycosis	Cat-scratch disease
Sarcoidosis	Anticonvulsant therapy
Syphilis	Vaccinations
Acquired immune deficiency syndrome	

MALIGNANT LYMPHORETICULAR DISORDERS

Adults	Children
Non-Hodgkin's lymphoma	Non-Hodgkin's lymphoma
Hodgkin's disease	Hodgkin's disease
Plasmacytoma	Neuroblastoma

METASTATIC CARCINOMAS AND SARCOMAS (PRIMARIES)

Adults	Children
Squamous: head and neck	Thyroid
Squamous: bronchogenic	Rhabdomyosarcoma
Thyroid	Ewing's sarcoma
Breast	
Gastrointestinal tract	
Lung: nonsquamous	
Kidney, testis, prostate	
Melanoma	

* Diagnosis by fine needle aspiration.

mined type. On reviewing the history, it was apparent that the patient had lost weight and was chronically ill. Examination revealed that the mass was partially fixed and did not move on swallowing. No lymph nodes were palpable. Examination of the breasts showed no abnormalities. A recent chest x-ray had two nodules suspicious for metastasis. The abdomen was flat. The liver was palpable at 3 cm and firm. Tattoo marks associated with radiation treatment were evident on the lower part of her abdomen. She stated that she had been treated for a pelvic condition, but she did not know the nature of it. On further investigation, it was determined that she had been treated for an endometrial carcinoma 5 years previously.

Fine needle aspiration of the mass yielded smears consistent with endometrial carcinoma. None of the usual thyroid tumors[42] could be identified from the smear. The patient subsequently died. Metastatic endometrial carcinoma was demonstrated at autopsy.

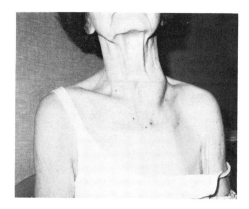

FIGURE 2-12: This patient was referred with a clinical diagnosis of thyroid tumor. Metastatic endometrial carcinoma was diagnosed by fine needle aspiration combined with clinical history.

Studies performed were history and physical examination, followed by fine needle aspiration of the neck mass.

Diagnosis was metastatic endometrial carcinoma.

Case 2-10

This patient (Fig. 2-13) visited the oncology clinic with a lump visible and palpable in his right lateral neck. It had been enlarging slowly and was asymptomatic. He had not seen a physician, but had been advised by a friend to attend the clinic. He was a smoker, but had no respiratory symptoms. He felt essentially well, had a normal appetite, and had not lost weight. On examination, the mass was fairly fixed and rubbery. No other nodes were palpable. His liver was not enlarged and no masses were palpable. No tumors were evident on rectal examination. The prostate was moderately enlarged and indurated. However, he had no urinary symptoms.

Fine needle aspiration of the cervical mass was performed as an initial study. Adenocarcinoma suggesting a prostate primary was considered. Prostate aspiration was performed immediately, and a moderately differentiated carcinoma with cytologic findings similar to the nodal smears was found.

Studies performed were history and physical examination, fine needle aspiration of the cervical mass, and fine needle aspiration of the prostate.

Diagnosis was metastatic prostate carcinoma.

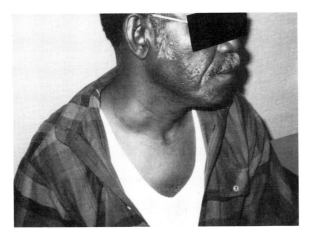

FIGURE 2-13: The lateral neck mass in this patient yielded adenocarcinoma on fine needle aspiration, suggesting a primary lesion in the prostate. This diagnosis was confirmed.

Enlarged Neck Nodes in Children

Enlarged neck nodes in children are a common clinical problem for which aspiration biopsy cytology is an important adjuvant procedure. Lymph nodes in children are extremely reactive and may enlarge rapidly to sizes that alarm parents and primary physicians. Referral for fine needle aspiration or even for surgical biopsy often is precipitated by anxiety. The great majority of enlarged nodes are nonspecific reactions to respiratory viruses and acute self-limited or treatable bacterial infections. They will regress after the antigenic stimulus has disappeared. Some will remain enlarged for days or weeks after the infection. Patients may be seen early or late in the course of the disorder and the clinical and cytologic findings will vary accordingly.

The most important and immediate determination is the separation of benign and malignant nodes. Although immediate aspiration may establish the diagnosis, it should be preceded by history and physical examination. Information so obtained will help reduce diagnostic possibilities for the clinician and should be submitted to the cytopathologist to aid cytologic differentiation.

Figure 2-14 illustrates a solitary node that was present for 3 months in a 3-year-old child. It was a residual swelling after an acute pharyngitis. However, its persistence was cause for parental anxiety, which led to a request for fine needle aspiration.

The cytologic report follows: ''A single smear consists of abundant lymphoid cells with a mixed pattern. There are numerous scattered transformed cells intermixed with both small and intermediate lymphoid cells.

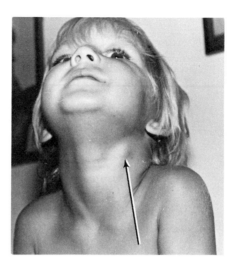

FIGURE 2-14: The solitary cervical node (*arrow*) in this patient yielded a reactive smear, which dictated delay in surgical biopsy.

There is an occasional neutrophil and plasma cell. Diagnosis: reactive lymphadenitis."

Fortified with a benign cytologic report, the clinician usually will be able to carry the family through this anxious period in anticipation of further, albeit slow, regression, and avoid surgery.

Outside of cancer centers or children's hospitals where pediatric tumors are concentrated, the primary diagnosis of a metastatic pediatric tumor from aspiration smears of cervical nodes is unusual. In 20 years of active oncologic practice, during which we have aspirated many cervical nodes in children, no metastatic tumors have been detected. However, primary lymphoma has been seen occasionally. The overwhelming majority of aspirations have yielded inflammatory or reactive smears, which have reduced the problem to separating the inflammation into specific types. Toxoplasmosis, for example, has been studied with the fine needle method,[1,2] and is discussed in detail in Chapter 7.

However, it is important to note that when toxoplasmosis is not associated with malignancy, adenopathy without fever is the most common presentation, and when toxoplasmosis is an opportunistic infection engrafted on underlying malignancy, adenopathy is rare.[29] The other important cause of pediatric cervical adenopathy is cat-scratch disease. History is important, with exposure to scratches by young cats a crucial feature. So-called oculoglandular disease with granuloma of the palpebral fissure and preauricular adenopathy occurs in a minority of cases of cat-scratch disease.[45] Cat-scratch disease also has been added to the list of non-neoplastic adenopathies that can histologically simulate lymphoma.[44] (See Chap. 8.) Exposure to pets is part of the history in both toxoplasmosis and cat-scratch disease. Clusters of granulocytes in smears, coupled with appropriate history, strengthens the diagnosis of cat-scratch disease.

A history of anticonvulsant therapy and vaccination, and a positive serologic test for infectious mononucleosis help confirm the respective diagnoses.

Non-Hodgkin's lymphoma with monomorphic smears is considered in Chapter 8. Such smears do not usually cause problems in differentiation from benign smears. The separation of benign hyperplastic smears from Hodgkin's disease may be a problem. The classical Sternberg–Reed cell is dramatic and diagnostic (see Fig. 2-10). Where the cytopathologist cannot specifically diagnose Hodgkin's disease, the clinician must rely on clinical criteria. The failure of nodes to regress with appropriate therapy or the passage of an appropriate amount of time must raise the question of surgical biopsy. In pediatric cases surgical biopsy to look for lymphoma should not be an early examination because of the low yield.

Nonepithelial Tumors of the Head and Neck

A variety of nonepithelial tumors of the head and neck must be kept in mind. They are discussed in previous publications. They include lymphomas (which are discussed under extranodal lymphomas in Chapter 9), plasmacytomas (see Case 2-2), fibrous histiocytoses, and smooth muscle, skeletal muscle, adipose, cartilaginous, osseous, and neural tumors. Case A-9 illustrates the importance of considering nonepithelial tumors.

Extracranial Meningiomas

The cytologic findings of meningiomas obtained from fine needle aspiration preparations are highly characteristic.[67] (See Case A-4.) Therefore, it is useful to be aware of potential sites of extracranial meningioma, which may present as lytic skull lesions (Case A-4), parotid tumors,[69] and tumors of the nasal cavity and paranasal sinuses,[15] orbit,[71] and skin.[50]

Summary

The head and neck region provides a wide variety of targets diagnosable by simple observation, palpation, and aspiration. In principle, almost all lesions are generic until cytology or pathology is examined under the microscope. There are a number of specialists in this area—general surgeons, otorhinolaryngologists, plastic surgeons, and oral surgeons—to whom a patient may be referred. The use of fine needle aspiration will often allow diagnosis on the initial visit and lead directly to therapy. An example is aspiration of pus from a suspected lymphomatous mass (see

Chap. 9). Case 2-5 illustrates the ease with which a patient may be victimized by the "shuttle syndrome."

The importance of preoperative diagnosis cannot be overstressed. Surgical biopsies of metastatic cervical nodes are never performed before the primary is controlled or at least discovered. In the absence of a primary, cytologic smears usually can place the origin above or below the clavicles. Also, not all enlarged neck nodes are metastatic, as has been demonstrated. Preoperative diagnosis of salivary tumors is equally useful, and helps to guide the extent of the surgery.

Finally, the application of fine needle aspiration will heighten the clinician's diagnostic sensibilities and greatly amplify his skill in differential diagnosis.

REFERENCES

1. Aisner SC, Aisner J, Moravec C et al: Acquired toxoplasmic lymphadenitis with demonstration of the cyst form. Am J Clin Pathol 79:125, 1983
2. Argyle JC, Schumann GB, Kjedlsberg C: Identification of a toxoplasma cyst by fine-needle aspiration. Am J Clin Pathol 80:256, 1983
3. Banfi A, Bonnadonna G, Carneval G et al: Lymphoreticular sarcomas with primary involvement of Waldeyer's ring. Cancer 26:341, 1970
4. Barrie JR, Knapper WH, Strong EW: Cervical nodal metastases of unknown origin. Am J Surg 120:466, 1971
5. Barton JH, Osborne BM, Butler JJ et al: Non-Hodgkins lymphoma of the tonsil: A clinicopathologic study of 65 cases. Cancer 53:86, 1984
6. Berge T, Söderström N: Fine-needle cytologic biopsy in diseases of the salivary glands. Acta Pathol Microbiol Scand 58:1, 1963
7. Bernier JL, Bhaskar SN: Lymphoepithelial lesions of salivary glands: Histogenesis and classification based on 186 cases. Cancer 11:1156, 1958
8. Bernstein A, Scardino PT, Tomaszewski M et al: Carcinoma arising in a branchial cleft cyst. Cancer 37:2417, 1976
9. Berthelsen A, Andersen AP, Jensen TS et al: Melanomas of the mucosa in the oral cavity and the upper respiratory passages. Cancer 54:907, 1984
10. Bhaskar SN, Bernier JL: Histogenesis of branchial cysts. Am J Pathol 35:407, 1959
11. Bill AH Jr, Vadheim JL: Cysts, sinuses and fistulas of the neck arising from the first and second branchial clefts. Ann Surg 142:904, 1955
12. Chaudhry AP, Gorlin RJ, Mosser DG: Carcinoma of the antrum: A clinical and histopathologic study. Oral Surg 13:264, 1960
13. Chen SY, Brannan RB, Miller AS et al: Acinic cell adenocarcinoma of minor salivary glands. Cancer 42:678, 1978
14. Comess MS, Beahrs O, Dockerty M: Cervical metastasis from occult carcinoma. Surg Gynecol Obstet 104:607, 1957
15. Coulson WF: Surgical Pathology. Philadelphia, JB Lippincott, 1978
16. Dolin S, Dewar JP: Extramedullary plasmocytosis. Am J Pathol 32:83, 1956
17. Eneroth CM, Zajicek J: Aspiration biopsy of salivary gland tumors. IV: Morphologic studies on smears and histologic sections from 45 cases of adenoid cystic carcinomas. Acta Cytol 13:59, 1969

18. Engzell U, Jakobsson PA, Sigurdson A et al: Aspiration biopsy of metastatic carcinoma in lymph nodes of the neck: A review of 1101 cases. Acta Otolaryngol (Stockh) 72:138, 1971
19. Engzell U, Franzen S, Zajicek J: Aspiration biopsy of the neck. II: Cytologic findings in 13 cases of carotid body tumor. Acta Cytol 15:25, 1971
20. Evans HL: Extranodal small lymphocytic proliferation: A clinicopathologic and immunocytochemical study. Cancer 49:84, 1982
21. Frable WJ, Frable MS: Thin-needle aspiration biospy: The diagnosis of head and neck tumors revisited. Cancer 43:154, 1979
22. Frable WJ: Thin-Needle Aspiration Biopsy. Philadelphia, WB Saunders, 1983
23. France CJ, Lucas R: The management and prognosis of metastatic neoplasms of the neck with an unknown primary. Am J Surg 106:835, 1963
24. Godwin JT: Cytologic diagnosis of aspiration biopsies of solid or cystic tumors. Acta Cytol 8:206, 1964
25. Godwin JT: Benign lymphoepithelial lesions of parotid gland (adenolymphoma, chronic inflammation, lympho-epithelioma, lymphocytic tumor, Mikulicz disease): Report of 11 cases. Cancer 5:1089, 1952
26. Gorlin RJ, Goldman H: Thoma's Oral Pathology, 6th ed. St. Louis, Mosby, 1970
27. Guepp DR, Chandler W, Hyams V: Primary Kaposi's sarcoma of the head and neck. Ann Intern Med 100:107, 1984
28. Grufferman S, Gillman MW, Pasternak LR et al: Familial carotid body tumors. Cancer 46:2116, 1980
29. Hakes TB, Armstrong D: Toxoplasmosis—problems in diagnosis and treatment. Cancer 52:1535, 1983
30. Hoffman E: Branchial cysts within the parotid gland. Am Surg 152:290, 1960
31. Hyman GA, Wolff M: Malignant lymphoma of the salivary glands. Am J Clin Pathol 65:421, 1976
32. Jacobs GH, Rippey JJ, Altini M: Prediction of aggressive behavior in basal cell carcinoma. Cancer 49:533, 1982
33. Jesse RH, Perez CA, Fletcher GS: Cervical lymph node metastasis: Unknown primary cancer. Cancer 31:854, 1973
34. Kasper CS, Schneider NR, Childers JH et al: Suprasellar germinoma. Am J Med 75:705, 1983
35. Katz AD: Unusual lesions of the parotid gland. J Surg Oncol 7:219, 1975
36. Khang-Loon H: Primary meningioma of the nasal cavity and paranasal sinuses. Cancer 46:1442, 1980
37. Khoory MS: Diseases of lymph nodes and spleen. In Linsk JA, Franzen S (eds): Clinical Aspiration Cytology, p 297–317. Philadelphia, JB Lippincott, 1983
38. King AI, Klima M, Johnson P: Sweat gland tumors of the head and neck. Arch Otolaryngol 108:48, 1982
39. Knowles DM, Jacobiec FA: Orbital lymphoid neoplasms: A clinicopathologic study of 60 patients. Cancer 46:576, 1980
40. Lack EE, Cabilla AL, Woodruff JM et al: Paragangliomas of the head and neck: A clinical study of 69 patients. Cancer 39:397, 1977
41. Levin PA, Falko JM, Dixon K et al: Benign parotid enlargement in bulimia. Ann Intern Med 93:827, 1980

42. Linsk JA, Franzen S: Clinical aspiration cytology. Philadelphia, JB Lippincott, 1983

43. Lipper S, Peiper SC: Sweat gland carcinoma with syringomatous features. Cancer 44:157, 1979

44. Luddy RE, Sutherland JS, Levy BE et al: Cat-scratch disease simulating malignant lymphoma. Cancer 50:584, 1982

45. Margolith AM: Cat-scratch disease: Nonbacterial regional lymphadenitis. Pediatrics 42:803, 1968

46. Martin H, Morfit HM, Ehrlich H: The case for branchiogenic cancer (malignant branchioma). Ann Surg 132:867, 1950

47. Mavec P, Eneroth CM, Franzen S et al: Aspiration biopsy of salivary gland tumors. I: Correlation of cytologic reports from 652 biopsies with clinical and histological findings. Acta Otolaryngol 58:471, 1964

48. Million RR: Management of neck node metastasis. JAMA 220:402, 1972

49. Nissenblatt MJ: Cyanotic heart disease: "Low altitude" risk for carotid body tumor. Johns Hopkins Med J 142:18, 1978

50. Nochomovitz LE, Jannotta F, Orenstein M: Meningioma of the scalp. Arch Pathol Lab Med 109:92, 1985

51. Persson PS, Zellergren L: Cytologic diagnosis of salivary gland tumors by aspiration biopsy. Acta Cytol 17:351, 1973

52. Perzin KH, Gullane P, Clairmont AC: Adenoid cystic carcinomas arising in salivary glands: A correlation of histologic features and clinical course. Cancer 42:265-282, 1978

53. Pollack PG, Koontz FP, Viner TF et al: Cervicofacial actinomycosis. Arch Otolaryngol 104:491, 1978

54. Redon H: Chirurgie des Glands Salivaires. Paris, Masson, 1955

55. Ree HJ, Rege VB, Knisler RE et al: Malignant lymphoma of Waldeyer's ring following gastrointestinal lymphoma. Cancer 46:1528, 1980

56. Rees WV, Robinson DS, Holmes EC et al: Altered lymphatic drainage following lymphadenectomy. Cancer 45:3045, 1980

57. Robertson ID, Cooney TP: Malignant carotid body paraganglioma: Light and electron microscopic study of the tumor and its metastasis. Cancer 46:2623, 1980

58. Rollo J, Rozenbom CV, Thawley S et al: Squamous carcinoma of the base of the tongue: A clinicopathologic study of 81 cases. Cancer 47:333, 1981

59. Rubin P: Cancer of the head and neck: Hypopharnyx and larynx. JAMA 221:68, 1972

60. Rubin P: Cancer of the head and neck: Nasopharyngeal cancer. JAMA 220:390, 1972

61. Rush BF: Familial bilateral carotid body tumors. Ann Surg 147:633, 1963

62. Saldana MJ, Salem LE, Travezan R et al: High altitude hypoxia and chemodectomas. Ann Pathol 4:251, 1973

63. Sismanes A, Merriam J, Yamaguchi KT et al: Diagnostic value of fine needle aspiration biopsy in neoplasms of the head and neck. Otolaryngol Head Neck Surg 89:62, 1981

64. Sjögren H: Zur kenntris der keratoconjunctivitis sicca. Acta Opthalmol (Suppl) 2:1–151, 1933

65. Spiro RH, Huvos AG, Strong EW: Malignant mixed tumor of salivary origin: A clinicopathologic study of 146 cases. Cancer 39:388, 1977

66. Von Mikulicz J: Concerning peculiar symmetrical disease of lachrymal and salivary glands. Med Classic 2:165, 1937

67. Willems J-S: Aspiration biopsy cytology of tumors and tumor-suspect lesions of bone. In Linsk JA, Franzen S (eds): Clinical Aspiration Cytology, pp 349–359. Philadelphia, JB Lippincott, 1983

68. Willis RA: Pathology of Tumours, pp 305–307. London, Butterworth, 1960

69. Wolff M, Rankow RM: Meningioma of the parotid gland: An insight into the pathogenesis of extracranial meningiomas. Hum Pathol 2:453, 1971

70. Zajicek J: Aspiration Cytology, Part I. Basel, S Karger, 1975

71. Zimmerman LE: Ophthalmic Pathology. In Anderson WAD, Kissane JM (eds): Pathology, pp 1181–1182. St. Louis, Mosby, 1977

3 Disorders of the Endocrine Organs

Endocrine disorders caused by increased secretion of hormones (including hyperparathyroidism, hyperthyroidism, and Cushing's syndrome) are seen uncommonly in general clinical practice. They have been detected more often since the widespread use of screening chemistry profiles, although it is likely that chemistry has been substituted for careful history and physical examination in many cases. Nevertheless, the diagnosis must be confirmed by chemical and hormonal studies. Fine needle aspiration has limited utility as a diagnostic aid. However, where the hormonal secretion is associated with tumor or hyperplasia of the endocrine organ, fine needle aspiration may be a useful diagnostic aid. Medullary carcinoma of the thyroid, in which calcitonin is secreted, is an example of this, and it is discussed later.

Endocrine glands are more often affected by nonsecreting disorders, such as chromophobe adenoma, Hashimoto's thyroiditis, and seminoma of the testis, some of which produce endocrine syndromes associated with underactivity of the gland. These disorders and most inflammations, hyperplasias, and tumors of the endocrine glands may become targets for fine needle aspiration.

Palpation may define the aspiration target in some disorders of the thyroid, testis, ovary, and adrenal gland, but imaging techniques including x-ray films (pituitary), scintigraphy (thyroid), computed tomography (adrenal), and ultrasonography (ovary) are often necessary.

How can the application of the techniques of fine needle aspiration shorten the diagnostic work-up and precisely identify the disorder? This will be considered for individual organs.

The Thyroid

Abnormalities of the thyroid gland are among the most common disorders seen in medical practice. Most of the major reports on the subject are published by referral institutions that have collected specific numbers of tumors and hyperplasias during defined time periods.[12,16,17,18,20,22,39,49,62,63] Referral centers by definition receive and report selected cases. Two major thyroid referral centers have had the opportunity to study the broad spectrum of thyroid abnormalities that physicians in any community clinic or office might see for diagnosis and treatment. These are the cytology laboratory of the Radiumhemmet in Stockholm where more than 25,000 pa-

tients with thyroid disease have been evaluated by fine needle aspiration*
and Henry Ford Hospital in Detroit.[49] Experience also has been collected
in a private office practicing internal medicine and oncology.

Many patients harbor thyroid swellings, nodules, or goiters, many of
which are under observation by a primary care physician without any
definitive diagnosis. This can be noted in any active clinic or office merely
by inspecting a patient's neck across the width of a desk. Many physicians
handle such abnormalities with benign neglect. Some request thyroid function studies, particularly $T_3T_4T_7$, and abnormal results may lead to immediate therapy or further testing. T_3 by radioimmunoassay (RIA) is useful
for borderline elevation, and thyroid-stimulating hormone (TSH) levels for
borderline depression of the $T_3T_4T_7$ thyroid function tests. Serologic studies
for autoimmune thyroiditis are requested often in thyroid clinics,[71] but
probably are requested infrequently in general clinical practice. Finally,
particularly with localized palpable abnormalities, radioactive scans are
requested. The significance of cold nodules can be defined further by (1)
ultrasonography, which distinguishes fluid from solid tissue,[59] and (2) thyroid suppression, which, by shrinking a cold nodule, confers a presumptive
diagnosis of benignity.[5]

Goiter

Any enlargement of the thyroid falls within the definition of goiter, although the term usually suggests prominent diffuse or nodular visible
enlargement. The normal thyroid gland is generally not visible. With the
exception of women with thin necks, visibility of the gland indicates a
pathologic process. Similarly, the normal gland most often cannot be defined by palpation.

Palpation of a visible mass or enlargement is not a problem, although
careful search of apparently normal portions of the gland to establish
multinodularity will help formulate a clinical diagnosis. Palpation of the
gland with alterations that are not visible is more of a clinical challenge.
Every physician will establish his own method of detection. Palpation while
standing behind the patient is traditional. Anterior palpation may be the
most useful for aspiration. When the patient's anterior cervical muscles are
relaxed, fingertip palpation will detect nodules as small as 1 cm (Fig. 3-1).
Lack of symmetry in resistance detected when gentle pressure is applied
alternately to each lobe may be sufficient to direct the needle. Of course,
outlining a distinct nodule is desirable, because it allows insertion of the
needle at various sites, including the center and periphery of the mass. The
formulation of a clinical diagnosis in physical examination is a useful
exercise. Size, texture, nodularity, fixation, movement, and tenderness are
all findings that enter into this formulation. However, the diagnosis remains

---

* Personal communication, T. Löwhagen.

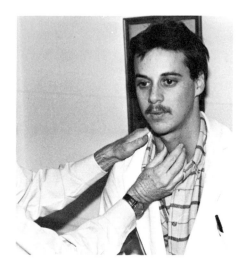

FIGURE 3-1: For small lesions, fingertip palpation is stressed. Superficial nodules less than 1 cm in diameter may be papillary carcinomas.

unknown until the target lesion finally is sampled. A fixed, hard gland may be due to thyroiditis, and a superficial small nodule may be a papillary carcinoma (see below).

Palpation of the neck to search for metastatic nodes is an essential adjuvant maneuver.

Figure 3-2 depicts the usual scientific methods, short of biopsy, of defining the pathologic condition of the thyroid. For functional disorders and Hashimoto's disease, these measures are useful, if not entirely precise. For solitary nodules, multinodular goiter, most diffuse enlargements, and cold areas seen on scan, examination of cells or tissue is essential.

Fine needle aspiration of a palpable abnormality, or less frequently, a nonpalpable cold area bypasses many of the diagnostic steps in Figure 3-3.

Most palpable thyroid abnormalities are observed first by family physicians, internists, and less often by endocrinologists. After the studies depicted in Figure 3-2, patients usually are referred to general surgeons. The application of the method of fine needle aspiration by the primary clinician will sharply reduce surgical intervention in benign disease. This has been clearly established in the thyroid clinics of Hamburger and co-workers,[22] at Karolinska,* and at other clinics.[18,50] (See section about the Economics of Fine Needle Aspiration.)

The sequence of diagnostic studies should be guided by the findings of

* Personal communication, T. Löwhagen.

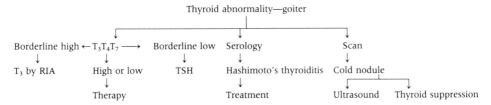

FIGURE 3-2: Methods for defining the pathologic condition of the thyroid.

the history and physical examination in conjunction with the following recommendations.

1. In the absence of clinical evidence of hyperthyroidism or hypothyroidism, the ritual requesting of thyroid function studies can be dispensed with.
2. The initial study in the presence of all palpable abnormalities is fine needle aspiration.
3. Scintigraphy may follow cytologic diagnosis to determine if there are additional nonpalpable cold areas.
4. If scintigraphy has been done as an initial procedure, fine needle aspiration of nonpalpable cold areas should follow immediately.
5. There is no indication for ultrasonography in the diagnosis of cystic thyroid masses. Computed tomography (CT) scans may be useful to the surgeon to define the extent of a tumor.
6. Fine needle aspiration of all cystic lesions must be followed by careful palpation for residual masses. Unless the cystic fluid is quite clear, it should be examined cytologically to exclude cystic carcinoma.
7. Positive antithyroid titers strongly suggest Hashimoto's thyroiditis, but fine needle aspiration is required for positive diagnosis and to exclude lymphoma.

Technique for Aspiration

The technique that we use and recommend for aspiration of cystic and solid lesions of the thyroid is designed to yield well-preserved, air-dried, and fixed smears. The use of such smears for rapid, atraumatic, inexpensive, direct outpatient diagnosis presupposes experience in reading the cytology. If the operator or pathologist does not have such experience, attempts at definitive diagnosis should be postponed until appropriate training and experience are obtained.

The smear method must not be confused with core biopsies (Vim–Silverman or Tru-cut needles), which provide the pathologist with accustomed histologic sections. Core biopsies are preferable to open biopsies. However, where local trauma[17] or needle implants of tumor have been

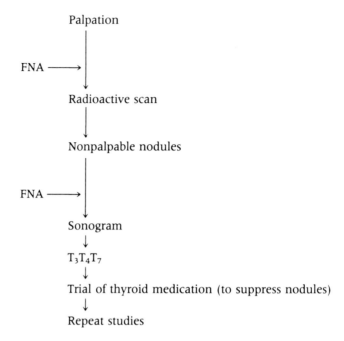

Palpation

FNA ⟶

Radioactive scan

Nonpalpable nodules

FNA ⟶

Sonogram

$T_3T_4T_7$

Trial of thyroid medication (to suppress nodules)

Repeat studies

Comment: FNA combined with clinical judgment
sharply reduces diagnostic testing, time, and cost.

FIGURE 3-3: Diagnostic schema for thyroid nodules, enlargements, and tumors.

reported, such biopsies have been used. Significant trauma and needle
implantation have not been seen with the fine needle method in our
experience. Furthermore, core biopsy lacks flexibility. It cannot be used for
multiple punctures and it is unsuitable for aspirating cysts. Small and
superficial lesions are poor targets.

Smaller needles cause less trauma and less morbidity. Needles measuring 0.7 mm outer diameter, 22 gauge, have been used at Radiumhemmet
for 30 years. There is no difficulty aspirating and emptying a cyst. The cell
yield from a solid mass is abundant and well preserved.

Aspiration is carried out as described in Chapter 1. The thyroid is fixed
firmly with one hand. If fluid is encountered, it is gently aspirated and the
cyst is compressed. The fluid is expelled on a watch glass. Any particles are
teased out and smeared. If it contains blood, or if color or texture differs
from the expected translucent brown, the fluid is drawn up, expelled into
a tube, and referred for cytologic examination.

If the mass is solid, it may be quite vascular. At the first appearance of
blood above the hub of the needle, discontinue the aspiration and withdraw
the needle while applying pressure. The contents of the lumen of the needle
will be adequate, but too much blood will dilute the specimen.

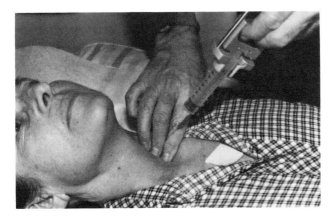

FIGURE 3-4: The carotid bundle is deflected laterally while the proposed target is fixed with the fingertips.

It must be noted that for masses near the midline, the carotid bundle should be deflected laterally to allow a clear medial puncture (Fig. 3-4).

If the needle penetrates a large vessel, pure blood will appear immediately in the syringe. The procedure should be repeated with greater care after pressure has been applied.

THYROIDITIS

Applying the techniques of fine needle aspiration to the diagnosis of thyroiditis of necessity will alter all statistics based on clinical evaluation of palpable disease and surgical experience, which is always selected. Experience based on careful palpation followed by immediate fine needle aspiration will heighten clinical skill in identifying Hashimoto's thyroiditis and subacute (de Quervain's) thyroiditis. Hashimoto's thyroiditis, described originally in 1912,[26] is now known to be an autoimmune disorder in which an immune process may invade a normal gland and a variety of thyroid pathologic processes. It has been associated with Graves' disease,[73] multinodular goiters, and solitary nodules.[8] Positive serologic tests are important identifying features, but are not pathognomonic.[71] The most significant correlation is with lymphoma, to be discussed later.

The following case illustrates clinical findings and the place of fine needle aspiration in diagnosis.

Case 3-1

The patient was a 43-year-old laboratory director who had been aware of a nodular thyroid enlargement for several years (Fig. 3-5). She had deferred examinations because of anxiety about possible surgery. A physician, impressed by its firm nodularity, insisted on a scin-

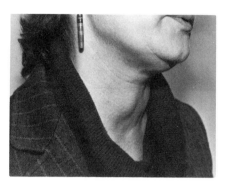

FIGURE 3-5: This patient's nodular thyroid was found to be Hashimoto's thyroiditis on fine needle aspiration.

tigram to assess iodine storage. There was an irregular cold area involving the right lobe, and surgery was recommended because of the strong possibility of carcinoma.

At this point, the patient agreed to fine needle aspiration. The yield consisted of abundant lymphoid cells intermixed with clusters of enlarged atypical epithelial cells cytologically diagnostic of Hashimoto's thyroiditis.

There was regression with thyroid medication and the patient remained under observation.

COMMENT It is important to note that although the thyroid gland usually presents as a diffuse firm enlargement, the enlargement may be irregular, multinodular, unilobular, or uninodular. Therefore, clinical diagnosis is only approximate. Thyroid function usually is depressed due to destruction of the functioning thyroid tissue. However, it is apparent that at the initiation of the autoimmune process a euthyroid or hyperthyroid state may be present and hypothyroidism supervenes as functioning thyroid is progressively depleted. Although lymphoid infiltration usually produces hyperplastic rubbery tissue, an atrophic gland may result. Fine needle aspiration of an atrophic gland, in which the needle sometimes reaches the thyroid cartilage, may yield characteristic smears diagnostic of Hashimoto's thyroiditis.

A word of caution is necessary. Patients with palpable abnormalities who are hypothyroid according to tests may be considered clinically to have thyroiditis, and they may be treated with thyroid medication without cytologic or histologic confirmation of the diagnosis. The following case illustrates this pitfall.

Case 3-2

The patient was a 61-year-old woman who had a nodular enlargement in the right lobe of her thyroid. Thyroid function tests demonstrated hypoactivity, and thyroid medication was started with the intention of observing the enlargement for regression. Over a period of 4 months, the gland appeared to the attending physician to have regressed somewhat.

While working as a salesperson, the patient abruptly developed diplopia and headache and was taken to a hospital. There was some proptosis of her right eye, and the ophthalmologic consultation recommended brain scan. In addition, on examination, there was a firm to hard nodular mass lying in the medial aspect of the right lobe of the thyroid very close to the trachea, which easily would have been missed without fingertip palpation.

Fine needle aspiration yielded a somewhat poorly differentiated follicular carcinoma. Two defects interpreted as metastatic nodules were evident on CT scan of the brain.

COMMENT Treating patients with thyroid medication in an effort to shrink a thyroid enlargement is fairly common practice that is successful in some cases. It is obvious that, without knowing the precise nature of the enlargement, risks are associated with this type of therapy. In this patient, the combination of the hard mass and the atypical follicular proliferation seen on smear was strong evidence for follicular carcinoma. The usual follicular carcinoma (see below) may not be differentiated easily from follicular adenoma.

Some cytologic findings should be of interest to the clinician. Two key cytologic alterations may be discussed usefully with the pathologist. One is enlarged, often atypical, epithelial cells, singly and in clusters, which are usually scattered in the lymphoid component. Epithelial cells may dominate, and with the characteristic atypia may be reported as an epithelial tumor of the Hürthle cell type. This is a diagnostic pitfall and should be discussed with the pathologist if other clinical evidence, particularly palpable and serologic, suggests Hashimoto's disease.

If the lymphoid component predominates, then there is a risk of considering a benign process to be a well-differentiated lymphoma. This is complicated by the fact that almost all lymphomas of the thyroid are associated with lymphoid thyroiditis.[8,11,77]

If the autoimmune process affects an overactive gland,[73] the epithelial component of the smear may exhibit the flaming alterations described in hyperthyroidism.[40]

Subacute (de Quervain's) thyroiditis in its acute phase is less likely to simulate the common neoplasms. For the clinician, the syndrome associated with subacute thyroiditis, including palpable enlargement, pain, tenderness, fever, and rapid sedimentation, is sufficiently suggestive to warrant a therapeutic trial of steroids. However, the differential diagnosis includes acute suppurative thyroiditis and rapidly evolving lymphoma or anaplastic carcinoma, all of which demand immediate precise diagnosis and therapy. Fine needle aspiration will produce purulent smears diagnostic of acute suppurative thyroiditis. The cytologic smears of large cell anaplastic carcinoma, also highly characteristic, will be discussed below. A lymphoid smear in the presence of painful swelling would suggest not Hashimoto's disease but lymphoma. The cytologic alterations of subacute thyroiditis have been presented in detail.[40] The presence of benign multinucleated giant cells is critical to the diagnosis.

In the postinflammatory phase, an indurated diffusely enlarged lobe that is cold on scintigram may be confused with neoplasm, and the cytologic yield will be extremely valuable in differentiation.[50] This is illustrated in the following case.

Case 3-3

The patient was an obese 76-year-old woman with a known diagnosis of non-Hodgkin's lymphoma in apparent remission. She had been treated 2 years previously with combined chemotherapy. She detected a firm mass in her right anterior neck, which had appeared gradually without any preceding inflammation or fever. It was cold on scintigram. She was referred for fine needle aspiration with a clinical diagnosis of probable lymphoma invading the thyroid. Aspiration yielded typical cytologic smears of subacute thyroiditis, and both hospitalization and radiotherapy were avoided.

COMMENT The above case is not an isolated instance. A firm to hard unilobular enlargement without significant or obtainable history of inflammation must include thyroiditis in the differential diagnosis before proceeding to surgery. Fine needle aspiration smears are usually decisive.

NODULAR GOITER

Careful palpation of the thyroid requires relaxation of the anterior cervical muscles, including the sternocleidomastoids. This is best accomplished with the patient supine. Apparent solitary nodules are often part of a multinodular gland,[2,39] and searching, gentle palpation may reveal other nodules. Although nodules smaller then 1 cm in diameter are considered impalpable for practical purposes,[56] detection of small, superficial nodules by stroking palpation may be highly significant (see Papillary Carcinoma). In general, multinodularity indicates a benign process, although studies of selected series report an incidence of 0.6% to 10% malignancy in resected glands.[36] Of course, such surgical series do not reflect the incidence of cancer in unselected multinodular goiters, which must be considerably lower. Nevertheless, it is important to palpate with great care to elicit multinodularity and to find all available targets for fine needle aspiration.

All discrete nodules should become separate targets for fine needle aspiration. This is illustrated in Case A-8 (see Appendix). The solitary nodule has been found to be malignant in 10% to 30% of several series of surgically selected cases.[56] Again, this does not reflect the incidence of carcinoma in an unselected population with uninodular goiter, since nodules with clinical evidence suggesting carcinoma (pain, growth, hardness, encroachment on speaking and swallowing) are more likely to have surgery.

Nodules that are found to be cold on scintigraphy are more likely to be malignant than warm or hot nodules are.[16,50] Again, such judgments are based on cases selected for surgery.[50] Fine needle aspiration has demonstrated effectively in our experience that the majority of cold nodules are degenerated colloid nodules, usually cystic. This confirms published evidence that sole reliance on scintigraphy as a guide to surgery is unacceptable.[65] For the clinician using fine needle aspiration to seek confirmation of a benign nodular goiter, several observations may be made.

1. After careful palpation, aspirate and smear all palpable nodules separately. Antecedent ultrasonography serves no purpose because cysts will be detected immediately by the aspiration. Ultrasonography is not used at Radiumhemmet (Karolinska Hospital, Stockholm) where 1000 thyroid aspirations are done yearly. Antecedent scintigraphy also appears to be superfluous in establishing morphologic diagnosis, although it may help identify nonpalpable masses.

2. Cystic fluid should be submitted for cytologic examination because of the possibility of cystic carcinoma. Benign cysts often present silently as an enlarging mass with no history of pain to suggest hemorrhage.

3. Smears may be made from particles teased out of the fluid on a watch glass.

4. Smears may be submitted air dried, or fixed, or both, according to prior arrangement with the cytopathologist.

5. Discuss smears with the cytopathologist to find out if colloid is present, strongly supporting a benign diagnosis. Also ask about granular debris and pigmented histiocytes, indicating prior hemorrhage into a benign degenerated nodule.

NODULE OR ADENOMA

Benign colloid nodules occur as a result of sequential hyperplasia and atrophy leading to sequestration of lobules of the thyroid gland by fibrous bands.[2] The histopathologic separation of such nodules from a true neoplasm (adenoma or carcinoma) is not always clear-cut.[2,10] For example, Coulson refers to macrofollicular adenomas in which follicles are distended with colloid.[10] If this is a true neoplasm, then separation cytologically from a colloid nodule would be impossible. However, in the overwhelming majority of instances, the cytologic smears can be read decisively and diagnosed as colloid nodule or adenoma.[39,40,49,72]

A diagnosis of adenoma, particularly in conjunction with a diagnosis of cold nodule on scintigraphy, usually will mandate surgery, although treatment with thyroid medication has been reported with some therapeutic response.[5,31]

It is recognized that adenomas may be difficult to distinguish from well-differentiated follicular carcinoma. Such specimens should be reported cytologically as follicular neoplasms. The clinician should alert the surgeon to the possibility of cancer even though the overwhelming majority of these tumors are benign adenomas. The final decision lies with the pathologist. The diagnosis of malignancy, short of electron microscopy or DNA studies, requires morphologic evidence of vascular or capsular invasion, which converts an apparently cytologically benign smear to a diagnosis of malignancy.

Of importance are the following caveats. The cytologist must separate benign nodules from follicular neoplasm.[48] The surgeon must carry out an appropriate procedure on all reported follicular neoplasms using the findings at surgery and frozen section, if necessary, to guide his work. The pathologist must identify cancer by appropriate criteria.

For the clinician, the following key elements in the smear will guide him and may be discussed with the pathologist. First, the presence of colloid identified by staining characteristics strongly, though not absolutely, confers a benign diagnosis. Second, pigmented histiocytes intermixed with clusters and loose sheets of small benign epithelial cells without intact follicles and solid papillary clusters favors a benign nodule. And finally, the presence of many microfollicles in the absence of colloid suggests a follicular neoplasm. Reviewing these components with the pathologist will encourage the clinician to note them in future reports.

FOLLICULAR CARCINOMA

Follicular carcinoma has been a source of much discussion and controversy. A major concern has been the question of its origin from adenoma versus a *de novo* origin. Problems arise because of the varying data bases from which conclusions have been drawn. These include selected surgical series[60,62] and autopsy series.[28] Well-defined and advanced tumors appearing in surgical series usually have obliterated any preexisting adenomas.

On the other hand, in sequential autopsy studies, thyroid dissection may be omitted, or it may not be carried out with thin serial sections.[62] There is evidence that at least some and possibly all differentiated follicular cancers arise in adenomas or at least have the initial appearance of adenomas.[62] There is also little doubt that follicular carcinomas, without transformation to anaplastic carcinoma, may kill the patient.

Because the histologic criteria of malignancy of well-differentiated carcinoma cannot be made evident by light microscopic examination of cytologic smears, concern has been expressed that fine needle aspiration will produce false-negative diagnoses that will lead to neglect of a lethal disease.[7,24] To no area of aspiration biopsy cytology do the following cardinal rules apply more than in this instance.

1. Smears of benign disorders, such as colloid cysts and thyroiditis, are not reported as "negative for cancer" but should specify the benign diagnosis.
2. Smears of follicular neoplasms may be reported as cancer if the cells are poorly differentiated with nucleoli[40] (see Case 3-2).
3. Smears containing well-differentiated monotonous follicles must be reported as "follicular neoplasm, malignancy to be determined by the pathologist after careful examination of the full surgical specimen."

Clearly, all well-defined palpable disease not treated surgically must remain under clinical observation. These rules also should eliminate any fears of malpractice suits, which pose a threat no greater in this instance than with any diagnostic procedure that results in a benign or negative report.

Since the precise preoperative diagnosis guides the clinician in choosing diagnostic measures (x-ray studies, scans, blood and bone marrow studies) and therapy (lobectomy versus total thyroidectomy; node dissection), it is important that the clinician discuss the cytologic findings with the pathologist reading the smears. Well-differentiated smears with monotonous microfollicles clearly indicate a well-differentiated neoplasm, which the pathologist ultimately will define as benign or malignant. Microfollicles with larger cells with prominent nucleoli indicate less differentiation, and require more intensive staging and appropriate therapeutic procedures.[40,41] Smears with combined follicular and papillary alterations address attention to regional nodes. Finally, poorly differentiated smears with a paucity of well-formed follicles and with larger atypical cells must be differentiated from the epithelial component of Hashimoto's thyroiditis. Such a tumor must be managed as a malignant tumor with metastatic potential. Total thyroidectomy and assessment of radioiodine uptake of skeleton and soft tissue are indicated.

The relationship of follicular neoplasms to anaplastic carcinoma is extremely important and is considered below.[1]

PAPILLARY CARCINOMA

Papillary carcinoma may present as a palpable mass that varies from a superficial nodule smaller than 1 cm in diameter to a hard, frankly malignant mass. Any papillary carcinoma can result in a fatal outcome.[70] Fine needle aspiration of small surface lesions may yield diagnostic smears if carried out carefully with short, fine needles (25 gauge). Sclerosing papillary carcinomas also occur as small (several millimeters in size) tumors that may be incidental findings in glands removed for other reasons. Such lesions do not become targets for fine needle aspiration.

Papillary tumors made up approximately 50% of all thyroid tumors seen in a 30-year period at the New England Deaconess Hospital,[45] and 25% of 254 cases reported by Selzer and co-workers.[60] They do not store iodine. Therefore, clinical suspicion of cold nodules should be high, and prompt, careful palpation of lateral cervical nodes, the common site of regional metastases, must be carried out.

The diagnosis is also complicated by the high incidence of cystic alteration (up to 47%)[45] leading to confusion with degenerated cystic colloid nodules. Cyst formation may be detected by aspiration of nodules 1 cm or smaller in diameter. This contrasts with the larger size of degenerated colloid cysts. Finding small cystic lesions should immediately arouse suspicion of papillary carcinoma. The cytologic report should reflect this (Fig. 3-6). Cyst formation also occurs in metastatic sites. The extraction of brown fluid from a lateral cystic lesion is almost pathognomonic of metastatic carcinoma. The color and texture of the fluid is significant, and it must be contrasted with branchial cleft cyst fluid, which is yellowish-gray and densely turbid. As noted previously, colloid fluid contains granular debris and numerous pigmented histiocytes (see also Case A-6). Clusters of atypical epithelial cells, sometimes forming papillary structures, are highly suggestive of papillary carcinoma. Such structures are shed from the often shaggy papillary lining of the cyst.

Aspiration of solid tumors will yield highly characteristic cytologic changes virtually pathognomonic of the tumor.[40,41] Such findings should be sought and reviewed by the clinician with the pathologist. Psammoma bodies are a fairly common, but extremely important, finding. They are identified easily. In smears, even a single calcific spherule (psammoma body) arouses high suspicion of carcinoma. In metastatic sites, differential diagnosis with ovarian carcinoma must be considered (see Case 9-13). Intranuclear inclusions described originally by Söderström are highly characteristic. Rare metastases of melanoma, hypernephroma, or hepatoma to the thyroid also may harbor intranuclear inclusions.[37,38] Finally, the absence of colloid and the presence of fingerlike papillary structures are important observations.[40,41,72] The presence of microfollicles indicates a mixed pathologic picture. Focal follicular change was noted in 39% of the Meissner series.[45] Sufficient follicular change, of course, will introduce characteristics of a follicular tumor, including iodine storage.

Cytologic Report

Patient __Johnson_____ Age __43__ Sex __F_____

Doctor __Lieberman_____ Date __12/20/84_____

Target Area: __Thyroid_____

REPORT:

    A nodule measuring 0.7 cm in the medial aspect of the right lobe was aspirated, yielding 0.5 cc of turbid brown fluid. No induration was detected post aspiration.

    Cytologic smears consist of clusters of atypical cells. Some form elongated structures. Nucleoli are prominent. Pigmented histiocytes are not evident.

DIAGNOSIS: Suspicious for papillary carcinoma.

NOTE: Surgery is recommended.

Joseph Linsk, M.D.

FIGURE 3-6: The cytologic report illustrates combined clinical and cytologic data.

THYROTOXICOSIS AND CANCER

Palpable alterations are suitable targets for fine needle aspiration regardless of the presence of hyperthyroidism. Carcinoma was found in 2% to 5% of several series of histologically studied thyrotoxic glands.[23,47,53] Although many of the cancers were nonpalpable and incidental,[53] cancer was clinically suspected because of nodule enlargement in six to ten cases harvested from 549 thyrotoxic glands.[23] The cancers are mainly differentiated follicular, papillary, or mixed histologic types and on fine needle aspiration will yield diagnostic smears. Smears of glands from patients with clinical hyperthyroidism will yield so-called flaming cells (also known as foaming cells or flare cells) on Romanowsky's stain. In the presence of nodular changes, repeat aspiration must be performed to rule out cancer.

Hyperthyroidism also may result from functioning follicular carcinoma,[15,47] which will produce a hot nodule on scintigram. If well differentiated, such a neoplasm cannot be labeled malignant without histologic analysis.

ANAPLASTIC CARCINOMA

The rapid, sometimes explosive growth of an anaplastic carcinoma arising apparently *de novo* is the singular characteristic aspect of this usually lethal tumor. In this rapid growth phase, it quickly overtakes a lobe or the entire gland and then can be confused with suppurative thyroiditis and subacute thyroiditis (see above).

The relationship of these tumors to preexisting well-differentiated carcinomas has been established by pathologic studies.[1,25,28] The preexisting tumor may be palpable or present but clinically not evident. The threat of this lethal tumor, particularly in older persons, is an additional mandate to identify all nodular disease by morphology and deal surgically with all neoplasms (in contrast with hyperplastic nodules).

In its earlier phases of growth, anaplastic carcinoma may be clinically indistinguishable from a more differentiated neoplasm. Therefore, it is es-

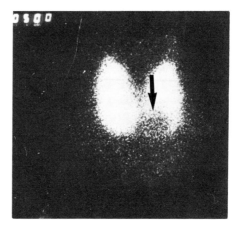

FIGURE 3-7: The "cold nodule" seen in this scintigram is entirely nonspecific. In this case it was due to anaplastic carcinoma.

sential to identify the tumor preoperatively, as illustrated in the following case.

Case 3-4

The patient was a 38-year-old woman who had noted a "lump" in her thyroid for about 1 year. She was prompted to see a surgeon because of a new subjective awareness of the mass, although she did not think it had enlarged. The surgeon ordered a scintigram, which revealed a cold area approximately 2 cm in diameter corresponding to the solitary, easily palpable, firm mass (Fig. 3-7). Fine needle aspiration was recommended to the surgeon, but he declined, considering it an unnecessary procedure because he was planning to proceed with surgery. He performed a lobectomy and isthmectomy. The nodule was an anaplastic carcinoma that recurred within weeks and invaded the neck, with fatal outcome, within 3 months.

At the Karolinska, thyroid surgery is never done before fine needle aspiration. Identification of anaplastic carcinoma is important because the treatment is not primarily surgery, but rather radiation and chemotherapy. Figure 3-8 illustrates a patient with a rapidly enlarging, firm to hard thyroid. Fine needle aspiration yielded findings typical of anaplastic carcinoma (Fig. 3-9). At the Karolinska, this patient would not be subjected to surgery initially. A reverse protocol with chemotherapy, radiation, and then surgery might alter the poor statistics for this tumor.

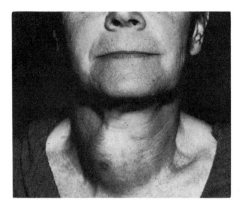

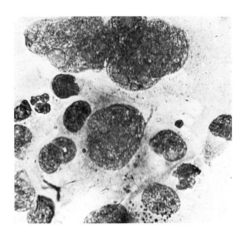

FIGURE 3-8: The clinical diagnosis of the thyroid enlargement in this patient included colloid goiter, thyroiditis, and carcinoma. Clinical history aids the diagnosis but fine needle aspiration is decisive. The diagnosis was anaplastic carcinoma.

FIGURE 3-9: Aspiration cytology is shown for anaplastic carcinoma of the thyroid. There is a mixed cell population with giant tumor cells.

Anaplastic carcinoma is recognized cytologically by the extensive necrosis, hemorrhage, and the giant anaplastic cells (see Fig. 3-9). Small cell anaplastic tumors are probably poorly differentiated lymphomas.[57] Cytologically, they have the appearance of poorly differentiated lymphomas seen in other areas.[40]

MEDULLARY CARCINOMA

Medullary carcinoma has been recognized as a separate histologic type of carcinoma only since 1951.[30] It was defined more fully pathologically in 1959.[27] Due to its origin from parafollicular cells (C cells), it has unique clinical characteristics and associations that separate it from the epithelial neoplasms (follicular and papillary).[67,76] Approximately one half of these tumors are sporadic in origin and present with palpable, radiographically cold masses indistinguishable clinically from other epithelial carcinomas. The other half are familial in type (see Case 5-2),[38] are often found at an earlier age, and may be occult tumors revealed by family history and calcitonin levels. Bilaterality is so common that surgery for cure should always be total thyroidectomy. Massive involvement of mediastinal and hilar nodes may occur.[35]

Medullary carcinoma is combined with bilateral pheochromocytomas in a small number of patients (4 out of 62),[76] and with cutaneous and gastrointestinal neuromas, parathyroid adenomas, and hyperplasia. Good medical practice dictates that pheochromocytomas be identified and removed before beginning thyroid surgery.[35]

There is no data that modest delay in surgically treating well-differentiated follicular and papillary carcinomas worsens the prognosis.[5] However, it appears logical that delay would be detrimental. Delay in treating medullary carcinoma, a progressive disease, should be discouraged strongly.[67] For that reason, palpable thyroid masses in patients with suspected medullary carcinoma, even if calcitonin levels are normal, should have immediate fine needle aspiration to establish a diagnosis. Case A-8 illustrates that medullary carcinoma can be associated with benign nodular disease (see Appendix). It also has been noted in a patient with Hashimoto's disease.[75]

These tumors are not cystic. Presumably, the aspirating needle may strike a calcium collection. The cytology has been described in detail.[40,66] A unique characteristic is the presence of fine reddish granulation on Romanowsky's stain, which is not seen in any of the other thyroid tumors, but is present in carcinoid, carotid body, and other tumors of the apudoma group.

LYMPHOMA OF THE THYROID

Lymphoma of the thyroid is an infrequent neoplasm. Clinical experience with these tumors by one observer in contrast with review of collected pathologic material is limited. The largest experience in which patients were examined physically and by modern diagnostic methods, including cytologic and histologic examination, was by Hamburger, Miller, and Kini reported in 1983.[22] Thirty patients were seen, and this group was 8% of a total of 382 neoplasms found among 4200 patients with thyroid nodules.[22] A clinical pathologic study of 245 cases submitted to the Armed Forces Institute of Pathology was reported by Campagno and Oertel.[8] Pathologic examinations were supplemented by reviewing clinical records and communicating with the physician whenever possible. Many similar observations were made by these observers and by others who had submitted previous studies.[11,64,77]

This tumor is not seen in children and is considered predominantly a disease of older patients. However, about 40% of the patients in several series are below 60 years of age.[11,22,64] Women are a substantial majority of most collected cases. There is general agreement that virtually all cases are associated with lymphoid thyroiditis (Hashimoto's disease), and where antibody studies have been carried out, a high percentage will yield positive findings.[22]

Smithers has reviewed the evidence, and it is not established that Hashimoto's disease is a precursor of lymphoma or carcinoma.[64] If that were the case, then all patients with Hashimoto's disease would require a thyroidectomy. Extensive experience with Hashimoto's disease at the Karolinska Clinic does not support that concept. Although lymphoma appears to occur in patients with Hashimoto's disease, it is rare compared with the incidence of the thyroiditis. The association of lymphoma with this benign lymphoid disorder suggests that the lymphoma arises from abnormal lymphoid proliferation within benign lymphoid tissue.[8] However, the rapidly fatal course of lymphoma associated with autoimmune disease is not seen in thyroid lymphoma.[42]

All observers agree that the omnipresence of lymphoid thyroiditis complicates the cytologic and histopathologic diagnosis of lymphoma. We agree with Hamburger and co-workers[22] that one cause of the problem in diagnostic differentiation is lack of experience. Equally important to experience in microscopy is the integration of clinical data into the final common pathway of diagnosis. The clinician's evaluation of the clinical problem precedes morphology and should guide the pathologist in distinguishing lymphoma from lymphoid thyroiditis.

History. The frequent association of Hashimoto's thyroiditis with lymphoma is confirmed by a history of thyroid enlargement preceding the more rapid development of an enlarging mass. The enlargement may occur rapidly over a period of several days or, more often, over a period of several weeks or months. This history must be elicited if the patient is unknown to the clinician. A history of underactive thyroid function is common.

Physical Examination. A solitary mass is most common. It may have enlarged to occupy an entire lobe. In the series of Campagno and Oertel[8] the size ranged from 1 cm (an incidental finding) to 14 cm. A massive, rapidly enlarging tumor that may be invading the tissues of the neck will override any equivocation concerning morphology. However, such tumors are usually poorly differentiated and rather clearly malignant.

Unfortunately, physical examination may reveal a multinodular goiter or diffuse enlargement that cannot be distinguished easily from benign processes.

In considering lymphoma, physical examination must include all nodal regions and the spleen. Fine needle aspiration of an enlarged lymph node in conjunction with a lymphoid thyroid smear may be decisive.

Isotopic Studies. Cold nodules that are not distinctive may be present. Poor scans are obtained in patients receiving thyroid therapy for hypothyroidism. Cold areas that do not correspond to palpable masses have been noted.[22,49,69]

Fine needle aspiration is carried out with all thyroid enlargements. All nodules and several areas of diffuse enlargements should be sampled. Smears should be made carefully because of the fragility of lymphoid cells.

Discussion with the pathologist should encompass the following cytologic principles.

1. Is the smear composed of monomorphic, poorly differentiated, fragile lymphoid cells accompanied by lymphoglandular bodies (fragments of cytoplasm)? This is the type that has been considered undifferentiated small cell carcinoma, a diagnosis that is no longer considered correct.[40,57]

2. Is the smear composed of differentiated lymphocytes? Are there clusters of atypical enlarged cells? Is the smear characteristic of Hashimoto's disease?

3. Is the smear composed of plasma cells? Plasmacytic and plasmacytoid lymphoma has been reported.[6,61]

4. Is there any evidence of Hodgkin's disease? Are there any Sternberg–Reed cells?

The majority of the tumors are non-Hodgkin's lymphoma arising primarily in the thyroid and extending to lymph nodes and other organs, including the gastrointestinal tract. Extension of extra thyroidal lymphoma to involve the thyroid is distinctly unusual. Involvement of the gastointestinal tract in patients with primary thyroid lymphoma has been summarized by Smithers.[64] It is present in 25% of thyroid lymphoma, but the most commonly involved organ is the kidney.[58]

The Economics of Fine Needle Aspiration of the Thyroid

Two areas of cost control in the diagnosis and treatment of thyroid disease are to be reviewed. Consideration must be given to the need for multiple expensive noninvasive studies that yield an inferential, but not a morphologic, diagnosis. Secondly, the question of unnecessary surgery for a benign disease must be addressed. The cost difference between conventional and aspiration biopsy methods of diagnosing a thyroid cyst has been presented graphically by Kaminsky.[33] The conventional method included office visit, isotopes, scan, ultrasonography, hospital admission, preoperative workup, surgery, anesthesia, pathology, and five days in the hospital: total cost, $4294.40. The aspiration biopsy method included office visit, isotope scan, ultrasonography, fine needle aspiration, and interpretation of smears: total cost, $534.64. In another study, noninvasive methods were used to select cold nodules for surgery.[5] This protocol included conventional laboratory studies, T_3, T_4, and TSH determination, antithyroid antibodies, isotopic scan, echography, suppressive therapy with liothyronine, monthly examinations, and several tracings of the nodule. At the end of 3 months, the echogram was repeated and a management decision was made. (See Case 3-2.)

At the Radiumhemmet of the Karolinska Hospital, about 1000 thyroid glands were aspirated each year. At this time almost 25,000 have been aspirated. All patients are coded and follow up is generally assured by the stable population and ready exchange of records and data. Experience has shown that preliminary studies, as discussed above, have not been necessary to arrive at a diagnosis. All palpable disease is punctured and immediate diagnosis is rendered on well-prepared smears. The use of isotopic scanning to detect nonpalpable disease is individualized. Echography is entirely unnecessary and is not done at Karolinska. The entire list of expensive visits, studies, and hospitalizations can be eliminated. This reduces the cost to include the services of the aspirating physician and the cytopathologist, if a different individual. The cost of slide preparation is negligible.

The implications of this for use in nonacademic, rural, and third world settings is apparent. Because of the frequency of undiagnosed benign tumors or goiters in thyroid disease, aspiration biopsy is particularly applicable. In addition, since fine needle aspiration is an office or clinic procedure, the patient can be spared travel and visits to unfamiliar doctors.

The savings in diagnostic studies, although significant, are less important than the reduction in surgery with its morbidity, mortality, and costs. The identification of benign disease including cysts, colloid nodules, and thyroiditis at the Radiumhemmet has resulted in a sharp reduction in surgical procedures for many years. Other reports confirm these observations. In 1978, Esselstyn and Crile described needle biopsy results in 460 patients.[17] Of this group, 393 were spared surgery, based on needle biopsy findings. Wang and co-workers reported that 725 patients were spared surgery based on needle biopsy reports.[74] Most of these biopsies yielded core rather than smear specimens, but the principle of sparing surgery because of the fine needle method applied equally. Miller, Hamburger, and Kini reported a 70% decrease in surgery for benign disease.[49]

As mentioned above (see Case 3-4), elimination of surgery for anaplastic carcinoma also can be effected by preoperative identification of the lesion.

The impact of these startling reductions in surgery at selected institutions is great. When the method is in general use worldwide, savings should be enormous.

Extrathyroidal Tumor

Metastatic Disease

Papillary carcinoma passes to regional nodes by way of the lymphatics. Large nodes may be present in the absence of a palpable primary. Formerly, these were termed *lateral aberrant thyroid.* Fine needle aspiration is diagnostic. Cystic metastases have been described previously. Distant metastases were reported in 7 of 89 cases.[46] Although this is an indolent tumor, in 70 fatal cases pulmonary metastases were found in 51.4% of the patients, osseous metastases in 25.7%, and brain metastases in 10%.[70]

Follicular Carcinoma

Follicular carcinoma invades locally and then tends to metastasize through the blood rather than the lymphatics to regional nodes. Initial findings may result from metastatic disease with inapparent primary, and include pulmonary, brain, and skeletal signs and symptoms. It may produce lytic bone lesions, which then form part of a differential diagnosis that includes myeloma, hypernephroma, and breast carcinoma. Intact and well-differentiated follicular structures similar to the primary lesion may be extracted and readily identified by fine needle aspiration.

Midline Thyroid Rests

The subject of midline thyroid rests has been reviewed by Smithers.[64] Twenty lingual thyroid tumors and 21 carcinomas of thyroglossal duct cysts and thyroglossal tracts were collected. Prognosis was poor for the lingual tumors, but only 1 of 29 thyroglossal duct tumors metastasized. Aspirated cyst fluid must be examined cytologically. Anaplastic carcinoma arising from a thyroglossal duct remnant has been reported.[52]

Substernal Thyroid

The identification of substernal thyroid is made easy by the fact that the great majority are extensions of a goiter. However, heterotopic thyroid is occasionally present. Distinction from other anterior mediastinal targets, particularly teratomas, usually is demonstrated conclusively by radioactive iodine uptake on scan.

Where a substernal mass produces compressive symptoms, it may be necessary to clarify the diagnosis by fine needle aspiration, particularly if it fails to store iodine. Needle aspiration may be carried out by a direct parasternal puncture. The aortic arch rises to the sternal angle and will be below a needle entering parallel to the manubrium. It also should be noted that there may be considerable space between the aorta and the sternum when a retrosternal mass is present. Needle puncture directly through the sternum is feasible (see Case 5-8 and Fig. 5-17). Puncture also has been performed successfully by angling down at the sternal notch.

A patient with follicular carcinoma in a retrosternal thyroid that eroded the sternum and presented presternally is presented elsewhere in a chapter on thyroid aspiration by Löwhagen and Linsk.[40]

Struma ovarii is a teratoma of the ovary that rarely may become malignant and metastasize.[13]

Secondary Tumors in the Thyroid

We have seen metastases to the thyroid from bronchogenic carcinoma,[40] hypernephroma,[37] melanoma, and breast carcinoma. All of these potentially may be identified by fine needle aspiration. There is a primary clear cell carcinoma of the thyroid that can be confused with a well-differentiated hypernephroma, clear cell type. Large cell bronchogenic carcinoma can simulate anaplastic carcinoma.[40]

Summary (Thyroid)

The impact of thyroid disease worldwide cannot be overestimated. The presence of goiter in endemic regions has been estimated to be 200 million people.[29] Such numbers together with the large numbers of sporadic cases encountered in practice add up to an enormous pool of clinical problems confronted by a small number of practicing clinicians.

For this reason, all physicians should be schooled and skilled in dealing with palpable thyroid disease. These problems are best dealt with rather than referred to remote thyroid centers, which cannot possibly manage the vast number of cases. Whereas core biopsies require specialized experience and may add complications, fine needle aspiration is relatively simple and atraumatic. The method should be wedded to clinical evaluation, and never should be substituted for careful follow up in patients whose conditions are deemed nonsurgical. Such follow up has been systematically adhered to at the Karolinska Hospital. It should be an important tool of all practicing physicians.

The Pituitary

Lesions of the pituitary produce three types of symptoms, any of which should prompt a consideration of immediate diagnosis by fine needle puncture. First, chromophobe adenoma may compress the normal pituitary and produce hypopituitarism with its accompanying end organ failures. Second, hypersecretion due to a functional adenoma may result in gigantism, acromegaly (in the adult), or, rarely, a variety of effects caused by thyrotropins, corticotropins, gonadotropins, and others. Finally, an enlarging tumor may produce local compressive effects with eye signs.[44]

The primary physician should retain an awareness of the usefulness of fine needle aspiration, which may spare the patient a formal surgical procedure to obtain a diagnosis. Regional or community hospitals may have radiotherapy units, but no expertise in puncture of the skull base. In such cases, the patient should be referred for cytologic diagnosis, and then return to the local hospital for treatment. This will spare him multiple visits to a distant center or the necessity of moving to that center for the extended weeks of therapy.

The other major lesion is craniopharyngioma. It can be diagnosed easily by puncture (see Case 3-5 below). Puncture of the skull base is discussed in Chapter 10.

Case 3-5

A 60-year-old Greek woman was referred for failing vision and an apparent intrasellar expanding mass. Transnasal fine needle aspiration (Fig. 3-10) yielded approximately 3 mL of brown fluid (Fig.

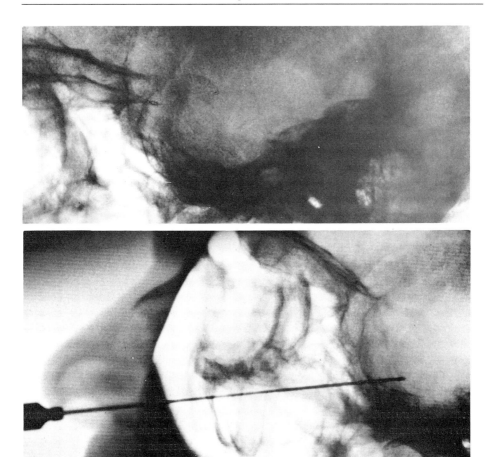

FIGURE 3-10: Transnasal puncture of the sella is illustrated. (Linsk JA, Franzen S: Clinical Aspiration Cytology, p 43. Philadelphia, JB Lippincott, 1983)

3-11,*A*). The cellular content was squamous (Fig. 3-11,*B*). The patient immediately experienced improvement in her vision and declined further therapy.

The Adrenal Gland

The adrenal gland and its lesions are infrequent targets for fine needle aspiration, primarily because adrenal tumors or masses are rare in general clinical practice and tend to be collected in large cancer institutes. From 1976 to 1981, 22 symptomatic and incidental adrenal masses were collected at the M.D. Anderson Hospital and Tumor Institute in Houston, Texas.[34] Of the 22, 13 were malignant tumors. Of the malignant tumors, seven were metastatic, two were neuroblastomas, and only four were primary adreno-

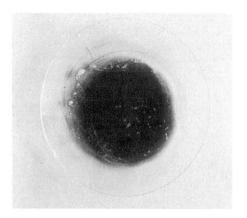 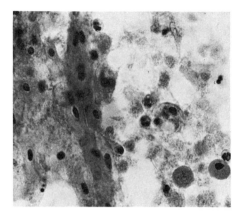

FIGURE 3-11: (*A*) Fluid obtained from a cystic craniopharyngioma. (*B*) Cytology shows atypical squamous cells.

cortical carcinomas. All were studied by fine needle aspiration and other confirmatory techniques. The incidence should be contrasted with the experience in the usual community or regional hospital where such lesions rarely are seen or recognized. This may change with the widespread, almost routine, use of CT scanning. It also should be contrasted with the enormous volume of major tumors (bronchogenic, breast, colon, and so forth). Nevertheless, the capability of identifying an adrenal mass cytologically is important. Seven of the patients in this study had prior documented carcinomas in other sites, and had presumed adrenal metastases that proved to be benign on fine needle aspiration. Of the nine patients with benign lesions, surgery was performed for tissue diagnosis in only three, illustrating again the value of the method for sparing surgery.

In a more recent study by Berkman and co-workers from Emory University, subtitled "An Alternative to Surgery in Adrenal Mass Diagnosis," biopsies were performed on 16 patients with adrenal masses, using CT guidance.[4] Adrenal adenomas, cysts, metastases, melanomas, and hemorrhage were identified. It is important to note that in nine patients with known extra-adrenal malignant tumors, four were found to have metastases, but five had other nonmalignant adrenal masses.

The cytology of benign and malignant adrenal masses falls into several distinct patterns that are recognizable with experience. Diagnosis should be rendered with caution in the absence of experience, and slides can be referred for consultation. Nevertheless, distinct recognizable patterns in conjunction with the clinical context will emerge from the study and leave a small number of difficult cases. Squamous or oat cell carcinoma extracted in a patient with a past or concurrent pulmonary lesion should be characteristic. Cystic material easily distinguishes solid and cystic (benign) lesions. However, diagnostic pitfalls include differentiation of melanoma, hepatoma, and hypernephroma, which may have similar cytologic patterns.

In infants and small children, recognition of neuroblastoma poses little problem, particularly in the appropriately studied clinical context. Lymphoma with intermediate cells is a leading consideration in cytologic differential diagnosis. In children, acute leukemia presenting as a mediastinal nodal mass in which neuroblastoma may be a consideration, yields blastic smears in cytologic contrast to neuroblastoma.

Pheochromocytoma, a secreting tumor of chromaffin tissue, most commonly of the adrenal, may be discovered as a result of hypertension investigation, incidentally at surgery, or as part of the multiple endocrine neoplasia syndrome. The last is of interest because of the ease of cytologic diagnosis of medullary carcinoma of the thyroid, which should mandate a study for pheochromocytoma (see above). Fifty-four cases, of which six were malignant, were reviewed at the Mayo Clinic by Sutton and co-workers.[68] The tumors varied in size from 0.5 cm to 18 cm, and from 600 mg to 3200 g. Therefore, they are suitable targets for fine needle aspiration, and may be defined by palpation rarely and by CT scan easily.

Pheochromocytoma yields atypical smears that, however, share the same morphologic pattern as the now well-established cytology of the carotid body tumor.[38] In fact, it is with experience and in the appropriate clinical context readily identified or strongly suspected.

Case 3-6 illustrates problems in diagnosis of adrenal tumors.

Case 3-6

A 70-year-old man presented with palpable scalp masses and underlying lytic lesion on skull films (Fig. 3-12). Aspiration biopsy yielded malignant cells of the clear cell type (Fig. 3-13), and a differential diagnosis of renal, adrenal, and primary hepatic carcinoma was of-

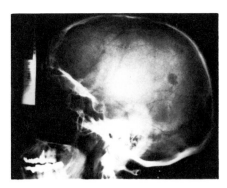

FIGURE 3-12: Lytic lesions are identified in the skull of a 70-year-old patient who had palpable scalp nodules.

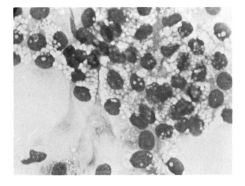

FIGURE 3-13: Aspiration cytology of a scalp nodule shows sheets of vacuolated cells. The differential diagnosis included hypernephroma, adrenal carcinoma, and hepatoma.

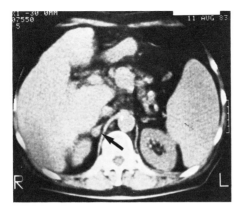

FIGURE 3-14: CT scan of the abdomen shows a 2-cm enlargement of the right adrenal gland (*arrow*). Fine needle aspiration with ultrasound guidance yielded cytologic smears identical to the scalp lesion in Figure 3-13.

fered. Surgical biopsy of the scalp lesion resulted in the same differential diagnosis.

A CT scan of the abdomen revealed a 2-cm swelling in the right adrenal gland (Fig. 3-14). Fine needle aspiration with ultrasound guidance secured smears identical to those from the scalp lesion.

The Testes

Long experience with fine needle aspiration of the testes has resulted in clinical perceptions somewhat at variance with the conventional approach to testicular disease, as illustrated below.

The identification of testicular, particularly germinal tumors, has become increasingly important in the past 10 years with the evolution of effective and curative chemotherapy protocols.[54,55] Although testicular tumors constitute only about 1% of male tumors, they cause 11% to 13% of the cancer deaths in young men.[9,14,21] This is clinically significant, because in this group preventive medicine and self-examination are infrequently pursued. As a result, testicular lesions that come to the surgical bench in pathology laboratories range from well-defined nodules to large masses that replace much or all of the testis. The earliest palpable alteration produced by testicular tumors is an ill-defined induration. It is curious that this pathologic change is so often not noticed by the patient. Testicular examination by the clinician (apart from urologists) often is omitted or is carried out perfunctorily. Of greater importance, however, is the moment of decision when the clinician does palpate a poorly defined area of induration and must consider whether it is significant. If the choice consists of observation on a return visit or immediate exploration and orchiectomy, a follow up often will appear desirable. It is precisely at this point that the utility of fine needle aspiration is most evident. In no other tumor does the triad of patient delay, doctor delay, and sometimes hospital delay play a greater role.

It is important to note that reliance on markers (alpha-fetoprotein and human chorionic gonadotropin) is not absolute and must give way to clinical and morphologic confirmation at all times.[32]

Diagnostic Delay

Diligent self-examination of the testes has not been emphasized as breast self-examination has been. This is dramatically evident in lecturing to resident physicians 25 to 35 years old, to whom the concept is entirely new. For the patient, painless enlargement, even if identified, is often ignored or considered a transient curiosity expected to subside spontaneously.

Patients may visit the physician with mild testicular pain and no grossly evident mass. In the presence of a variocele or a history of straining, this might be dismissed with scrotal support and application of heat. At this point, careful examination of the testes, checking for early, often subtle, parenchymal alteration or induration is essential. It is most important that any area of induration, nodularity, or irregularity should be considered a tumor (see below).

A painful scrotal mass may be attributed to trauma, epididymitis, epididymo-orchitis, or torsion, and dismissed as a benign lesion. This produces marked delay. Failure to carry out follow up palpation after the pain has subsided adds to the delay.

In the absence of a preoperative diagnosis obtained by fine needle aspiration, inappropriate initial treatment may follow. Trans-scrotal surgery yielding a malignant tumor then may require further surgery to sterilize the operative field (wide local excision of scrotal incision) and removal of all the ipsilateral scrotal contents by an inguinal incision. Fine needle aspiration allows definitive surgical planning and reduces hospital delay.

Not all palpable masses are germinal tumors. Leydig cell tumors, lymphomas, adenomatoid tumors of the epididymis, epididymo-orchitis, granulomatous orchitis, both specific and nonspecific (tuberculosis, gumma), all provide cytologic smears with a high specificity.[38] Preoperative identification has obvious advantages, since radical inguinal orchiectomy is not the procedure of choice for these entities.

Physical Examination

Massive intrascrotal masses that fill the sac, stretching the scrotal skin, are self-evident. Well defined nodular masses within the body of the testicle also present no problems of identification. A mass that can be separated from the main body of the testis is never a germinal tumor. This applies particularly to the epididymis and its lesions. The epididymis is draped linearly along the posterior surface of the testis. The head is the wider, superior portion. It can be separated by palpation. Where it is thickened and blends with the testis and particularly if the vas deferens is thickened, this is strong presumptive evidence of inflammation and against tumor.

Between the easily palpable and identifiable masses and nonpalpable tumors found only at the surgical bench, which may have produced generalized metastasis, are the subtle changes that challenge the clinician's skill. If such changes are detected, the most important rule to keep in mind is to avoid a return visit to recheck the area.

What Is Obtained by Fine Needle Aspiration?

FERTILITY STUDIES

Male infertility may be caused by testicular failure or blockage of the ejaculatory ducts. Cytologic smears obtained by direct trans-scrotal puncture reveal the source of this problem quickly. In testicular atrophy, the germinal cells are absent, leaving Sertoli's and interstitial cells, which presents a fairly characteristic cytologic picture. With blocked ducts, the smears contain a full distribution of germinal cells from primary spermatogonia to spermatozoa.

GERMINAL TUMORS

All tumor masses, nodules, nodularities, indurations, and subtle changes in testicular parenchyma should be punctured by trans-scrotal fine needle aspiration. (See Inhibitory Factors, below). The sensitivity of the method is almost 100%. Individual cell types (for example, seminoma as opposed to embryonal cell type) have high degrees of specificity.[38]

LEYDIG'S CELL TUMORS

A nongerminal testicular nodule may be clinically indistinguishable from a germinal tumor. Three percent of testicular masses fall in this group. The cytology is highly specific. Both air-dried and Papanicolaou's smears should be obtained, and preoperative identification should forestall radical orchiectomy.

LYMPHOMA

Germinal tumors are uncommon beyond the fourth decade and are rare in the older age group. The dominant tumor in this group is lymphoma, previously designated reticulum cell sarcoma because of its immature cytology. Differentiation of lymphoma and seminoma may be a problem, but the experience of the clinician and the age of the patient are decisive factors.

The recognition of occult testicular leukemia in children in complete remission from acute lymphocytic leukemia has prompted a recommendation for routine bilateral surgical wedge biopsy of the testis.[3] Fine needle aspiration of the testis in this clinical context has been carried out satisfactorily for a number of years at the Karolinska. The procedure is done in conjunction with sampling of the cerebrospinal fluid under light anesthesia.

OTHER APPLICATIONS

ADENOMATOID TUMORS

Adenomatoid tumors of the epididymis should be recognizable by findings on palpation coupled with characteristic cytology.[38] Preoperative identification should forestall radical orchiectomy.

EPIDIDYMO-ORCHITIS

Epididymo-orchitis will produce a confluent mass consisting of the epididymis and testis. The cytology, particularly if granulomatous, is identifiable with experience.[38] Granulomatous stroma of seminoma may be a source of confusion. All such lesions must be evaluated clinically. Evaluation should include age of the patient, length of time the mass has been present, and palpatory findings. Most will be managed surgically even with a benign diagnosis.

FLUID-FILLED SACS

Fluid-filled sacs often are punctured for examination of the fluid. This often is preceded by transillumination. Spermatoceles yield milky fluid that is easily identified microscopically by the large number of non-motile spermatozoa. Hydrocele usually contains clear yellow fluid. Five percent to ten percent of hydroceles appearing suddenly in young men are associated with germinal tumors.[49] Hemorrhagic fluid is highly suspicious.

Technique of Puncture

With a readily accessible target, puncture poses few difficulties. A 22-gauge or 23-gauge needle attached to a one-handed syringe may be thrust easily through the scrotal skin into the mass without anesthesia (Fig. 3-15). Firm

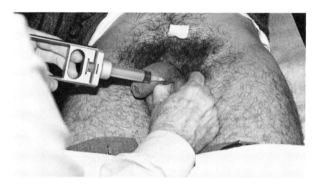

FIGURE 3-15: The testicle is grasped firmly and the needle is inserted briskly into the fixed target.

grasp of the testis or mass is crucial. The puncture is relatively painless. For large masses, the needle should be directed to sample several areas because of the possibility of necrosis. There should be no hesitation in repeating the puncture. If fluid is evacuated, careful palpation for residual induration and repeat puncture is indicated.

Inhibitory Factors

Although puncture of fluid-filled sacs is carried out regularly, there are numerous warnings in the literature concerned with violation of the scrotal barrier, local implantation, and dissemination of tumor.[43,51] The only published series that has studied the problems failed to show any adverse effects of trans-scrotal puncture with a fine needle.[78] It must be stressed that core biopsy of suspected testicular tumors should be avoided because local scrotal implantation is possible. This parallels the experience with core biopsy in other areas.

Summary (Pituitary, Adrenal, and Testes)

The facility with which the skull base can be punctured (see Chap. 10) brings the pituitary within reach of rapid diagnosis, often at the community or regional level. Separation of craniopharyngioma and adenoma cytologically should be relatively easy. With further study and collection of data, separation of the epithelial tumor may be achieved.[19]

Recent experience has shown that the use of CT scanning will reveal an increased number of adrenal masses. Most of these will be benign or metastatic masses, since primary malignancy of the adrenal is rare. Nevertheless, awareness of the utility of fine needle aspiration will lead to earlier, more specific diagnoses. The cytology of adrenal carcinoma can be confused with that of hypernephroma and hepatoma, and therefore all clinical data and clinical judgment must be used and exercised.

The testis is one of the last frontiers for aspiration cytologic diagnosis. (The brain is also in this category; see Chap. 11.) The limiting factors are two. First, there is a failure of early detection because of a lack of diligent clinical and self-examination. This problem requires educational efforts by clinicians and the lay public. Second, there is a widespread and traditional sense of caution on the part of clinicians, particularly urologists. This will have to await published studies or larger series confirming the value of the technique. In the meantime, the clinician should be alert to early, often unobtrusive changes in the testicle, which in fact may be signs of a lethal tumor.

REFERENCES
1. Aldinger KA, Samaan N, Ibanez M et al: Anaplastic carcinoma of the thyroid. Cancer 41:2267, 1978
2. Anderson WAD, Kissane JM: Pathology. St. Louis, Mosby, 1977

3. Askin FB, Lund VJ, Sullivan MP et al: Occult testicular leukemia: Testicular biopsy at 3 years continuous complete remission of childhood leukemia. Cancer 47:470, 1981

4. Berkman WA, Bernardino ME, Sewell CW et al: The computed tomography-guided adrenal biopsy: An alternative to surgery in adrenal mass diagnosis. Cancer 53:2098, 1984

5. Blum M, Rothschild M: Improved nonoperative diagnosis of the solitary "cold" thyroid nodule. JAMA 243:242, 1980

6. Buss DH, Marshall RB, Holleman IL et al: Malignant lymphoma of the thyroid gland with plasma cell differentiation (plasmacytoma). Cancer 46:2671, 1980

7. Christopherson WW: Cytologic detection and diagnosis of cancer: Its contributions and limitations. Cancer 51:1201, 1983

8. Campagno J, Oertel JE: Malignant lymphoma and other lymphoproliferative disorders of the thyroid gland. Am J Clin Path 74:1, 1980

9. Collins DH, Pugh RCB: Classification and frequency of testicular tumours. Br J Urol (suppl) 36:1, 1964

10. Coulson WF: Surgical Pathology. Philadelphia, JB Lippincott, 1978

11. Crile G Jr: Lymphosarcoma and reticulum cell sarcoma of the thyroid. Surg Gynecol Obstet 116:449, 1963

12. Crile G Jr, Hawk WA: Aspiration biopsy of thyroid nodules. Surg Gynecol Obstet 136:241, 1973

13. Dalley VM: Struma ovarii. In Smithers D (ed): Tumours of the Thyroid Gland, pp 162–168. London, Livingstone, 1970

14. Drain LS: Testicular cancer in California from 1942–1969: The California tumor registry experience. Oncology 27:45, 1973

15. Egmark A, Larson LG, Liljestrand A et al: Iodine-concentrating thyroid carcinoma: A report of three cases. Acta Radiol (Stockh) 39:423, 1953

16. Einhorn J, Franzen S: Thin-needle biopsy in the diagnosis of thyroid disease. Acta Radiol 58:321, 1962

17. Esselstyn CB, Crile G Jr: Needle aspiration and needle biopsy of the thyroid. World J Surg 2:321, 1978

18. Frable WJ: Thin-needle aspiration biopsy. Philadelphia, WB Saunders, 1983

19. Gandolfi A: Cytology of a chromophobe pituitary adenoma. Acta Cytol 27:521, 1983

20. Gharib H, Goellner JR, Zinsmeister AR et al: Fine needle aspiration biopsy of the thyroid: The problem of suspicious cytologic findings. Ann Intern Med 101:25, 1984

21. Gordon-Taylor G, Wyndham NR: On malignant tumours of the testicles. Br J Surg 35:6, 1957

22. Hamburger JI, Miller JM, Kini SR: Lymphoma of thyroid. Ann Intern Med 99:685, 1983

23. Hancock BW, Bing RF, Dirmikis SM et al: Thyroid carcinoma and concurrent hyperthyroidism. Cancer 39:298, 1977

24. Hajdu SI, Melamed MR: Limitation of aspiration cytology in the diagnosis of primary neoplasms. Acta Cytol 28:337, 1984

25. Harada T, Ito K, Shimaoka K et al: Fatal thyroid carcinoma; anaplastic transformation of adenocarcinoma. Cancer 39:2588, 1977

26. Hashimoto H: Zur Kenntanis der lymphomatosum verandring der schild-

ruse (struma lymphomatosa). Arch F Klin Chir 97:219, 1912

27. Hazard JB, Hawk WA, Crile G Jr: Medullary (solid) carcinoma of the thyroid: A clinico-pathological entity. J Clin Endocrinol Metab 19:152, 1959

28. Heitz P, Moser H, Straub JJ: Thyroid cancer: A study of 573 thyroid tumors and 161 autopsy cases observed over a thirty-year period. Cancer 37:2329, 1976

29. Hoffenberg R: Thyroid disorders. In Weatherall DJ, Ledingham JGG, Warrell DA (eds): Oxford Textbook of Medicine. Oxford, Oxford University Press, 1983

30. Horn RC Jr: Carcinoma of the thyroid. Cancer 4:697, 1951

31. Ingbar S, Woeber K: Diseases of the thyroid. In Isselbacher KJ, Adams RD, Braunwald E et al (eds): Principles of Internal Medicine. New York, McGraw-Hill, 1980

32. Javadpour N, Soares T: False positive and false negative alpha fetoprotein and human chorionic gonadotropin assays in testicular cancer. Cancer 48:2270, 1981

33. Kaminsky DB: Aspiration Biopsy for the Community Hospital. New York, Masson, 1981

34. Katz RL, Patel S, MacKay B et al: Fine needle aspiration cytology of the adrenal gland. Acta Cytol 28:269, 1984

35. Keiser HR, Beaven MA, Doppman J et al: Sipples syndrome: Medullary thyroid carcinoma, pheochromocytoma and parathyroid disease. Ann Intern Med 78:561, 1973

36. Lahey FH, Hare HF: Malignancy in adenomas of the thyroid. JAMA 145:689, 1951

37. Linsk JA, Franzen S: Aspiration cytology of metastatic hypernephroma. Acta Cytol 28:250, 1984

38. Linsk JA, Franzen S: Clinical Aspiration Cytology. Philadelphia, JB Lippincott, 1983

39. Löwhagen T, Granberg P-O, Lundell G et al: Aspiration biopsy cytology in nodules of the thyroid gland suspected to be malignant. Surg Clin North Am 59:3, 1979

40. Löwhagen T, Linsk JA: Aspiration biopsy cytology of the thyroid gland. In Linsk JA, Franzen S (eds): Clinical Aspiration Cytology, pp 61–83. Philadelphia, JB Lippincott, 1983

41. Löwhagen T, Sprenger E: Cytologic presentation of thyroid tumors in aspiration biopsy smear. Acta Ctyol 18:192, 1974

42. Lukes RJ, Collins RD: New approach to the classification of the lymphomata. Br J Cancer (Suppl 2) 31:1–28, 1975

43. Markland C, Kedia K, Fraley EE: Inadequate orchiectomy for patients with testicular tumors. JAMA 224:1025, 1973

44. Mackinnon PCB: Introduction to Endocrinology. In Weatherall DJ, Ledingham JGG, Warrell DA (eds): Oxford Textbook of Medicine. Oxford, Oxford University Press, 1983

45. Meissner WA, Adler A: Papillary carcinoma of the thyroid. Arch Pathol 66:518, 1958

46. McDermott WV Jr, Morgan WS, Hamlin E Jr et al: Cancer of the thyroid. J Clin Endocrinol Metabol 14:1336, 1954

47. McLaughlin RP, Scholz DA, McConahey WM et al: Metastatic thyroid

carcinoma with hyperthyroidism: Two cases with functioning metastatic follicular thyroid carcinoma. Mayo Clin Proc 45:328, 1970

48. Miller JM: Carcinoma and thyroid nodules: The problem in an endemic goiter area. N Engl J Med: 252:247, 1955

49. Miller MJ, Hamburger JI, Kini S: Diagnosis of thyroid nodules: Use of fine-needle aspiration and needle biopsy. JAMA 241:481, 1979

50. Miller JM, Hamburger JI, Mellinger RC: The thyroid scintigram. II: The cold nodule. Radiology 85:702, 1965

51. Mostofi FK, Price EB: Tumors of the Male Genital System. Washington DC, Armed Forces Institute of Pathology, 1973

52. Nussbaum M, Buchwald RP, Ribner A et al: Anaplastic carcinoma arising from median ectopic thyroid (thyroglossal duct remnant). Cancer 48:2724, 1981

53. Olen E, Klinck GH: Hyperthyroidism and thyroid cancer. Arch Pathol 81:531, 1966

54. Patton JF, Hewitt CB, Mallis N: Diagnosis and treatment of tumors of the testis. JAMA 117:2194, 1959

55. Einhorn LH, Donohue JP, Peckham MJ et al: Cancer of the testes. In DeVita VT, Hellman S, Rosenberg SA (eds): Cancer: Principles and Practice of Oncology, pp 979–1011. Philadelphia, JB Lippincott, 1985

56. Perlmutter M, Slater SL: Which nodular goiter should be removed? N Engl J Med 255:65, 1956

57. Rayfield EJ, Nishiyama RH, Sisson JC: Small cell tumors of the thyroid. Cancer 28:1023, 1971

58. Richmond J, Sherman RS, Diamond HD et al: Renal lesions associated with malignant lymphomas. Am J Med 32:184, 1962

59. Salzman AJ: Imaging techniques in aspiration biopsy. In Linsk JA, Franzen S (eds): Aspiration Cytology. Philadelphia, JB Lippincott, 1983

60. Selzer G, Kahn LB, Albertyn L: Primary malignant tumors of the thyroid gland: A Clinico-pathologic study of 254 cases. Cancer 40:1501, 1977

61. Shimaoka K, Galani S, Tsukada Y et al: Plasma cell neoplasm involving the thyroid. Cancer 41:1140, 1978

62. Silverberg SG, Vidone RA: Adenoma and carcinoma of the thyroid. Cancer 19:1053, 1966

63. Smithers DS: Tumours of the Thyroid Gland. Edinburgh, E & S Livingstone, 1970

64. Smithers DS: Malignant lymphomas of the thyroid gland. In Smithers DS (ed): Tumours of the Thyroid Gland, pp 141–154. Edinburgh, E & S Livingstone, 1970

65. Stavric GD, Karanfilski BT, Kalamaras AK et al: Early diagnosis and detection of clinically non-suspected thyroid neoplasia by the cytologic method. Cancer 45:340, 1980

66. Söderström N, Telenius-Berg M, Ackerman M: Diagnosis of medullary carcinoma of the thyroid by fine needle aspiration biopsy. Acta Med Scand 197:71, 1975

67. Stepanas AV, Samaan NA, Hill CS Jr et al: Medullary thyroid cancer: Importance of serial serum calcitonin measurement. Cancer 43:825, 1979

68. Sutton MG St J, Sheps SG, Lie JT: Prevalence of clinically unsuspected pheochromocytoma. Mayo Clin Proc 56:354, 1981

69. Ternvall J, Cedarquist E, Moller T et al: Preoperative scintigraphy with correlation to cytology and histopathology in carcinoma of the thyroid. Acta Radiol [Oncol] 22:183, 1983

70. Tollefsen HR, DeCosse JJ, Hutter RV: Papillary carcinoma of the thyroid: A clinical and pathologic study of 70 fatal cases. Cancer 17:1035, 1964

71. UCLA Conference: Autoimmune thyroid disease: Graves' and Hashimoto's. Ann Intern Med 88:370, 1978

72. UCLA Conference: The thyroid nodule. Ann Intern Med 96:221, 1982

73. Volpe R, Farid NR, Van Westtarp C et al: A viewpoint: The pathogenesis of Graves' disease and Hashimoto's thyroiditis. Clin Endocrinol 3:239, 1974

74. Wang C, Vickery AL Jr, Maloof F: Needle biopsy of the thyroid. Surg Gynecol Obstet 143:365, 1976

75. Weiss LM, Weinberg DS, Warhol MJ: Medullary carcinoma arising in a thyroid with Hashimoto's disease. Am J Clin Pathol 80:534, 1983

76. Williams ED: The origin and association of medullary carcinoma of the thyroid. In Smithers DS (ed): Tumours of the Thyroid Gland, pp 130–140. Edinburgh, E & S Livingstone, 1970

77. Woolner LB, McConahey WM, Beahrs OH et al: Primary malignant lymphoma of the thyroid: Review of forty-six cases. Am J Surg 111:502, 1966

78. Zajicek J: Aspiration Biopsy Cytology. Part 2, Cytology of Infradiaprhagmatic Organs. Basel, S Karger, 1979

4 The Breast: Diagnosis and Management

Diagnosis of breast disease by fine needle aspiration is the most important area of study in the entire range of application of the method. Historically, the breast was the first region to which pioneers in the method addressed their efforts.[34,50,53] It is usually the first area in which the examining physician, surgeon, oncologist, or radiotherapist will be prompted to or will be called upon to utilize the fine needle method. This is due in part to the frequency of palpable malignant tumors, but more commonly is due to the vast numbers of anxious patients with lumpy, nodular, or tender breasts with benign disease. The method has long existed in Europe. With its popularization in the United States, patients will be requesting the procedure specifically as an initial step before undergoing surgical biopsy. The success of new imaging methods combined with fine needle aspiration for nonpalpable disease will familiarize the public further with the efficacy of fine needle aspiration.[16,26,38]

Indications for Aspiration Biopsy

Why subject the patient to an additional procedure and additional cost together with the inconvenience of setting up appointments, possibly traveling, and meeting yet another physician? Why do this when traditional wisdom dictates surgery for palpable disease? What is gained by cytologic diagnosis when it must be reaffirmed by histopathologic analysis of the surgical specimen?

It is stated repeatedly in this book and in other publications[31,53] that a negative cytologic report must be evaluated critically from a clinical viewpoint. More specifically, this means that negative reports do not exclude cancer, because of the possibility of missing the target or misinterpreting the cytologic report (false-negative). In dealing with breast disease, however, a negative report is not simply null data, since positive diagnoses of benign disease are made frequently.

The clinical evaluation of breast disease, as with all other pathologic procedures, includes the age of the patient, history (particularly of the family), and physical findings. *There is enormous variation in an individual clinician's perception of breast disease, as illustrated in the following case.*

Case 4-1

A 27-year-old pregnant woman was observed in an obstetrical clinic in a regional hospital. In the seventh month of pregnancy, she discovered a globular, somewhat tender mass in the upper outer quadrant of her right breast. It measured 2 cm by 3 cm. She was examined by her obstetrician (a woman), who advised her that the mass was related to prelactation breast tissue proliferation and that she would reexamine after delivery of the baby. Following delivery, the mass persisted and the patient reported to a surgical clinic where fine needle aspiration was carried out, yielding a diagnosis of ductal carcinoma. Mastectomy was done 5 months after the initial discovery.

The obstetrician subsequently reported to the surgical clinic for evaluation of tender nodularity in her right breast. On examination, there was no definite mass but rather a more generalized fibronodularity. Fine needle aspiration of the most prominent area was performed with a 25-gauge needle, primarily to relieve the well-controlled anxiety of the patient/physician.

Clinical perception becomes a most important aspect of initiating the diagnosis of significant breast disease. There is little controversy about the majority of dominant masses; they demand a morphologic diagnosis and appropriate therapy. However, as Case 4-1 illustrates, in girls, elderly women, and patients with severely debilitating unrelated illness or metastatic tumors arising in nonmammary primaries, the demand for traditional surgical biopsy with or without frozen section may be modified. In all of these exceptional circumstances, fine needle aspiration is an excellent, expeditious method of obtaining a diagnosis, which may or may not be acted upon. Sometimes the clinical decision to perform surgery will be aided by knowledge of the morphologic diagnosis, for example, in a chronically ill 90-year-old woman. At the very least, it will allow intelligent discussion with the patient. Aspects of managing these nonrepresentative lesions will be discussed later.

In the more usual breast mass presenting as a dominant lump in an otherwise healthy mature woman, fine needle aspiration continues to be questioned in the face of traditional, "foolproof" frozen section. As experience with the method has deepened, multiple justifications have been accepted increasingly and are listed as follows:

To distinguish breast cellulitis or abscess from inflammatory carcinoma
To identify fat necrosis, which can simulate carcinoma (see Case 4-3)
To identify hematoma, which may simulate a solid mass
To specifically identify the following benign lesions, which may present

as apparently solid masses: cysts, fibroadenoma, granular cell myoblastoma,[9] lipoma, gynecomastia (in men)

To identify the following malignant tumors, which may guide or modify the surgical procedure: lymphoma, lobular carcinoma, inflammatory carcinoma, Paget's disease of nipple, subareolar carcinoma

To present the surgeon with a preoperative diagnosis, which will eliminate frozen section and up to 20 or more minutes of anesthesia,
and allow him to plan alternate procedures.[7]

Cellulitis, fat necrosis, and hematoma can be treated with antibiotics
and local applications, and observed. Cycsts may be evacuated, followed
by careful palpation for residual tumor. Surgery is often eliminated.

Discovery of the Lesion

It is difficult to establish precisely how often a suspicious abnormality is
discovered initially by the patient. Self-examination has been advocated.
Education by the American Cancer Society and other organizations, as well
as individual instruction by physicians, has resulted in a growing selected
group of women in whom self-discovery of the lesion is far more likely
than would be expected on random or chance discovery in women who
have not been instructed.[19] Chance discovery occurs particularly during
showering and bathing, when the soaped skin heightens the tactile sense
because surface friction is reduced (see below). Even without palpation,
women may experience sensitivity, tenderness, or fullness in an affected
breast. A cardinal rule in breast evaluation is *listen to the patient.* Experience
has shown that she will point to the site of disease not detectable on casual
examination (Fig. 4-1). (This is also illustrated later in Case 4-10.)

There are three types of examinations that may reveal breast disease.
Physicians often see patients specifically for breast examination at regular
intervals, because of known risk factors or because of previously noted
suspicious findings. Such findings include atypical mammography, previous
biopsies with benign epithelial proliferations, previous fine needle aspiration with varying degrees of mammary dysplasia,[31,53] and previous examinations with slightly suspicious findings deemed insufficient for intervention. Risk factors include prior mastectomy in the patient and carcinoma
in her mother or sisters. (See Case 4-9 later.) Such historic factors demand
regular examination and mammography.

Probably the most common breast examination is carried out by gynecologists in the process of obtaining a cervical smear for Pap examination,
which usually occurs annually. Breast and other examinations are included
in this gynecologic checkup. A busy gynecologist may examine 20 to 40
women daily.

Finally, breast examination is, or should be, part of any general examination by family practitioners, internists, and general surgeons. Although there are physicians who compulsively examine patients rather

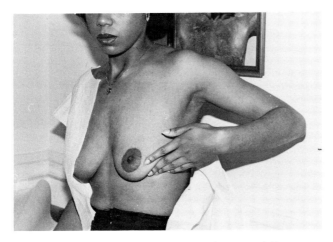

FIGURE 4-1: The patient is indicating the area of discomfort in her breast. This may pinpoint the disease process and should not be ignored. (See Case 4-10.)

completely, often for minor or local disorders, others still persist in forgetting breast examination.

The Examination

The initial step in the examination is asking the patient for her appraisal. Always listen to the patient, who may point out an area of tenderness or vague discomfort, a mass, or an area of nodularity.

Inspection in the sitting position (Fig. 4-2) seeks retractions, asymmetries, edema, discoloration, and nipple retraction (see below). Inspection continues while the patient elevates her arms. In the patient shown in Figure 4-3, retraction can be detected in the undersurface of the right breast. This is more evident with external compression (Fig. 4-4). Retraction is quite evident in another patient (Fig. 4-5). Palpation continues with an examination of the axillae (Fig. 4-6). The patient's arm should be in a relaxed position. The axilla is described below.

The supraclavicular space is palpated with the patient's head flexed (Fig. 4-7). Nodes sometimes can be detected on the inner surfaces of the clavicles.

With the patient supine, the breasts are examined by palpation with the flat fingers (Fig. 4-8). Fingertip sensitivity is important, and it is heightened by repeating the examination after soaping the breast (Fig. 4-9). Liquid soap (Fig. 4-10) breaks surface tension, revealing abnormalities not previously noted. The examination should be accompanied by instructions in self-examination.

Masses and nodules are sometimes palpable in the sitting position but not with the patient supine. This was illustrated in a previously reported

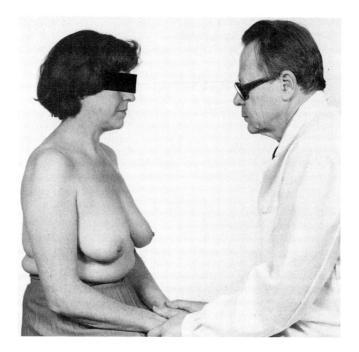

FIGURE 4-2: Inspection in the sitting position will reveal subtle asymmetries of the breasts.

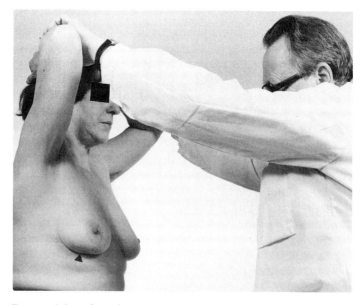

FIGURE 4-3: When the patient elevates her arms, retraction can be detected in the undersurface of the right breast (*arrowhead*).

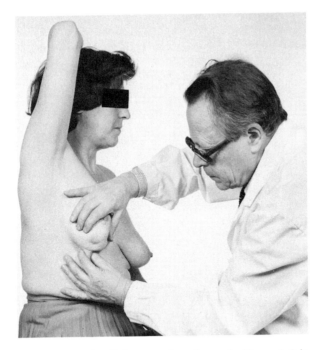

FIGURE 4-4: The slight retraction shown in Figure 4-3 is made evident by external compression.

case[31] (see Case 7-1). It may be useful to maintain contact with the mass while the patient moves from the sitting to the lying position.

The examination is carried out systematically. Nipples are inspected for eczema (Paget's disease) and the areolae are compressed to express secretion. The breast is examined in quadrants, with particular attention to the upper outer quadrant, which is the location of the majority of carcinomas. This area includes the tail of the breast. Palpation extends to all lateral margins, including the parasternal intercostal spaces, subclavicular space, inframammary fold, and anterior axillary fold.

Grasping the full thickness of the breast may reveal masses, sometimes large, deep within the substance of the breast.

Suspected but ill-defined lesions are sometimes outlined more easily by switching the palpating hand, changing the patient's position, or changing the position of the palpating hand.

The yield by palpation includes small firm nodules (fibroadenomas), globular masses (cysts), well-defined firm masses (carcinomas), and ill-defined often irregular lesions (mammary dysplasia).

The Irradiated Breast

Irradiation of the breast may follow lumpectomy (excision of the palpable mass) or wedge biopsy of the mass, which is then left *in situ*. Removal of

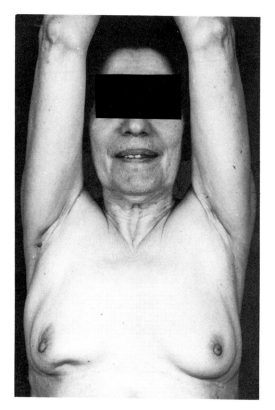

FIGURE 4-5: Retraction is more prominent in this 65-year-old woman (different patient).

tissue, even though a firm cytologic diagnosis has been made, is necessary for estrogen receptor studies in most laboratories. However, this procedure has been performed successfully on cellular material obtained by aspiration.[45]

The decision for limited surgery followed by radiation may result from exercising a therapeutic option that yields cure rates equal to mastectomy,[5,15,28] inoperable status because of mass size, associated medical disorder, or age of the patient. In all cases, surgery is preceded by aspiration biopsy cytology, which establishes the diagnosis and helps guide the decision. This is illustrated in the following case.

Case 4-2

The patient was a 72-year-old woman referred for aspiration of a 4-cm breast mass that was clinically suspicious for carcinoma. On immediate examination, the smears were composed of a monomorphic pattern of intermediate lymphocytes. At this point, a more searching

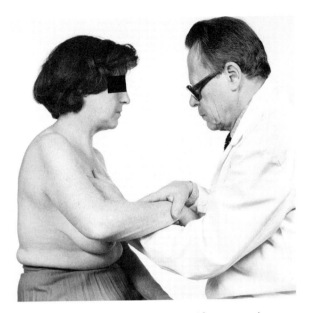

FIGURE 4-6: Palpation continues with an examination of the axilla. The patient's arm is relaxed, and rests on the examiner's arm.

examination revealed palpable lymph nodes in the posterior cervical triangle. The white blood count was 11,000 with 62% lymphocytes. Further studies, including a bone marrow examination, established the presence of a lymphoproliferative disorder. The breast mass was an extranodal manifestation and prompted considerable discussion before initiating radiation therapy.

Depending on mass size and surgical technique, residual induration may remain following surgery alone. Irradiation of the whole breast following lumpectomy or wedge resection, however, often results in a general thickening, increase in density, and loss of elasticity (Fig. 4-11), but more specifically there may be a linear induration at the site of excision. Where a biopsy of the mass is done but the mass is left *in situ*, irradiation leaves fibrotic induration with ill-defined margins. This may be palpated deep within the breast depending on the site of the original tumor.

Follow-up examinations of the intact breast require, in particular, careful palpation with measurement and topographic recording of the shape of residual indurations, as well as assessment of their texture. During and following radiation, these parameters may undergo change. There is no

(Text continues on p. 110.)

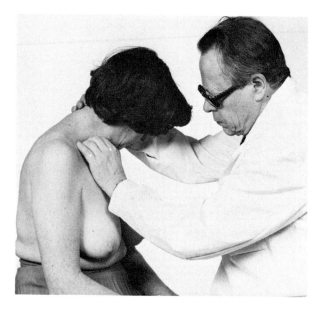

FIGURE 4-7: The supraclavicular space is palpated with the patient's head flexed and the shoulder elevated to relax the fascia.

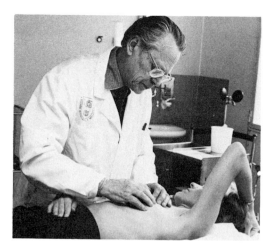

FIGURE 4-8: With the patient supine, the breast is examined with flattened fingers and fingertips.

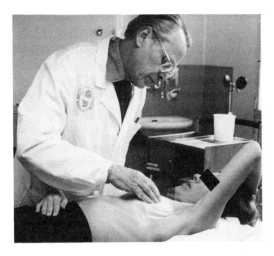

FIGURE 4-9: The examination is repeated after soaping the breast.

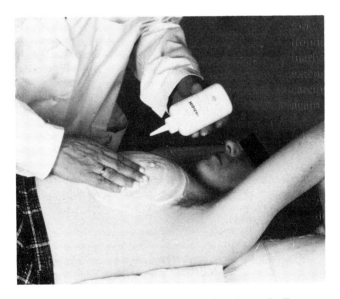

FIGURE 4-10: Liquid soap can be used with good effect. The examination should include instructions to the patient about self-examination.

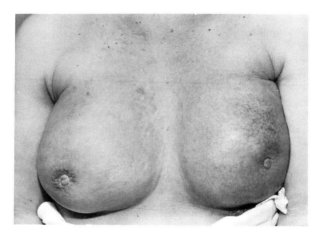

FIGURE 4-11: Both breasts have received irradiation. Loss of elasticity and mobility has occurred. The left nipple is retracted.

more suitable method to evaluate indurated portions of the irradiated breast than fine needle aspiration.

In Figure 4-12, there is marked contraction of the irradiated breast. The shrunken breast is firm to hard. Careful physical examination together with fine needle aspiration provides the best approach to follow up.

Figure 4-13 illustrates post-irradiation induration and fibrosis in the intermammary tissue following mediastinal radiation for bronchogenic carcinoma. There are parallel firm ridges extending into both breasts. Local nodularity was palpated in the inner quadrant of the right breast and aspiration yielded carcinoma cells. This proved to be a second primary on follow up.

Aspiration sometimes will require a somewhat forceful entry of the needle into fibrotic tissue. A firm grasp of the full thickness of the breast may be necessary to immobilize dense residual tissue after irradiation of a large tumor mass.

As a rule, recurrent tumor will readily yield diagnosable material with ample cellularity. However, the earliest yield may be a drop of thin tissue fluid that may contain a few distorted tumor cells. Cell viability then becomes a consideration. Intact, recognizable cells, even if sparse, must be viewed with suspicion. Clinical evidence of an enlarging mass coupled with the presence of cancer cells should be sufficient evidence of viable tumor. An *in vitro* method of evaluating cancer cells harvested from a treated area utilizing cell culture technique has been presented.[17] However, determination of viability still remains a practical clinical problem.

Fat necrosis following both implant therapy and external radiation may present as a recurrent breast mass.[47] This mass cannot be readily discriminated from carcinoma by mammography. In a series of eight pa-

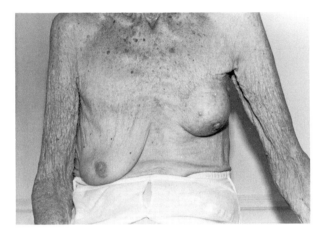

Figure 4-12: The left breast is contracted and hard after irradiation. Follow-up includes fine needle aspiration to detect recurrence.

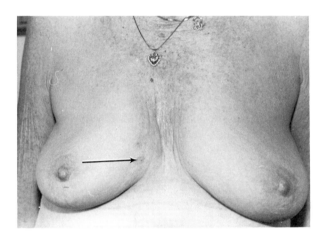

Figure 4-13: The intermammary skin is thickened with linear, post-irradiation wrinkling. Induration of the lower inner quadrant of the right breast (*arrow*) was due to a second primary carcinoma.

tients, clinical presentation varied from ill-defined induration to a painless discrete mass without overlying dimpling. These findings contrast somewhat with post-traumatic fat necrosis (see below).

Rises of carcinoembryonic antigen (CEA) during the follow-up period in the absence of obvious metastatic disease should prompt breast aspiration. Patients with CEA levels remaining above 2.5 mg (Roche) after mastectomy had a more rapid recurrence rate, and such patients should be aspirated more freely during the posttreatment period.[49]

Interpretation of the post-irradiation mammogram is difficult. False-positive patterns are more likely to occur in the irradiated breast than in the untreated breast.[30] A baseline mammogram should be obtained immediately after irradiation so that future progressive changes may be evaluated. It is not unusual to detect masses on mammography that are not palpable because of skin thickening, fibrosis, and distortion. The mammogram may guide fine needle aspiration where the size of the residual mass changes.[30,41] Fine needle aspiration adds another parameter that should reduce the margin of error, just as the triple method of diagnosis (palpation, mammography, and aspiration biopsy cytology) has done in the pretreatment breast.[26] (See below.)

Post-Traumatic Fat Necrosis

Most traumatic fat necrosis as traditionally reported[27] (see Case 4-3) simulates carcinoma clinically. More recently, it has been found to simulate it radiographically.[3] Most often, it occurs in obese patients with pendulous breasts within 1 year of trauma, but it may occur some years later. Of particular interest is the fact that there may be an enlarging mass, attachment to the chest wall and the skin, and nipple retraction (see below).[1] Liquefied material may be extracted. Smears provide fairly characteristic and useful data that must be considered in conjunction with clinical, historic, and radiographic findings in deciding an appropriate therapy. Dystrophic calcification (in contrast with microcalcification, which occurs regularly in malignancy) occurs irregularly.[6] Where the area of fat necrosis is extensive, sampling several areas with the fine needle is suggested. Because carcinoma may occur adjacent to fat necrosis, all nonmalignant smears again must be evaluated on clinical grounds.

Case 4-3 illustrates the importance of identifying the nature of a generic "tumor."

Case 4-3

A 66-year-old woman was referred for aspiration of a fairly well-defined mass in the upper outer quadrant of her right breast. She had declined surgical biopsy because of experience with postoperative bleeding following minor procedures in the past.

On inspection, there were several ecchymotic areas on her breast and she stated that they occurred periodically in other parts of her body after minor trauma.

Fine needle aspiration yielded evidence of old hemorrhage and fat necrosis. The mass regressed on several follow-up examinations. Hematologic evaluation revealed a diagnosis of von Willebrand's disease.

Regions of the Breast

The Nipple

Alterations in the nipple, areola, and subareolar tissues invite cytologic evaluation. Consideration should be given to nipple secretions, nipple retraction, Paget's disease, and palpable masses.

The cytology of nipple secretions is described in reviews of exfoliative cytology.[25] Intraductal papilloma producing serous greenish black or bloody secretions may be nonpalpable, or may be up to several centimeters in diameter (see below). On careful observation, secretion may be seen to emerge from a single duct. The secretion of cells by ductal or papillary carcinoma is distinctly unusual,[39] but malignancy must be considered in every case. In the absence of a palpable mass, reliance must be placed on radiographic techniques.[23]

Nipple retraction is often a striking finding noted by the patient and usually detected by the examining physician. It is most often due to carcinoma evident on palpation. Senile duct ectasia may produce a subareolar mass with nipple retraction and inflammation, which suggests inflammatory carcinoma. Nipple retraction also occurs with fat necrosis. Fine needle aspiration will help identify these lesions, but the final therapeutic decision is multifactorial. The presence of cancer cells obviously settles the issue.

Nipple retraction should not be confused with nipple inversion. The patient is usually aware of longstanding nipple inversion.

Paget's disease is characterized by eczematoid changes of the nipple. The changes may be subtle, and minor changes should not be ignored.[2] Dermatitis of the areola without nipple change does not result from Paget's disease. Diagnosis is determined rapidly by scraping the nipple and smearing the superficial layer, which is invaded by ductal carcinoma cells. The use of a scalpel blade to obtain material is illustrated in Figures 4-14 and 4-15. Palpable tumors are undetected in a large percentage of cases, but mammograms may be positive.[6] The diagnostic sequence should include detection of early or well-defined changes on physical examination, preparation of cytologic smears from scraping, and mammography. The presence of cancer cells is sufficient indication for therapy even with negative mammography.

Palpable masses in the region of the nipple are as follows:

Papillary nipple adenoma
Fat necrosis
Duct ectasia
Carcinoma associated with Paget's disease
Intraductal papilloma
Tubular adenoma
Papillary carcinoma
Ductal carcinoma

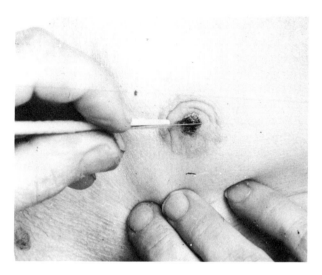

FIGURE 4-14: The nipple is scraped to obtain material for a smear when Paget's disease is suspected. (Linsk JA, Franzen S: Clinical Aspiration Cytology, p 109. Philadelphia, JB Lippincott, 1983)

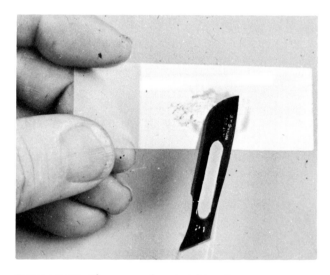

FIGURE 4-15: The smeared material has the same morphologic characteristics as aspirated cells have. (Linsk JA, Franzen S: Clinical Aspiration Cytology, p 109. Philadelphia, JB Lippincott, 1983)

Although specific cytologic diagnosis on fine needle aspiration may be difficult, particularly in distinguishing benign papilloma from papillary carcinoma, material should be obtained. It may yield an unequivocal diagnosis or provide some guidance for the surgeon. Cytologic diagnosis of a tubular adenoma supported by electron microscopy (EM) studies was reported recently.[36] The cytology of papillary lesions has been presented,[31] but there is no definitive study of a large number of these lesions to date.

Metastatic Tumors

A metastatic tumor in the breast cannot be clinically distinguished from a primary tumor. History of a previous or concurrent cancer should alert the examining physician, although second or even third independent malignancies are not rare.[4] The most common metastases to the breast arise from carcinoma of the opposite breast.[4,44] It may be difficult or impossible to distinguish primary from metastatic masses both cytologically and histopathologically. On the other hand, there are cytologically distinct breast carcinomas that may allow the distinction. A case has been reported of a patient with ductal carcinoma, not otherwise specified (NOS) of the right breast, which was resected in 1967, in whom a new, cytologically apocrine carcinoma was identified in the left breast in 1980.[31] Specific cytologic types that may be identified are as follows:

Apocrine carcinoma
Carcinoma with magenta bodies[31]
Colloid carcinoma
Medullary carcinoma
Adenoid cystic carcinoma
Squamous carcinoma

Identification of cell type and distinction of metastatic from primary tumors, where feasible, guides therapy.

Other metastatic masses that may be specifically identified cytologically are as follows:

Renal cell carcinoma
Melanoma
Lymphoma
Dysgerminoma

Signet cell carcinoma of the gastrointestinal tract may be confused with primary signet cell carcinoma of the breast. It is also difficult to distinguish squamous carcinoma, most adenocarcinomas, adenoid cystic carcinoma, and carcinoid as to point of origin.

The Upper Outer Quadrant

Palpable alterations in the upper outer quadrant of the breast provide the major diagnostic problem for the examining physician. Both mammary

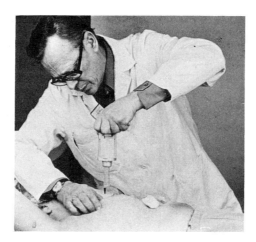

FIGURE 4-16: If it appears suspicious, the conglomerate thickening of the upper outer quadrant of the breast is grasped with full thickness for aspiration.

dysplasia and breast carcinoma are found more commonly in this area than any other breast region. Palpable tissue structures, often radiating with a linear architecture from the nipple, may be grasped as a conglomerate mass of fibroductal and glandular tissue with suspicious irregularities (Fig. 4-16). There also may be discrete fibronodular lumps that most often yield fat with or without clusters of benign epithelium and scattered, oval, naked nuclei on fine needle aspiration. Macrocysts presenting as rather discrete globular masses, which may be mistaken for solid tumors, also occur. Clinical clues of malignancy including evident dimpling, or skin retraction on compression of an ill-defined mass, are useful and help direct the needle (see Fig. 4-4).

A lesion in the tail of the breast may be difficult to distinguish from metastatic nodes. The presence of lymphocytes mixed with carcinoma in the smear may help identify the lymph node origin.

The Margins

Extensions of glandular breast tissue reach to the parasternal, subclavicular, anterior axillary, and inferior fold margins of the breast topography.[11] As a result, fibronodular alterations of mammary dysplasia and carcinomas may be found at all these sites and in the main mass of the breast. It is necessary to palpate the parasternal intercostal spaces in the sitting as well as the supine positions (see The Examination, above). Small nodules may be palpated at the anterior axillary curve of the ribs. In a thin patient, these nodules do not differ from chest wall nodules and may not be separated from the underlying muscle by breast fat. Such nodules should be aspirated with care using a 0.5-in, 25-gauge needle. Hazards are illustrated in the following case.

Case 4-4

The patient was a 31-year-old, thin, tense woman referred by a gynecologist for aspiration of a firm, 0.6-cm nodule that could be palpated within the lateral substance of the breast when the patient was seated. When the patient was supine, the nodule could be felt just under the skin. In spite of reassurance, the patient moved abruptly as the needle entered the nodule, and the needle passed momentarily between the ribs, with a resulting pneumothorax.

A subclavicular mass is illustrated by the following case.

Case 4-5

The patient was a 28-year-old woman with stage IIA Hodgkin's disease, and enlarged right supraclavicular and mediastinal nodes. Following radiation therapy to the mantle, a rubbery, firm, right subclavicular skin mass was palpated. It appeared to be within the superior, thin portion of the breast. On fine needle aspiration, smears were diagnostic of Hodgkin's disease, and further radiotherapy was elected.

The Lumpy Breast

There are several varieties of lumpy breast that may become suitable targets for fine needle aspiration in diagnosis. In the fat-depleted breast, particularly in girls and young women, firm, irregular glandular tissue may be palpated and consideration given to neoplastic proliferation. With the accumulation of fat, Cooper's ligaments divide the fat layer into lobules that the experienced palpator recognizes as fatty lobules, but that a patient or a less experienced physician may perceive as breast lumps requiring investigation.

Fibrocystic disease is responsible for the major diagnostic problems in women, particularly in younger women. These alterations, often, but not necessarily, bilateral, produce irregularities varying from quite small (0.5 cm to 1 cm), fibronodular masses to large, usually ill-defined tissue aggregates that demand clarification. As noted above, the larger mass of this dysplastic tissue is found in the upper outer quadrant. It is precisely in dealing with these elusive masses that palpation of the soaped breast is most useful (see Figs. 4-9 and 4-10). Macrocystic disease is part of the mixed pathology of mammary dysplasia and is usually a movable, globular mass, easily evacuated by a fine needle. There is no necessity to use a needle larger then 22 gauge. Also, ultrasonography has been suggested as an adjuvant procedure to identify cysts.[37] In our experience, palpable disease does not require adjuvant methods. Evacuation of cysts is a regular procedure usually carried out by surgeons. The clinician should be prepared to aspirate a solid mass when he fails to extract fluid freely. As with all cysts, evacuation must be followed by palpation for residual masses and aspiration if masses are present.

Although fibroadenoma is usually a solitary, firm, mobile mass found in young women, multiple fibroadenomata produce one form of discretely lumpy breast. Proliferation of fibroadenomata may be so profuse that multiple excisions are impracticable, and fine needle aspiration of selected lesions to establish the diagnosis[32] may be all that can be done.

The major question in dealing with all varieties of lumpy breast is when to biopsy. The clinician's perception of the importance of, and his approach to palpable breast disease, have been noted previously in Case 4-1 and in the sections on discovery and examination of breast lesions. Decision making is also complicated by the medico-legal climate, particularly in the United States.

Several options can be considered:

1. Dismiss the findings as insignificant.
2. Request repeat examination 1 week after the end of menses.
3. Refer the patient for a second opinion.
4. Refer the patient for mammography.
5. Refer the patient for local excision.
6. Refer the patient for frozen section and radical mastectomy.
7. Refer the patient for fine needle aspiration, or perform it himself.

The combination of mammography and aspiration biopsy cytology[26] cannot be stressed too strongly. Normal mammography in the presence of a palpable lesion must be followed by aspiration biopsy. Eleven of sixteen normal mammograms were reported in patients with palpable breast carcinoma.[10] Particularly with the Wolfe "Dy" pattern,[51,52] it appeared obvious that reliance on mammography alone was "extremely hazardous." In the presence of palpable disease, aspiration should precede mammography.[10] An attempt should be made to reduce surgical biopsy to a minimum because it distorts mammographic findings and may interfere with future clinical evaluation. Where surgery is deemed necessary, however, it should be preceded by a baseline mammogram.

If the fine needle aspiration yields characteristic cytology of mammary dysplasia,[31,32] this added data may enable the physician more objectively to reserve surgery and place the patient in a follow-up program. When all factors, including cytology and mammography, are evaluated with prudence, a significant number of surgical procedures can be eliminated in our experience and that of others.[24] Particularly in women under the age of 30, in whom only 1% to 3% of breast cancers are found,[35] as many as 30 surgical biopsies are performed for each carcinoma diagnosed.[20,29,43]

Nonpalpable lesions may be discovered by mammography carried out routinely or for some palpable or symptomatic abnormality. There are numerous reports on lesion localization and wide excision of the region, which have been summarized by Levy.[29] Fine needle aspiration using a computerized stereotactic method of needle placement has been employed with good results.[37] (See Case 4-8 later.) Adequate cytologic preparations also can be obtained with localization using needles in two planes, guided by mammography.[16]

Carcinoma

The dominant lump or surgical mass is detected easily. Although skin dimpling, retraction, and peau d'orange are useful additional findings, the frank palpation of a mass with well-defined margins is enough evidence for immediate fine needle aspiration. There are no contraindications to this procedure, which will yield a diagnosis in well over 90% of these masses. Palpation of the mass eliminates the immediate need for mammography and all ancillary tests and examinations. Identification of the cancer by fine needle aspiration will more efficiently point the way to further studies, or will suggest that further studies are not necessary. The latter would occur, for example, if the cytologic diagnosis is granular cell myoblastoma[9] or lipoma.[53] On the other hand, a lymphoid mass (as described in Case 4-2) will suggest further studies. The diagnosis of carcinoma requires a searching examination of the axillae and the supraclavicular regions. Preoperative diagnosis confirms the possible need for (1) mammography, (2) bone scan, and (3) selected studies for metastatic disease. It also answers questions, relieves anxiety in some patients, and allows planning of therapy.

Inflammatory carcinoma presenting as a tense, hyperemic, inflamed area simulating cellulitis is an ideal lesion for aspiration biopsy diagnosis. Suitable diagnostic material can be obtained with a small needle inserted tangentially under the skin. (See Fig. 9-23.) It will extract cells from dermal lymphatics. Unequivocal cancer cells, dispersed and in groups, are diagnostic of this lesion and therapy can proceed without incisional biopsy. Failure to obtain cancer cells on superficial puncture should prompt a deeper puncture possibly to obtain acute inflammatory exudate from an abscess, mixed round cell exudate from plasma cell mastitis, or granular necrotic material with phagocytic histiocytes from fat necrosis.

Aspiration of the Male Breast

Gynecomastia is a frequent finding from puberty to old age. It is rare to find carcinoma in clinically suspected gynecomastia in the younger age group. Unilateral or bilateral gynecomastia in the postpuberty period is attributed to physiological hormone stimulation. Fine needle aspiration rarely is indicated. In the third or the early part of the fourth decade, gynecomastia should suggest examination of the testes for hormone-producing tumors. Measurement of the beta subunit of chorionic gonadotrophin is indicated. However, primary carcinoma cannot be excluded, as demonstrated in the following case.

Case 4-6

The patient was a 28-year-old man who had a unilateral breast mass. He was receiving no medication. Testes examination was normal. General history and results of physical examination were normal. Fine needle aspiration yielded typical ductal carcinoma. In spite of this, local excision was performed and the diagnosis was carcinoma. Radical mastectomy followed and all nodes were negative.

The benign tissue of gynecomastia may be densely applied to the skin of the areola, and it moves with the skin on palpation. Careful palpation will determine that carcinoma is often separate from the areolar subepithelial tissue. Abnormalities of the nipple including crusting ulceration, discharge, and retraction are more obvious manifestations of carcinoma and are not easily confused with gynecomastia. There are, however, carcinomas that cannot be clinically distinguished from benign gynecomastia, and fine needle aspiration is usually decisive.

Etiologies of gynecomastia include drugs (digitalis preparations and spironolactone [Aldactone]),[33] inflammations and neoplasms,[12,48] bilharziasis with liver disease, hyperestrogenism, Klinefelter's syndrome,[13] and hormone therapy. In prostate carcinoma, gynecomastia secondary to estrogen therapy is a site of primary carcinoma.[22] Hormone-producing tumors of the testes are clinically important causes of gynecomastia,[21] and careful examination is necessary.

The Axilla

The axilla is a pyramidal space containing lymph nodes, fat, vessels, and nerves. The apex extends to the supraclavicular space. Lymph nodes palpable in the supraclavicular space may be an extension of the axillary apical nodes. Palpation with the patient in the sitting position is carried out by supporting the patient's arm with one hand and reaching high into the axilla with the other (see Fig. 4-6). The patient's arm must be lowered to relax the axillary fascia and allow deep palpation starting at the apex and capturing all palpable nodes against the chest wall. (Figure 8-4 illustrates pinioning a lymph node for aspiration.) The axillary fold and the medial surface of the upper arm should be palpated. When the patient is supine, again palpation must be carried out with the axillary fascia relaxed.

In the presence of known breast carcinoma, palpable axillary nodes ultimately are determined to be falsely positive for cancer in 24% to 29% of several series.[14] Clinical staging is converted to preoperative pathologic staging by fine needle aspiration of palpable nodes.

The presence of metastatic axillary nodes with an unknown primary is an important diagnostic problem. The breast is the most common site of origin, but melanoma, bronchogenic carcinoma, and less frequently a variety of primary adenocarcinomas may be the sites of origin.

Specific cytologic types of breast carcinoma (see above) and a cytologic diagnosis of melanoma will establish the diagnosis. Aspiration of small cell undifferentiated carcinoma will suggest oat cell carcinoma of the lung, which may be present as an occult lesion in a patient with a normal chest film. However, adenocarcinoma from most sites is indistinguishable from the usual breast carcinoma designated NOS.[8] The occult primary lesion may be noninvasive.[42]

The Aspiration Technique

The aspiration technique is the same as described in Chapter 1. Because the breasts are mobile, particular attention must be paid to fixation of the mass. With appropriate preliminary explanation to the patient, local anesthesia is not necessary. It may distort the landmarks, and if it is injected too close to the lesion, may cause osmotic distortion of the cells.

For superficial small nodules, a useful technique consists of inserting the needle first so that it transfixes the mass (Fig. 4-17, *left*). Then, the syringe is attached and aspiration is performed without oscillating the needle beyond the mass (Fig. 4-17, *right*).

For deeper masses, initial penetration of the needle through the skin, followed by a thrust into the fixated mass is suggested. A difference in texture between breast fat and the firmer tumor tissue can be noted.

In Figure 4-18 (*left*), a moderate-sized mass palpable beneath the skin is fixated. The needle is thrust directly through the skin into the mass in a continuous movement. It has been observed that blood usually will emerge from the puncture site in cases of carcinoma but not with benign disease (Fig. 4-18, *right*).

Aspiration of small skin deposits in the postmastectomy follow-up examination (Fig. 4-19) is best accomplished with a 25-gauge needle inserted tangentially into the lesion (see Chap. 9).

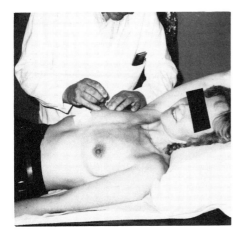 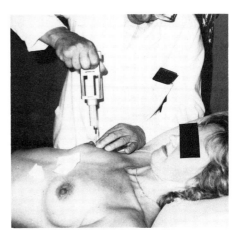

FIGURE 4-17: (*Left*) Small lesions, which are often detected by fingertip examination, may be transfixed for greater control by manually inserting a small needle. (*Right*) This is followed by attachment of a syringe, and aspiration.

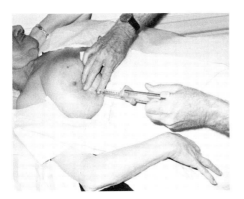 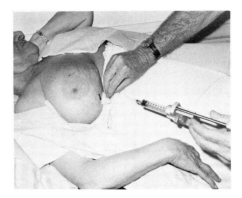

FIGURE 4-18: (*Left*) Masses that are palpable beneath the skin are transfixed and entered with a direct puncture. (*Right*) Prompt return of blood at the picture site suggests malignancy.

The Triple Diagnostic Method

Diagnosis of breast lesions by practicing clinicians is quite variable, and depends very much on the clinician's attitudes and perceptions. This is illustrated in Case 4-1.

Examination of the same patient by more than one clinician often will result in more than one diagnosis and plan of management. As a result, second opinions have been required by some third party payers.

A triple diagnostic method of breast diagnosis originally was suggested by Kreuzer and co-workers.[26] The triple diagnostic method attempts to objectify the diagnosis. It consists of three steps:

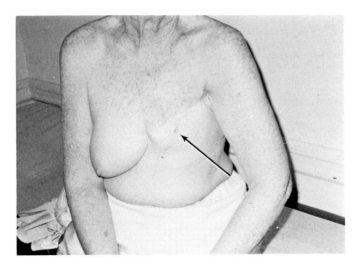

FIGURE 4-19: Biopsies of small deposits in the skin (*arrow*) are easily done by tangential aspiration with a small needle.

Clinical examination
Mammography
Aspiration biopsy

The steps are complementary. One or more may be positive, and the others may be negative. The application of the method is illustrated in the following cases and is depicted in Figure 4-20.

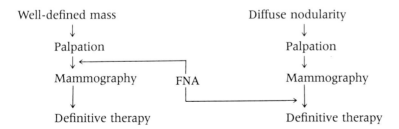

Comment: Well-defined palpable masses should be aspirated for diagnosis and bilateral mammography carried out to detect other nonpalpable disease.

Nodular breasts without a dominant lump should have mammography first, which may direct FNA or require a stereotactic approach.

FIGURE 4-20: Diagnostic schema for breast tumors.

Case 4-7

The patient was a 36-year-old woman who regularly jogged in the park. She was asymptomatic. Following her exercise, it was her habit to take a shower during which she soaped her torso, including her breasts and axillae. Unexpectedly, she felt an asymmetry under her soaped fingers not previously noted. It prompted a visit to her doctor, and she pointed out to him a superficial nodule smaller than a grain of rice in the lateral surface of the left breast (Fig. 4-21). No other masses were palpable.

Mammography was normal.

Fine needle aspiration yielded a cellular smear diagnostic of colloid carcinoma. The smear was composed of masses of mucin intermixed with clusters of tumor cells (Fig. 4-22).

Local excision was carried out. Multiple sections were made of the surgical specimen without detecting cancer (Fig. 4-23). Review of the smear prompted further sections (see Fig. 4-23), and a colloid carcinoma measuring 3 mm by 7 mm was identified (Fig. 4-24). Figure 4-25 illustrates the patient's presurgical appearance with the puncture site. Figure 4-26 illustrates the patient's postoperative appearance. There was no further therapy.

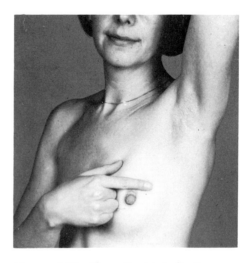

FIGURE 4-21: The patient is indicating a minute nodule in the superficial tissues of her breast. She detected the nodule while soaping herself in the shower.

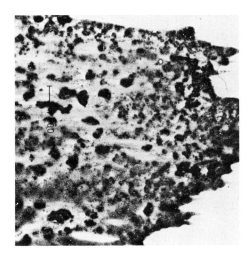

FIGURE 4-22: Low-power view of fine needle aspirate of breast nodule. The dark masses are composed of tumor cells and the background is stained purple with May–Grünwald–Giemsa stain. The cytologic diagnosis is colloid carcinoma.

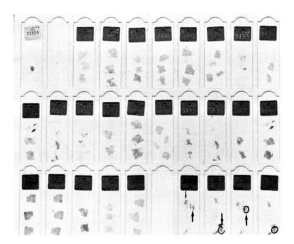

FIGURE 4-23: These slides contain multiple sections of the excised mass, initially negative for cancer. After the smears were reviewed, further sections (*arrows*) were taken and carcinoma was identified.

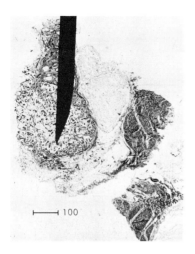

FIGURE 4-24: Tissue section of a colloid carcinoma measuring 3 mm × 7 mm is shown with superimposed needle point.

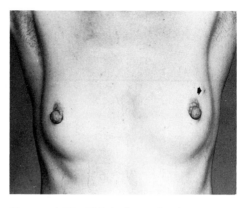

FIGURE 4-25: This is the patient's preoperative appearance with the puncture site (*arrow*).

In this patient, results of the clinical examination were positive, mammography was negative, and fine needle aspiration was positive.

Case 4-8

A 40-year-old woman had a screening mammography. A complex lesion consisting of an apparent fibroadenoma and an adjacent suspicious cluster of microcalcifications was reported by the radiologist (Fig. 4-27). On clinical examination, no mass could be palpated.

The patient was referred for stereotactic fine needle biopsy using the Nordenström technique (Fig. 4-28). In Figure 4-29, separate guide needles can be seen within the larger benign lesion and the smaller suspicious cluster of microcalcifications.

On fine needle aspiration, the benign lesion yielded the typical cytologic changes of a fibroadenoma.[32] The needle entering the microcalcifications produced a frankly malignant smear. Contrasting cells of the two lesions are seen in tissue section (Fig. 4-30).

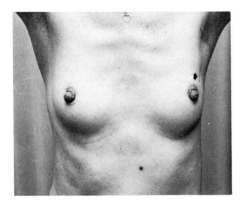

FIGURE 4-26: This is the patient's post-operative appearance with the incision site (*arrow*).

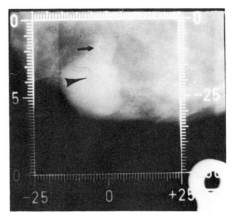

FIGURE 4-27: Mammogram. The large triangular arrow identifies a fibroadenoma. The small barbed arrow is pointing at microcalcifications associated with cancer.

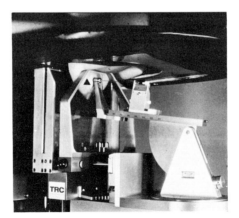

FIGURE 4-28: This apparatus was invented by Dr. B. Nordenström to carry out stereotactic biopsies with mammographic guidance. The triangular arrow indicates the fixed dependent breast with the needle entering.

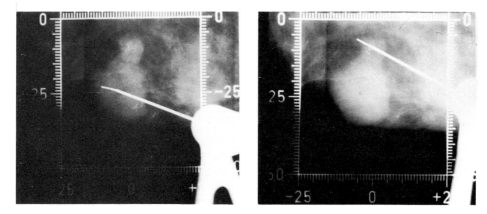

FIGURE 4-29: Mammogram. (*Left*) The needle guide has entered the fibroadenoma and the fine needle is seen protruding. (*Right*) The needle has punctured the area of microcalcification.

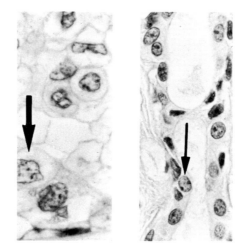

FIGURE 4-30: Tissue section of cancer and fibroadenoma. On the left is a cancer cell with an enlarged, irregular nucleus (*thick arrow*). This contrasts with a cell from the fibroadenoma (*thin arrow*).

In summary, with the triple diagnostic method, there were negative results from clinical examination, positive mammography, and positive cytology.

Case 4-9

A 36-year-old woman visited her physician with anxiety concerning breast cancer. She had a strong family history with cancer present in her mother and two of three older sisters. Careful clinical examination including breast palpation with soaped fingers failed to detect any abnormalities. The patient was referred for mammography. A small area of clustered microcalcifications was observed (Fig. 4-31).

Stereotactic fine needle biopsy was carried out using the Nordenström computerized technique. Only a small cluster of apocrine cells was obtained; therefore, surgery was performed.

In Figure 4-32 are x-ray films of several slices of the surgical specimen. The arrow indicates the identifying calcification. In Figure 4-33, a 1-mm carcinoma is identified. Magnified at higher power, microcalcification was seen within the carcinoma.

This patient had a strong family history. Results of clinical examination were negative, mammography was positive, and fine needle aspiration was negative. Treatment was local excision only.

Case 4-10

A healthy woman, 30 years old, reported to her gynecologist for a routine check-up. She told him she had discomfort in the lateral portion of her left breast. It was vague, but there was a distinct difference in her awareness of her two breasts. The sensation was new. After careful examination, finding nothing, but impressed with the atypical localized symptoms, the gynecologist referred her for further breast evaluation and possible biopsy.

On examination, the patient pointed out the area of discomfort in her breast (Fig. 4-34). There were no findings on palpation with or without soaped fingers. Because of her apprehension and insistence, a fine needle aspiration was carried out precisely in the area indicated.

Surprisingly, a cell-rich smear was obtained diagnostic of ductal carcinoma (Fig. 4-35).

Mammography was then ordered. In Figure 4-36, asymmetry and density of the pattern in the left breast is seen, but this is not diagnostic of cancer.

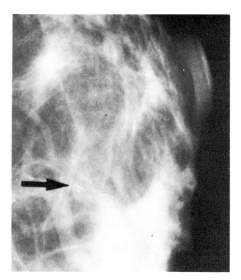

FIGURE 4-31: Mammogram. There is a small area of microcalcification (*arrow*).

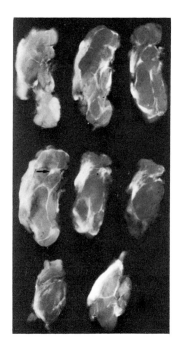

FIGURE 4-32: X-ray film of surgical specimen. Multiple slices are made and microcalcifications are identified in one slice (*arrow*), indicating that excision has been successful.

Local excision and node dissection followed. The tumor measured 9 mm. It was intraductal, but diffusely spreading through all the observed ducts on several sections. Postoperative radiation was therefore administered. In Figure 4-37, the patient is seen 1 year later.

In summary, results of the clinical examination were negative, the mammography was positive, but nondiagnostic for tumor. The aspiration was positive.

Case 4-11

A 60-year-old woman reported for a routine examination including mammography. A mastectomy had been performed on her right breast 5 years earlier (Fig. 4-38). Clinical examination was negative. On mammography, a small lesion rich in calcification was demonstrated (Fig. 4-39).

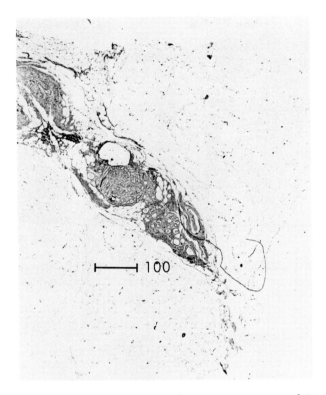

FIGURE 4-33: Tissue section. The carcinoma measured 1 mm in diameter.

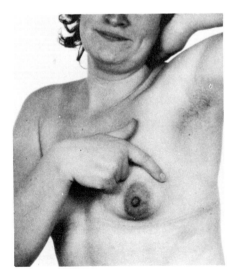

FIGURE 4-34: The patient is pointing to an area of discomfort in her left breast.

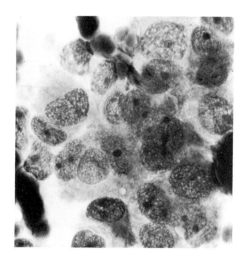

FIGURE 4-35: This smear of aspirate from the left breast is crowded with carcinoma cells.

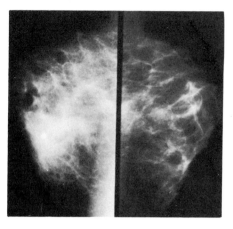

FIGURE 4-36: Mammogram reveals asymmetry with a dense area in the left breast (*white marker*), but no microcalcifications or spiculations. The right breast is unremarkable.

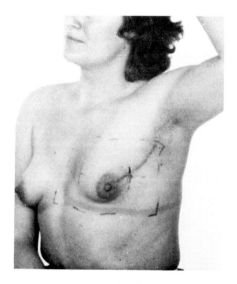

FIGURE 4-37: A satisfied patient is seen 1 year after local excision of a 9-mm tumor, followed by radiation.

Stereotactic biopsy using a screw needle and the Nordenström technique (Fig. 4-40; see also Fig. 4-28) yielded amorphous calcareous masses together with abnormal epithelium, with a cytologic diagnosis of ductal carcinoma.

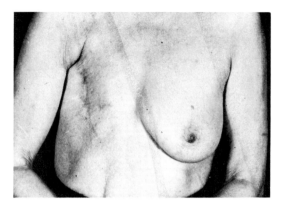

FIGURE 4-38: Sixty-year-old woman 5 years after mastectomy.

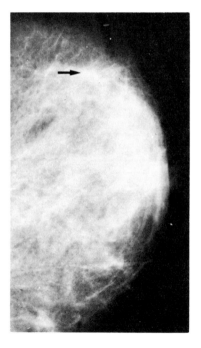

FIGURE 4-39: Mammogram. The arrow indicates a cluster of micro-calcifications.

A radical mastectomy was done, and the histologic diagnosis confirmed the cytology. The triple diagnostic method in this case consisted of negative palpation, positive mammography, and positive cytology.

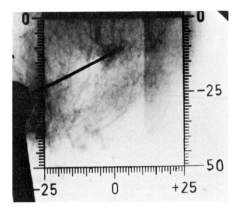

FIGURE 4-40: Mammogram. Needle biopsy of the lesion was done using the Nordenström technique and the screw needle, which extracts minute fragments.

Case 4-12

A 35-year-old woman had a large mass in her right breast and a small palpable mass in her left breast (Fig. 4-41). Mammography of the right breast demonstrated only increased density without any structure (Fig. 4-42).

The left breast was punctured without the syringe (illustrated in Fig. 4-17). This provides greater sensitivity and control in reaching a small lesion. After the needle is implanted, aspiration is carried out. The right breast was aspirated with ease, and ample material was obtained for estrogen receptor analysis.[45] Both aspirations demonstrated carcinoma (Fig. 4-43).

In summary, this patient had a clinically apparent carcinoma with inconclusive mammography on the right and a small palpable mass with normal mammography on the left. Cytologic analysis was positive from both lesions. The triple diagnostic method yielded positive clinical examination results, negative mammography, and positive cytology.

Breast Biopsy

The frozen section biopsy, a one-stage procedure, is still the standard methodology in many if not most surgical arenas. Adherence to the method has been based primarily on tradition rather than on controlled data demonstrating its superiority in terms of metastatic spread and longevity. In 1960, the necessity for frozen section was questioned.[40] The reliability of the

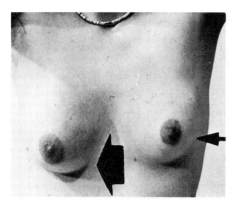

FIGURE 4-41: There is a large visible mass in the right breast (*thick arrow*) and a small palpable mass in the left breast (*thin arrow*).

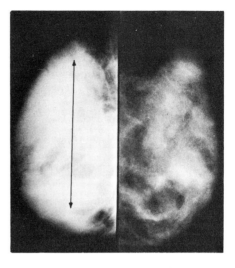

FIGURE 4-42: Mammogram. The right breast shows increased density (*arrow*), but none of the cardinal signs of cancer. The left breast is unremarkable.

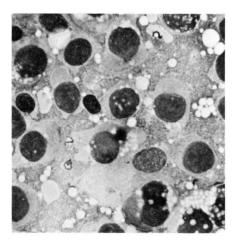

FIGURE 4-43: Aspiration cytology smear. There are dispersed cells characteristic of the monolayer pattern of breast carcinoma.

method was subjected to scrutiny in 1962.[46] Perhaps the most important conclusion was that the procedure reached its highest level of exactness in the hands of competent pathologists and surgeons with the most experience and skill. Exacting quality control is critical.[18]

In 1982, critical evaluation of the one-stage frozen section, mastectomy, had evolved to a point where two procedures were advocated as the safest, most rational method.[14] This was partly a result of the facility with which outpatient surgical biopsy could be arranged and performed. It has resulted also from the widespread use of preoperative diagnosis utilizing needle biopsy, both core biopsy and aspiration biopsy. Preoperative diagnosis by fine needle aspiration is now standard procedure in many of the major centers in Europe and some in the United States. Again, experience and competence are prerequisites, as well as an understanding of the clinical aspects discussed in this chapter. Having achieved these qualities, the exclusion of unnecessary surgery and the saving in money, time, and anesthesia yield important dividends.

Recurrent Carcinoma

Local recurrence will appear initially as a minute dermal or subcutaneous nodule in the incisional scar or adjacent skin, both radiated and nonradiated. The curious development of multiple metastatic cutaneous implants confined within the radiation portals has been observed occasionally.

Postmastectomy follow-up examination should include stroking palpation of the entire anterior and axillary thoracic topography.

The smallest skin elevation (see Fig. 4-19) can be aspirated carefully with a 25-gauge needle and yield a few cancer cells sufficient for diagnosis or recurrence. This is illustrated in the following case.

Case 4-13

The patient was a 78-year-old woman with bilateral mastectomies, one done in 1934 and the other in 1936. The records were in accessible, and her memories of the events were vague. In 1974, she presented for examination and was found to have a dermal nodule (with intact epithelium) precisely within the thin scar of the second (1936) mastectomy. The nodule measured 4 mm in diameter. Fine needle aspiration yielded a small cluster of atypical epithelial cells and several dispersed cells. A diagnosis of recurrent ductal carcinoma 38 years after mastectomy was made. Surgical biopsy confirmed the presence of carcinoma consistent with ductal carcinoma, invading the dermis. The patient died of disseminated disease in 1975 and no other primary was found at autopsy.

Identification of cell type is useful and was reported in a 59-year-old woman found to have mucinous carcinoma in a lytic lesion of the right tibia. A small nodule in the scar of a mastectomy done 11 years previously yielded mucinous cells of the same type (colloid carcinoma).[31]

Local regional recurrence may appear in the supraclavicular fossa and on any surface of the pyramidal axillary space, including the medial aspect of the upper arm.

Further regional evolution of the tumor may occur in the form of lymphatic permeation of the entire extremity on the operated side. Dense swelling of the arm after mastectomy that responds poorly to elevation and compressive sleeves should be palpated carefully for nodules. Random subcutaneous puncture has yielded cancer cells in three cases in our experience. The tumor had penetrated to the forearm in one case.

Conclusion

Breast disease presents broad opportunities for the primary clinician, medical or surgical, to engage the clinical problem. Instant referral to a subspecialist authority should not be necessary until the problem has been analyzed. This includes a satisfactory history, careful examination stressing searching palpation, and a consideration of the options specified above, including fine needle aspiration, mammography, and surgical biopsy. With the data recorded from these studies in mind, the clinician can aspirate or refer appropriately for aspiration, incorporating in his referral note his observations and the point of aspiration. This has been marked by application of adhesive tape in some cases in our experience.

Attention to clinical aspects places breast disease well within the province of primary care physicians and at a minimum will encourage physicians to examine the breasts, and ideally, to examine with care. It also schools the physician in responding to the many questions raised by anxious patients.

As with all aspects of fine needle aspiration, good smears are critical, and smears negative for tumor cells do not exclude cancer. Clinical decisionmaking retains its primacy.

REFERENCES

1. Adair F, Munzer J: Fat necrosis of the female breast. Am J Surg 74:117, 1970
2. Ashikar R, Park K, Huvos AG et al: Paget's disease of the breast. Cancer 26:680, 1970
3. Bassett L, Gold R, Cove A: Mammographic spectrum of traumatic fat necrosis: The fallibility of "pathognomonic" signs of carcinoma. Am J Roentgenol 130:119, 1978
4. Charache H: Metastatic tumors in breast. Am Surg 115:42, 1942
5. Clark RM, Wilkinson RH, Mahoney LJ et al: Breast cancer: A 21 year

experience with conservative surgery and radiation. Int J Radiat Oncol Biol Phys 8:967, 1982

6. Coulson WF: Surgical Pathology. Philadelphia, JB Lippincott, 1978
7. Fisher B, Montagne E, Redmond C: Comparison of radical mastectomy with alternative treatments for primary breast cancer: A first report of results from a prospective randomized clinical trial. Cancer 39:2827, 1977
8. Fisher ER, Gergario RM, Fisher B: The pathology of invasive breast cancer. Cancer 1:1, 1975
9. Franzen S, Stenkvist B: Diagnosis of granular cell myoblastoma by fine-needle aspiration biopsy. Acta Pathol Microbiol Scand 72:391, 1968
10. Frazier TG, Rowland CW, Woolery CL et al: Aspiration cytology: The step before mammography. Today's Clin 2:21, 1978
11. Haogensen CD: Disease of the Breast, 2nd ed. Philadelphia, WB Saunders, 1971
12. Hardy HD: Gynecomastia associated with lung cancer. JAMA 173:1462, 1960
13. Harndern DG, Maclean N, Langlands AO: Carcinoma of the male breast and Klinefelter's syndrome. J Med Genet 8:460, 1971
14. Hellman S, Harris JR, Canellos GP et al: Cancer of the breast. In DeVita VT Jr, Hellman S, Rosenberg SA (eds): Cancer: Principles and Practice of Oncology. Philadelphia, JB Lippincott, 1982
15. Hellman S, Harris JR, Leverne MB: Radiation therapy of early carcinoma of the breast without mastectomy. Cancer 46:988, 1980
16. Henning K, Johansson J, Rimsten A et al: X-ray and fine-needle biopsy in diagnosis of non-palpable breast lesions. Acta Cytol 19:1, 1976
17. Herman CJ, Pelgrim O, Kirkels WJ et al: "Viable" tumor cells in post therapy biopsy specimens. Arch Pathol Lab Med 107:81, 1983
18. Holaday WJ, Assor D: Ten thousand consecutive frozen sections. Am J Clin Path 61:769, 1974
19. Huguley CM Jr, Brown RL: The value of breast self examination. Cancer 47:989, 1981
20. Hunt TK, Cross RA: Breast biopsies on outpatients. Surg Gynecol Obstet 141:591, 1975
21. Hunt VC, Budd JW: Gynecomastia associated with interstitial cell tumor of the testicle. J Urol 42:1242, 1939
22. Jakobsen AHI: Bilateral mammary carcinoma in male following stilbestrol therapy. Acta Pathol Microbiol Immunol Scand 31:61, 1952
23. Kalisher L, Rickert RR: Intraductal papilloma. Breast 6:7, 1980
24. Kline TS, Neal HS: Needle aspiration of the breast: Why bother? Acta Cytol 20:324, 1976
25. Koss L: Diagnostic Cytology and Its Histopathic Bases, 3rd ed. Philadelphia, JB Lippincott, 1979
26. Kreuzer G, Boquoi E: Aspiration biopsy cytology, mammography and clinical exploration: A modern setup in diagnosis of tumors of the breast. Acta Cytol 20:319, 1976
27. Lee BJ, Adair F: Traumatic fat necrosis of the female breast and its differentiation from carcinoma. Ann Surg 72:188, 1920
28. Levene MD, Harrn JR, Hellman S: Treatment of carcinoma of the breast by radiation therapy. Cancer 39:2840, 1977
29. Levy MD: Indications for breast biopsy: A review. Breast 7:8, 1981

30. Libshitz HI: Diagnostic Roentgenology of Radiotherapy Change. Baltimore, Williams & Wilkins, 1979
31. Linsk JA, Franzen S: Clinical Aspiration Cytology, p 108. Philadelphia, JB Lippincott, 1983
32. Linsk JA, Kreuzer G, Zajicek J: Cytologic diagnosis of mammary tumours from aspiration biopsy smears: Studies of 210 fibroadenomas and 210 cases of benign mammary dysplasia. Acta Cytol 16:130, 1972
33. Mann NM: Gynecomastia during therapy with spironolactone. JAMA 184:778, 1963
34. Martin HE, Ellis EB: Biopsy by needle puncture and aspiration. Ann Surg 92:109, 1930
35. Moore SW, Lewis RJ: Carcinoma of the breast in women 30 years of age and under. Surg Gynecol Obstet 119:1253, 1969
36. Moross T, Lang AP, Mahoney L: Tubular adenoma of breast. Arch Pathol Lab Med 107:84, 1983
37. Muller JW: Ultrasound in the diagnosis of cystic disease in young women. Breast, Discovery of the Breast 7:18, 1981
38. Nordenström B, Zajicek J: Stereotaxic needle biopsy and preoperative indication of nonpalpable mammary lesions. Acta Cytol 21:350, 1977
39. Papanicolaou GN, Holmquist DG, Bader BM et al: Exfoliative cytology of human mammary gland and its value in diagnosis of cancer and other diseases of breast. Cancer 11:377, 1958
40. Parker ML, Rubenstone AI: Editorial: Diagnosis from FS on lesions of the breast. Am J Surg 100:661, 1960
41. Paulus DD, Libshitz HI: Breast. In Libshitz HI (ed): Diagnostic Roentgenology of Radiotherapy Change. Baltimore, Williams & Wilkins, 1979
42. Rosen PP: Axillary lymph node metastasis in patients with occult noninvasive breast carcinoma. Cancer 46:1298, 1980
43. Saltstein EC: Outpatient breast biopsy. Arch Surg 109:287, 1974
44. Sandison AT: Metastatic tumors in the breast. Br J Surg 47:54, 1959
45. Silverswärd C, Humla S: Estrogen receptor analysis on needle aspirates from human mammary carcinoma. Acta Cytol 24:54, 1980
46. Sparkman RS: Reliability of frozen sections in the diagnosis of breast lesions. Ann Surg 155:924, 1962
47. Stefanik DE, Brereton HD, Lee TC et al: Fat necrosis following breast irradiation for carcinoma: Clinical presentation and diagnosis. Breast 8:4, 1982
48. Summerskill WH, Adrian MA: Gynecomastia associated as a sign of hepatoma. Am J Dig Dis 7:250, 1962
49. Wang DY, Bulbrook RD, Haywood JC et al: Relationship between plasma carcinoembryonic antigen and prognosis in women with breast carcinoma. Eur J Cancer 11:615, 1975
50. Webb AJ: Through a glass darkly (the development of needle aspiration biopsy). Br Med J 89:59, 1974
51. Wolfe JN: Risk for breast cancer development determined by mammographic parenchymal pattern. Cancer 37:2486, 1976
52. Wolfe JN: Breast patterns as an index of risks for developing breast cancer. Am J Roentgenol Radiol Ther Nuclear Med 126:1130, 1976
53. Zajicek J: Aspiration Biopsy Cytology. Part I: Cytology of Supra-Diaphragmatic Organs. New York, S Karger, 1974

5 Diagnostic Problems of the Chest

The chest is probably the major site of significant problems dealt with by the general clinician in daily patient encounters. Cardiovascular and diffuse pulmonary disorders generally do not provide targets for fine needle aspiration. However, all palpable and structural abnormalities detected by clinical and imaging examinations are potential targets. Obvious acute pneumonic processes usually are not approached by the aspiration method, but there are distinct inflammatory disorders (for example, abscess) that may yield rapid diagnosis by aspiration when other methods fail. This is illustrated in the following case.

Case 5-1

The patient was a 73-year-old retired waitress who was admitted to the hospital with a diagnosis of acute cavitary tuberculosis. Two years earlier, a diagnosis of stage III ovarian carcinoma had been established at laparotomy. The patient underwent treatment with irradiation and chemotherapy and was free of disease for 8 months. She developed intestinal obstruction, and tumor implants were found at laparotomy. Again, chemotherapy produced complete clinical remission.

One month before admission, the patient developed an upper respiratory infection with low-grade fever. Admission was prompted by hemoptysis and an initial x-ray film diagnosed directly as acute cavitary tuberculosis (Fig. 5-1). Three samples of sputum were negative for acid-fast bacteria. On bronchoscopy, bronchial stenosis at the site of the lesion was detected. Specimens, including biopsy, were negative for acid fast bacilli (AFB) but culture was positive for *Pseudomonas*.

Fine needle aspiration was carried out under fluoroscopy by a posterior approach. Air was aspirated and the needle advanced to the wall of the cavity. Inflammatory smears were obtained and the material was negative for acid-fast bacilli. The cavity regressed during a 6-week course of antibiotic therapy.

COMMENT After negative sputa and bronchoscopic study in the face of a compelling x-ray picture, consideration was given to the history of ovarian carcinoma or even a new primary, but radiographically

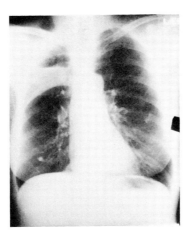

FIGURE 5-1: This film was identified categorically as cavitary tuberculosis in a patient with known prior metastatic ovarian carcinoma. On cavitary puncture it proved to be a nontuberculous abscess.

such diagnoses were unlikely. Fine needle aspiration, negative for both acid-fast bacilli and tumor cells, helped settle the issue and antibiotic treatment could proceed with some security.

Carcinomatous abscess must be included in the differential diagnosis,[51] and diagnosis by fine needle aspiration will again be the method of choice. Fungal lesions are noted below.

The direct approach to palpable masses is self-evident, but pulmonary and mediastinal masses demonstrated by imaging techniques until recently have been approached traditionally by indirect methods, as illustrated in the following case.

Case 5-2

The patient was a 62-year-old man with a moderate productive cough and weight loss. Chest x-ray films revealed a posterior right lung mass with moderate surrounding infiltration and a pleural effusion (Fig. 5-2).

Three carefully obtained sputa were submitted, and 24 slides screened were negative for tumor. Bronchoscopy demonstrated extrinsic compression, but biopsy and washings were negative for tumor. Pleurocentesis yielded exudate, but there were no cancer cells

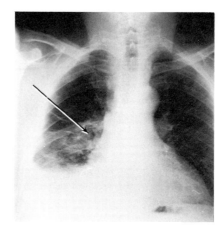

FIGURE 5-2: There is a mass (*arrow*) in the posterior portion of the right lower lobe and a pleural effusion. Fine needle aspiration by posterior approach yielded oat cell carcinoma.

or tuberculosis on smear. This was followed by mediastinoscopy in search of metastasis, but this was negative for tumor. Time spent in the hospital pursuing this workup was 1 month.

Fine needle aspiration carried out at the bedside using a posterior approach at a premarked point on the chest wall yielded oat cell carcinoma. Time for the procedure and reading could be measured in minutes.

False-negative results in this context are rare, and all of the foregoing procedures could have been eliminated.

Bedside punctures of thoracic tumors are accomplished easily, depending on the size and location of the mass.[26]

Discovery of the Lesion and Sources of Cytologic Material

Patients may present for examination because they have discovered a mass, irregularity, or asymmetry of the chest wall, clavicles, or supraclavicular regions. Alternatively, patients may be referred by a primary physician to a surgeon, oncologist, or interventional radiologist because a fresh lesion was found on examination or an x-ray abnormality was reported. Finally, aspiration may be requested after multiple prior diagnostic procedures (see Case 5-2).

From the standpoint of aspiration biopsy, the thorax may be viewed as a topographic unit that includes the ribs and intercostal structures, the sternum, the spine, the clavicles, and the supraclavicular and suprasternal spaces. Lesions in all of these regions may be palpable, or they may be identified by point tenderness or by imaging evidence of a skeletal lesion. Intrathoracic structures consist of the lungs, pleura, and mediastinum. For the most part, potential targets are revealed by chest films.

The Chest Wall

Asymmetries of the chest wall are often smooth elevations appearing slowly and unobtrusively. They may be noted by a family member rather than by the patient. They are often painless masses with ill-defined borders (Figs. 5-3 and 5-4). The most common pathological lesion is carcinoma, both local extension of bronchogenic tumors and metastatic deposits from multiple primaries. The following case is illustrative.

Case 5-3

The patient was a 72-year-old man seen 1 year after receiving 6000 rads to a squamous carcinoma of the midportion of the esophagus. Diagnosis had been established by endoscopy and biopsy. There was no evidence of local recurrence of the lesion. He noticed a swelling in the right posterior axillary line, which had appeared slowly over an estimated period of 4 weeks. The mass was nontender, 5 cm by 6 cm, with intact skin. The ribs were intact on x-ray films. Fine needle aspiration yielded squamous carcinoma. The disease progressed in spite of further radiation, and the patient died. At autopsy, no other primary was found.

COMMENT In this case, there was no subpleural mass or evident rib involvement. This appeared to be a hematogenous spread of the esophageal carcinoma. Fine needle aspiration yielding squamous carcinoma was considered diagnostic in the presence of a normal chest film and negative head and neck examination. A similar problem involving ribs is noted below.

Direct extension of bronchogenic carcinoma producing a chest wall mass is usually in continuity with a subpleural or peripheral lung mass. Portions of ribs may be inapparent on x-ray films (Fig. 5-5). The peripheral lung carcinoma that might invade the chest wall is usually adenocarcinoma.

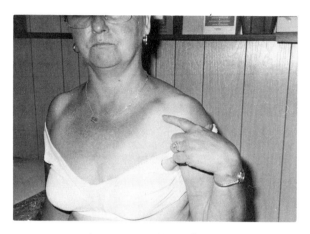

FIGURE 5-3: This 48-year-old woman is pointing to a subclavicular swelling that she detected. She had a history of bronchogenic carcinoma.

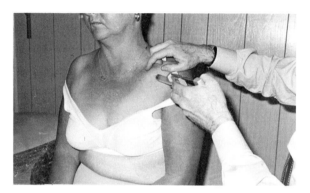

FIGURE 5-4: Fine needle aspiration is carried out in the physician's office.

Fine needle aspiration of a chest wall mass most often will yield adenocarcinoma. In addition to bronchogenic carcinoma, common origins of metastatic masses are the breast, the pancreas, and the gastrointestinal tract. Cytologic distinction of these primaries may be difficult, although breast cytology may be identified. (See Chap 4.)

Renal cell carcinoma also metastasizes to the chest wall. Metastasis may be the initial presentation of hypernephroma in as many as 50% of cases.[25] The cytology is distinctive, and ordinarily is not confused with other adenocarcinomas. Figure 5-6 shows a massive implantation tumor in a 45-year-old man, 1 month after thoracotomy for a nonresectable large cell poorly differentiated carcinoma. A mass underlying the incision (im-

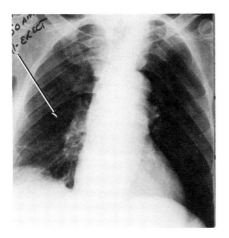

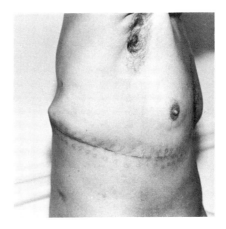

FIGURE 5-5: A segment of the sixth rib (*arrow*) is not seen. Without history, this was read as a surgical defect (see Fig. 10-5). Fine needle aspiration yielded squamous carcinoma, metastatic to the rib.

FIGURE 5-6: There is a massive incisional thoracic wall implantation of a large cell bronchogenic carcinoma.

plantation tumor) is evident. (An implantation mass is seen also in Figure 10-15.)

Mesothelioma has become a prominent clinical entity in the past few years.[23] It may present as a smooth chest wall mass indistinguishable from any of the above adenocarcinomas. On aspiration, the epithelial component may simulate adenocarcinoma.[24]

Subcutaneous and dermal masses involving the skin of the thorax are not distinctive for this topographic region with the exception of local breast recurrence (see Chaps. 4 and 9). Fibrosarcoma presenting as a bulge in the chest wall was illustrated recently.[24]

The Ribs

Lesions of the ribs are occasionally painful, even without fracture, and are often tender and infrequently palpable. A painful, tender, nonpalpable lesion is illustrated in Case 5-4, which follows.

Case 5-4

The patient was a 63-year-old man with a basosquamous cell carcinoma diathesis of the skin. A number of basal cell and two squamous cell carcinomas had been treated over a 10 year period in this patient. One squamous carcinoma of the forehead required fairly extensive plastic surgery. He now had an infiltrated ulcerated lesion at the left angle of the jaw, and another plastic surgical procedure was contemplated. He also had a nonpleuritic painful area in the left posterolateral region at the level of the sixth rib. On examination, there was tenderness along the course of the palpable sixth rib for a distance of 4 cm. On chest x-ray films (Fig. 5-7) the posterolateral sixth rib was not seen as an ossified structure. The remaining lung fields were clear. Fine needle aspiration of the rib was carried out with fluoroscopic control. Because the scapula covered the area, the needle had to be inserted tangentially under the scapula and into the rib. Squamous carcinoma was obtained.

COMMENT This was considered a metastasis from the cutaneous lesion of the face. A peripheral bronchogenic carcinoma producing a subpleural mass and rib invasion seemed less likely because peripheral, particularly subsurface, lesions are usually adenocarcinomas. Initial therapy consisted of excision of the skin mass and radiotherapy to the rib lesion.

PUNCTURE OF THE RIB

A lytic lesion in a readily accessible rib identified clearly by point tenderness may be punctured in the office or at the bedside. (See Case 10-4.) When there is doubt as to the precise location, or if the lesion is inaccessible to direct puncture (see Case 5-4), fluoroscopy will be a necessary aid.

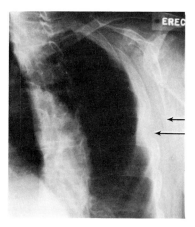

FIGURE 5-7: In oblique view, the normal contour of the rib is absent (*bottom arrow*). The lytic lesion extends under the scapula (*top arrow*).

Single plane fluoroscopy should be satisfactory. A small-caliber needle pointing at the lesion is a satisfactory marker. Local anesthesia will distort landmarks and is not necessary. Both surfaces of the rib should be palpated and the aspirating needle should be kept on target. It is easy to slip over the edge of the rib (see Chap. 1, Pneumothorax), and to penetrate both cortices and enter the lung. A needle varying from 19 gauge to 22 gauge may be satisfactory depending on the amount of deossification. The needle is advanced gently with a twisting motion. It may be held directly or attached to the aspirating syringe. It is best to enter the rib tangentially (Fig. 5-8). Precisely targeting the lesion usually will yield abundant material. Perfectly characteristic and normal marrow aspirate may be obtained if the needle misses the lesion. Desmoplastic reaction seen with some lymphomas and carcinomas may result in a scanty yield, although even a few carcinoma cells may be diagnostic.

Rib lesions also are discovered on routine chest x-ray films or films obtained as part of a staging examination in the presence of a known primary. Lesions may be lytic or blastic.

Isolated lytic lesions in the absence of known primary result from plasma cell myeloma, eosinophilic granuloma, Ewing's sarcoma, and metastatic carcinoma with an unknown primary. Fine needle aspiration will identify most of these. Diagnosis of myeloma and eosinophilic granuloma should suggest further studies, including a skeletal survey in search of other deposits. The usual studies for myeloma include bone marrow puncture (sternal, iliac) and protein measurements of serum and urine.

As a rule, metastatic lytic lesions will be identified by aspiration cytol-

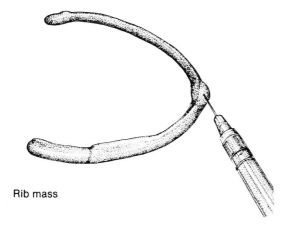

Rib mass

FIGURE 5-8: The rib must be entered with care. A fine needle can ordinarily penetrate without difficulty. (Linsk JA, Franzen S: Clinical Aspiration Cytology, p 142. Philadelphia, JB Lippincott, 1983)

ogy combined with a history of breast, kidney, lung, thyroid, or gastoin-testinal neoplasm.

Blastic lesions are the usual finding in prostate carcinoma. Hodgkin's disease is also an occasional primary. Mixed blastic lytic lesions are frequent findings with most carcinomas. Aspiration of blastic lesions may require an 18-gauge or 19-gauge bone marrow needle. Lesions of the clavicles, sternum, and scapulae are dealt with in similar fashion. (Details of bone lesions are reviewed in Chap. 10.)

Pleural Disease

The pleura is ordinarily not a target for fine needle aspiration. Biopsy in the presence of pleural effusion usually is carried out with a Cope needle, which is used to obtain tissue for histopathologic study. However, pleural masses (Fig. 5-9) are quite suitable targets. Aspiration is carried out with a short (2-cm to 3-cm), fine needle using landmarks determined from films and topography or with fluoroscopic control. A pleural mass may be impossible to distinguish from a contiguous parenchymal lung mass. (See Case 5-6 later.) An inadvertent or even deliberate pneumothorax will separate the surfaces and localize the mass.

The major primary pleural tumor is mesothelioma.[23] Diagnosis initially becomes evident by chest film. Radiographic distinction between primary pleural and metastatic tumor is difficult. Fine needle aspiration may yield a spindle cell smear highly suggestive of mesothelioma, particularly if there is history of exposure to asbestos.[50] On the other hand, an epithelial smear

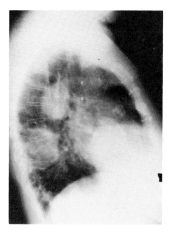

FIGURE 5-9: Multiple pleural masses. Fine needle aspiration carried out with fluoroscopic control yielded lymphoid smears.

may not be distinguishable from metastatic adenocarcinoma, particularly of the pancreas, gastrointestinal tract, and ovary.[23]

Pleural disease is illustrated in the following case report.

Case 5-5

This female patient was admitted for evaluation of a pleural mass (Fig. 5-9) at age 69. At age 61, she had sustained a severe myocardial infarction resulting in a ventricular aneurysm. Shortly after this, she underwent aneurysmectomy and implantation of a pacemaker. During a subsequent cardiac evaluation, a pelvic mass was detected. She then underwent hysterectomy and bilateral salpingo-oophorectomy for well-differentiated bilateral papillary serous cyst adenocarcinoma of the ovaries, stage IIA. No postoperative radiation therapy or chemotherapy was given.

One year before admission, pleural thickening and a widened mediastinum were detected (Fig. 5-10). The widening proved to be an anterior mediastinal mass on computed tomographic (CT) scan (Fig. 5-11). Mediastinoscopy with biopsy was carried out. The pathologic condition was reported as "atypical lymphoid hyperplasia," and because of the patient's limited cardiac reserves, further diagnostic measures were not pursued at that time.

Progression of the pleural disease was detected by x-ray, and although the patient was quite asymptomatic, she was readmitted on

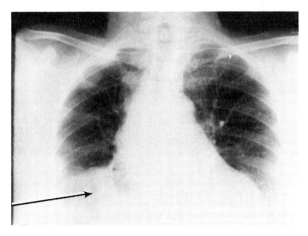

FIGURE 5-10: A lower lobe mass (*arrow*) proved to be a pleural thickening.

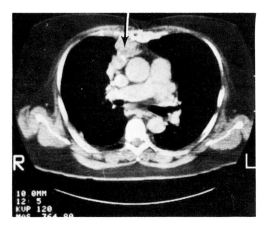

FIGURE 5-11: The anterior mediastinal mass (*arrow*) in this CT scan proved to be a thymoma.

this occasion for fine needle aspiration of one of the pleural masses. Lymphoid smears were obtained, and a diagnosis of lymphoma was considered.

Because questions still remained about the diagnosis, the patient was referred to a major cancer center where, after review of the case findings, thoracotomy was recommended in spite of her cardiac disorder.

The patient delayed, and on her subsequent return for follow up, films demonstrated additional pleural masses and thickening of the previous masses. At this point, fine needle aspiration with CT guidance (Fig. 5-12) yielded mixed lymphoid and epithelial cells diagnostic of thymoma.[10,41] In retrospect, epithelial clusters were present in the original pleural aspiration. She was treated with irradiation.

COMMENT There are several features of interest. Most important was the failure to recognize earlier the clinical complex of anterior mediastinal mass, pleural masses, and lymphoid smears. Secondly, the cytologic condition required more intensive scrutiny, and a clinician faced with this clinical picture should persist in requesting careful review of the morphology. Finally, the cancer center immediately leaped to thoracotomy in a cardiac patient before pursuing the cytologic route more diligently. The extension of thymoma to the pleura is a common development, and was present in 24 of 54 thymomas.[3]

Further problems relating to pleural masses are illustrated in the following interesting and complex case.

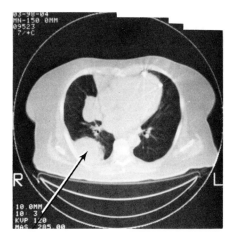

FIGURE 5-12: This CT scan clearly demonstrates the pleural mass, which was
entered easily and yielded diagnostic
smears.

Case 5-6

The patient was a 59-year-old woman who presented herself directly
to a surgeon because of a mass in the upper portion of her left
breast. It was large, ill-defined, and did not appear to be entirely
within the breast. The patient was admitted for frozen section and
possible mastectomy. However, the admission chest x-ray revealed a
pleural mass (Fig. 5-13) interpreted as probably metastatic from the
breast lesion. For that reason, a wedge biopsy for estrogen receptors
was carried out. However, the pathology report was "spindle cell tumor suggesting mesenchymal origin." Slides were referred for consultation.

At this point, the oncologist was asked to see the patient. Under
fluoroscopic control, it was evident that the "pleural" mass was within
the lung parenchyma. Fine needle aspiration yielded smears diagnostic of hypernephroma. In addition to the usual large rounded cells,
there were also some elongated cells, and the suggested diagnosis
was hypernephroma with sarcomatoid changes and metastases to
lung and breast.

An intravenous pyelogram confirmed the presence of a large
mass in the upper pole of the right kidney. On further discussion
with the pathologist, the original breast sections were deemed quite
compatible with renal origin.

COMMENT This patient would have been better managed with a preoperative fine needle aspiration of the "breast" mass. The "pleural"

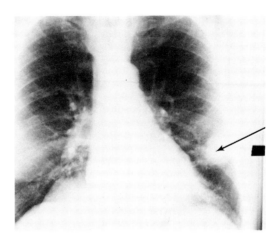

FIGURE 5-13: The "pleural" mass (*arrow*) proved to be pulmonary on fluoroscopy. Fine needle aspiration was carried out without pneumothorax.

mass (x-ray interpretation) was better defined as a parenchymal pulmonary lesion with fluoroscopy. Distinguishing between pleural and parenchymal masses may be difficult. Pneumothorax after lung puncture may settle this issue.

The Lungs

INTRATHORACIC LESIONS

The clinician presented with a localized lesion discovered on chest film must review the diagnostic options (Fig. 5-14). Rapid, specific diagnosis is desirable. Traditional methods are encompassed in Case 5-2. A review of lung carcinoma classification is useful.[55]

In Case 5-2, although the diagnosis may have become apparent at any one of the series of procedures, it is clear that the diagnostic sensitivity overall is low. On fiberoptic endoscopy, direct visualization of pulmonary lesions is successful in 50% to 60% of patients.[56] In one series, 49% of endobronchial and 21% of transbronchial biopsies were diagnostic.[18] The results are improved when the procedures are performed by highly experienced operators.[13,56] In a study comparing transthoracic needle biopsy and bronchoscopic biopsy, the former clearly gave superior results.[9]

Sputum examinations for central lesions are outpatient, noninvasive diagnostic tools, the use of which should be encouraged. However, depending on the clinical context, definitive therapy (surgery, radiation, and chemotherapy) may not be rendered by the treating physician without the

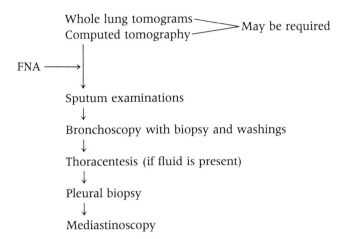

Chest x-ray

Whole lung tomograms⟶
Computed tomography⟶ May be required

FNA ⟶

Sputum examinations
↓
Bronchoscopy with biopsy and washings
↓
Thoracentesis (if fluid is present)
↓
Pleural biopsy
↓
Mediastinoscopy

Comment: FNA may eliminate prolonged hospitalization (Case 5-1), in addition to reducing time and cost.

FIGURE 5-14: Diagnostic schema for lung and mediastinal tumors.

more specific evidence provided by a biopsy. The patient who is a long-term smoker with potentially extensive squamous metaplasia and often focal dysplasia of the mucosa of the upper oropharyngeal and respiratory passages easily may harbor a squamous carcinoma that sheds positive cells and could be confused with a primary epidermoid carcinoma of the lung. For peripheral lesions, the yields of both sputum and endoscopic examinations are poor, and with the availability of fine needle aspiration, there appears to be no reason to request them. Fine needle aspiration as an initial procedure gradually has achieved acceptance for almost all such lesions. Its diagnostic sensitivity is over 90%.[32,47,48] In a comparison of transthoracic needle biopsy and sputum examination in 125 patients with histologically proved pulmonary lesions, 93% were diagnosed by aspiration and 64% by sputum cytology.[8]

As with all procedures, the frequency of use will depend on the interest of the cooperating physicians—radiologists, thoracic surgeons, and pathologists. Clinicians requesting the procedure should seek their cooperation. Once the procedure is routine, it rapidly will become the initial step in evaluating coin lesions, peripheral lesions of all kinds, and subpleural lesions.[48] With further experience, central and apical targets are diagnosed initially with the fine needle. The need for endoscopic study should be individualized.

An elderly patient with chronic obstructive pulmonary disease (COPD) and a large posterior basal lesion may be punctured to exclude oat cell carcinoma. Finding a non-oat cell lesion may and probably should result in a recommendation for no further studies and no specific therapy (surgery, radiation, chemotherapy). The difficulties posed by a small hilar lesion may exceed the capabilities or experience of the local institution. Other methods, including surgical exploration of an unknown mass, may be necessary. It is also possible to transfer the patient to a regional center where the appropriate, experienced practitioners are available. This is, of course, true of all procedures, including endoscopy.

Finally, and perhaps most important, fine needle study will exclude from surgery a significant number of solitary lesions traditionally treated by extirpation with little dissent. In studies of large numbers of solitary lesions, up to 60% are reported benign.[47]

THE MEDIASTINAL AND HILAR REGIONS

The mediastinum is anatomically divided into superior, anterior, middle, and posterior regions. Lesions that provide the dominant target for fine needle aspiration are listed below.

Superior
Substernal thyroid
Thymoma (thymic cyst)
Lymphoma
Metastatic carcinoma

Anterior
Lymphoma
Thymoma (thymic cyst)
Teratomas and germinal tumors
Metastatic carcinoma
Extension of bronchogenic carcinoma

Middle
Lymphoma
Extension of bronchogenic carcinoma
Sarcoid
Metastatic carcinoma

Posterior
Neurogenic tumors
Lymphomas
Extension of bronchogenic carcinoma

Primary mediastinal tumors are rare,[46] and it is obvious that the major targets presented for evaluation, particularly in regional (nonreferral) hospitals, are lymphomas or carcinomas (metastatic or by extension). Nevertheless, the large number of tissue types and structures within the region, all of which are potential sources of congenital and neoplastic masses and cysts, must be considered in diagnostic evaluation and must challenge the imaginations of radiologists and aspiration cytologists.

The most common presentation is the discovery of a silent lesion on chest film. Although malignant tumors often may be discovered by the onset of symptoms (*e.g.*, compression of superior vena cave, tracheobronchial structures, and esophagus), most commonly they are found in association with a known primary or peripheral neoplasm (*e.g.*, bronchogenic carcinoma, lymphoma). It is the usual medical practice in that case to unify the changes into one pathologic group. The classic example is that of a nodular sclerosing Hodgkin's disease diagnosed on cervical or supraclavicular node biopsy coupled with a wide mediastinum. Without further biopsy, the patient's disease is preliminarily staged as II. In the absence of disease below the diaphragm, excluded by special studies (CT scan, lymphangiogram, sometimes laparotomy), the patient will be treated with radiation (mantle, with or without chemotherapy).

Unilateral hilar or mediastinal node enlargement in the presence of a diagnosed peripheral bronchogenic carcinoma may mandate inoperability depending on size and other radiologic characteristics. However, biopsy procedures (mediastinoscopy, aspiration biopsy) often are pursued. Mediastinoscopy is hazardous in lesions on the left side, and fine needle aspiration, if feasible, should be performed.

Significant bilateral hilar adenopathy with clear lung fields suggests sarcoidosis, lymphoma, and metastatic carcinoma. Evaluation includes detailed history and physical examination, indirect studies such as skin tests, and biopsy procedures. Depending on the site and distribution of the nodes, fine needle aspiration may be performed easily, and will yield a prompt diagnosis. An example is the following case.

Case 5-7

A 56-year-old nonsmoking bus driver was found to have massive bilateral hilar nodes (Fig. 5-15). He had a mild cough and minimal chest discomfort. Results of examination were negative for any obvious primary tumor, but the presence of an abdominal scar helped to elicit a history of colon resection 7 years previously. Puncture of the nodes was carried out at the patient's bedside, and yielded considerable necrosis intermixed with strips of tumor cells with columnar configuration. The diagnosis was metastatic colon carcinoma, and further search for a primary was deemed unwarranted.

Hilar nodes in the presence of an extrathoracic primary cannot be assumed to be metastatic from that primary. This is illustrated in the next case.

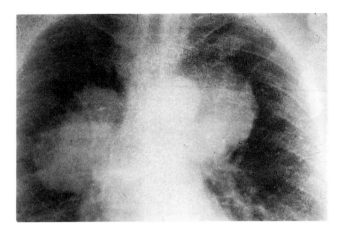

FIGURE 5-15: Massive bilateral hilar nodes were punctured easily with a parasternal approach at the patient's bedside. Puncture yielded necrosis and columnar cells diagnostic of metastatic carcinoma of the colon.

Case 5-8

A well-differentiated psammomatous papillary carcinoma of the ovary, stage IA, was extirpated in a patient whose preoperative chest film demonstrated bilateral hilar adenopathy. The radiographic diagnosis was sarcoid or lymphoma.

Fine needle aspiration was carried out postoperatively with mediastinoscopic guidance and yielded poorly differentiated carcinoma quite different from the ovarian carcinoma. It was obviously a metastatic deposit from another primary, site unknown. The patient died with brain metastasis that proved to be of bronchogenic origin.

All anterior mediastinal masses should be evaluated by thorough physical examination. Lymphoma may be accompanied by lymphadenopathy or hepatosplenomegaly. In contrast, thymoma rarely metastasizes, but extends to the pleura and the pericardium (see Case 5-5). Testes, pelvis, and retroperitoneum must be evaluated by careful and deep palpation when consideration is given to germinal tumors. Radioactive studies will identify mature substernal thyroid masses, but non-iodine-storing tumors (*e.g.,* papillary tumors, anaplastic carcinoma) may not be identified.

All imaging techniques are used, including chest films, CT scans and fluoroscopy. In Figure 5-16, a large anterior mediastinal mass evident on CT scan was diagnosed easily by parasternal puncture as a poorly differentiated non-Hodgkin's lymphoma. Subsequent anterior thoracotomy and histopathologic study established that the morphology was poorly differ-

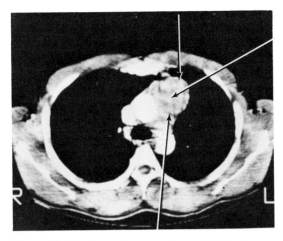

FIGURE 5-16: A massive anterior mediastinal mass was punctured easily by parasternal approach (*short arrow*). (The two long arrows indicate the center of the mass.) Diagnosis was non-Hodgkin's lymphoma.

entiated and diffuse. The patient was treated with combined chemotherapy (CHOP) and was free of disease at 2 years.

Problems of anterior mediastinal masses are illustrated further in the following case.

Case 5-9

The patient was a robust, 35-year-old construction worker, shown in Figure 5-17 after therapy. He originally had stage III, lymphocyte-poor Hodgkin's disease with massive mediastinal enlargement. Treatment consisted of three cycles of chemotherapy (MOPP), which markedly reduced the size of the mediastinal mass. The patient then received total nodal irradiation, including 3600 rads to the center of the chest. On follow-up examinations, he appeared to be in complete remission with no evidence of lymphadenopathy and a normal chest x-ray. Two years after treatment, the patient was referred for CT scan of the chest and abdomen as a follow-up measure.

Impression was as follows: "There is a 4 cm by 5 cm soft tissue mass in the anterior mediastinum. While this could represent fibrosis in a previously radiated Hodgkin's disease, the presence of active disease cannot be completely excluded."

At this time, the patient had no symptoms and appeared as shown in Figure 5-17.

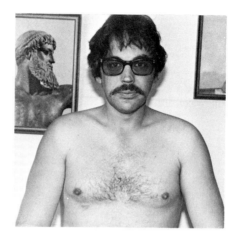

FIGURE 5-17: This patient is shown 2 years after receiving radiation for stage III lymphocyte-poor Hodgkin's disease.

Under fluoroscopic control, a bone marrow needle was inserted through the sternum (Fig. 5-18), penetrating the posterior cortex. A fine needle was then passed through the bone marrow needle and into the mediastinal tissues. Several aspirations were obtained. The aspiration yielded only tissue fluid, and a few fibrocytic cells and inflammatory cells. The diagnosis was scar tissue. The patient remained well 1 year later.

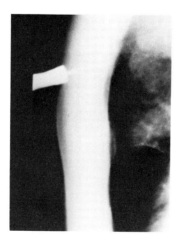

FIGURE 5-18: Puncture of the sternum. The needle penetrates both cortices and becomes a guide for fine needle aspiration.

COMMENT Tissues of the anterior mediastinum are a considerable distance from the vital structures of the chest, and fine needle aspiration can be performed with a certain amount of facility. Where the tumor is directly behind the sternum with no parasternal extension, fine needle aspiration is probably the most efficient way to make a diagnosis. Midline germinal tumors may be diagnosed by this method with high specificity, and radiotherapy can proceed without surgical intervention.

As shown in Figure 5-15, tumors may be approached by direct parasternal puncture, and the needle may be angled down at the suprasternal notch.

In the middle mediastinum, lymphoma and metastatic carcinoma (usually bronchogenic) must be considered. The approach is tangential, originating several centimeters from the sternal border.

The dominant lesion in the posterior mediastinum is a neural tumor. The approach should be through the posterior thoracic wall. Fluoroscopy and CT scanning allow easy access.

Cytologic identification of mediastinal masses is highly specific. Surgical biopsy is rarely required, as illustrated in Table 5-1.

The cytology of these tumors has been presented in a number of published sources cited in Chapter 1.

TABLE 5-1: Cytologic Identification of Mediastinal Masses

Tumor	Cytology
Germinal	Highly specific
Thyroid	Highly specific
Thymoma	Strongly suggestive
Lymphoma	Strongly suggestive
Carcinoma	Highly specific
Neurofibroma	Highly specific

The Lung Puncture

For the clinician, the first encounter with the diagnostic lung puncture may be somewhat forbidding. Violation of the parietal pleura to drain pleural fluid has been an accepted procedure for decades. Puncture of the visceral pleura, however, raises questions of pneumothorax, bronchopleural fistula, and empyema, and puncture of tumors adds the possibility of tumor implantation. Experience has shown that the fine needle as a practical matter may produce pneumothorax in variable percentages in different reported series, but that none of the other hazards is of practical significance. Pneumothorax, discussed below, is an acceptable risk in most cases. It occurs so frequently that it no longer is considered a complication, but an anticipated part of the procedure.

The procedure is simply reduced, then, to slipping a fine needle between the ribs with or without local anesthesia with the patient in apnea. For deeper lesions, the patient may breathe gently while the needle is advanced. Problems of localization remain, but they have been managed in most instances by diagnostic radiologists practicing intervention radiology very effectively. Techniques vary from the most sophisticated, designed to reach small central lesions using specialized techniques, to straightforward visualization with biplanar fluoroscopy,[7,47,48] to unipolar fluoroscopy,[19] to direct bedside puncture.[26] Figure 5-19 illustrates a massive tumor that was punctured easily at bedside to confirm metastasis from a previously diagnosed sarcoma in a patient with a newly discovered breast cancer.

The entire procedure may be carried out by a radiology team,[22] a pathologist and a radiologist, and clinicians (thoracic surgeons, pulmonologists, oncologists) and radiologists.[19,26] With appropriate experience and preparation, any clinician can team with a hospital radiologist who will assist in localization, and carry out a variety of punctures. Extensive technical details are available in several pertinent publications.[7,19,57]

Frequent pneumothorax, tension pneumothorax, hemorrhage, and tumor implantation occur most readily with thicker needles, which produce greater tissue trauma.[20,30,54] The tools necessary are 22-gauge needles rang-

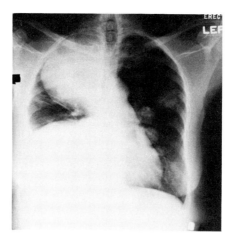

FIGURE 5-19: This huge mass in the upper lung was punctured easily at the patient's bedside. Puncture yielded a diagnosis of sarcoma.

ing from 3 cm to 9 cm or more. We have found a stylet useful, because it lends stability to the longer needles. It may help avoid the rare complication of air embolism resulting from connection of a large vein with the atmosphere. Placement of a large-caliber needle (18 gauge or 19 gauge) through the chest wall to the parietal pleura allows repeated passes of the fine needle without repeated puncturing of the chest wall tissues. We generally advance the needle by hand, remove the stylet, attach the syringe, and aspirate, oscillating the needle tip through the mass. Steel rods with screw tips have been used by Nordenström[35] with singular success. The lesional material is scraped onto a slide. It is particularly useful for fibrous and cartilaginous nodules like hamartomas.[11]

Deaths that have been reported with this procedure because of hemorrhage or air embolism have occurred only with cutting needles.[57]

HOW TO PROCEED

The initial step in fine needle aspiration of the lungs is reviewing the films with the radiologist. Posteroanterior and lateral views usually will localize the lesion in its three-dimensional position. It is important to note whether it is obscured by a bony structure such as the scapula (see Case 5-4). This will modify the direct puncture. The radiologist will best be able to indicate a fruitful approach and point it out topographically on himself or on the operating physician. Most of the reports in the literature emanate from referral centers where skilled radiographic teams have been successful in obtaining diagnostic material from relatively early (small) lesions. In the community hospital the clinician is often presented with a large lesion (Fig. 5-19), usually inoperable, which for practical purposes should be diagnosed and referred for treatment in a local or regional hospital.[26] Central lesions often will yield positive sputum or bronchoscopy washings. In conjunction with other clinical findings, this may be decisive, obviating a variety of adjuvant procedures. However, the sensitivity of sputum and bronchial wash cytology in diagnosing cancer varies greatly with the reporting laboratory and depends to some extent on the intensity of the search.[36,38] In one series, six to ten consecutive morning deep cough samples were collected and at least eight slides were prepared from each specimen.[17] Screening 48 to 80 slides for each case is clearly beyond the practical capability of the majority of hospital laboratories. Time spent collecting specimens, including the frequent rejection of unsatisfactory ones, should direct the clinician's attention to immediate direct puncture and diagnosis.

Having reviewed the film, it may be determined that the tumor can be reached easily at the bedside. This would apply to large central, basal, and apical masses as well as pleural-based masses that are sufficiently large and topographically identified.[26] Bedside puncture offers speed, efficiency, and cost-effectiveness. Perhaps more important is convenience and comfort to the patient, who is spared yet another ride on a stretcher, shift to a hard, cold fluoroscopy table, and a wait before returning to his bed. Before all punctures, the procedure is discussed in a reassuring manner with the patient. The possibility of pneumothorax (air leak) is reviewed, as well as the unlikelihood of damaging the heart.

Where the lesion is small and is not pleural based, the approach is discussed with the radiologist. Punctures are carried out by intervention radiologists in many hospitals or by the clinician, as noted above.

Several rules of puncture are useful.

1. Select the chest wall closest to the lesion.
2. The needle should pass over the superior edge of the lower rib.
3. Avoid the heart and major vessels.
4. Approach subscapular lesions anteriorly, tangentially, or laterally, and approach apical lesions posteriorly.
5. A posterior approach may be necessary to reach lesions behind the clavicle and anterior first rib.
6. The puncture is best done at right angles to the anterior or posterior chest surface with the patient supine or prone.

The best results are obtained when carefully prepared smears are examined immediately after one of the quick stains.* This is achieved when the clinician is also skilled in microscopy or when the cooperation of a pathologist is enlisted. This helps solve the problem of negative smears because of failure to reach the target.[22] It is much easier, psychologically, to proceed with an immediate repeat puncture than to dismiss the patient and then ask for a repeat in the following days. Also, if the material is unexpectedly inflammatory (abscess) appropriate cultures can be requested.

Following the puncture, the patient should be clinically appraised for the rapid evolution of tension pneumothorax, a rare but alarming complication. Rapid insertion of a tube with underwater drainage or Heimlich valve is indicated.[57]

In the absence of acute dyspnea, an immediate follow-up chest film may reveal an early pneumothorax, which requires close clinical observation. The procedure may be performed in an outpatient setting. Subpleural masses do not pose a problem of pneumothorax. Patients with emphysema or deep lesions probably should be kept under observation overnight, or at least should be individualized.

Before lung puncture, there are two important clinical considerations. A thorough physical examination may disclose an enlarged lymph node, subcutaneous mass, or liver, which will usually become a preferential, less hazardous target. Fine needle aspiration of this target together with other clinical data may be decisive in rendering a diagnosis and may eliminate a lung puncture. Secondly, identification of a pulmonary lesion is important only if the information will be useful in deciding clinical management of the patient.

* Diff-Quick, Papanicolaou's, hematoxylin.

Application of Fine Needle Aspiration to the Diagnosis of Pulmonary Lesions

Questions frequently are raised concerning the necessity of lung puncture because clinical context, radiographic findings, sputum, and sometimes bronchoscopy have provided sufficient data to allow exploratory thoracotomy and resection therapy for many surgeons and for several decades. This is particularly the case for solitary peripheral coin lesions, which provide strong temptation to proceed at once with resection. In a review of 955 patients with coin lesions in whom thoracotomy was performed, 51% were benign.[49]

This has been changed by the recognition that oat cell carcinoma is a nonsurgical lesion (see below). Also, increasing numbers of immunosuppressed patients have lung lesions that require identification before surgery. Hamartomas and granulomas present as solitary lesions also are identifiable by fine needle aspiration.[28,52]

General rules are difficult to establish because decisions are modified by the patient's age, pulmonary function, and medical status. The following lists summarize the application of fine needle aspiration to the diagnosis of lung lesions.

For *apparently operable* lesions, perform fine needle aspiration to:

1. Identify oat cell carcinoma.
2. Identify hamartomas and carcinoid lesions.
3. Identify an inflammatory lesion.[15]
4. Identify a metastatic lesion (see Case 5-6),[5] such as hypernephroma or melanoma.
5. Establish a diagnosis of inconclusive radiographic lesion that might incorrectly be kept under observation rather than treated.
6. Obtain a preoperative diagnosis for the surgeon to guide his procedure.

For *apparently inoperable* lesions, perform fine needle aspiration to:

1. Obtain morphologic diagnosis for radiotherapy.
2. Identify oat cell carcinoma.
3. Clarify an apparent metastatic lesion or a possible second primary[37,44] (see Case 5-8).
4. Identify a lymphocytic tumor.

A request for fine needle aspiration of pulmonary lesions sometimes is submitted in an effort to complete the record. Many physicians abhor a diagnostic vacuum. Many pursue diagnosis as though they were on a safari or on a treasure hunt, regardless of the effect on the patient. This invasive procedure and many other types of invasive and noninvasive diagnostic studies serve no purpose and may endanger the patient when the result will add nothing to the management of the illness. Therefore, fine needle aspiration should not be performed on a suspected pulmonary tumor in an elderly or medically disabled patient who is not a candidate for surgery, radiation, or chemotherapy.

Observations on the Cytologic Differentiation of Lung Tumors

A classification of pulmonary tumors based on aspiration cytology has been proposed[25] and is shown in part in the accompanying chart.

Cytologic Classification of Primary Pulmonary Carcinoma.*

Squamous
Adenocarcinoma
   Bronchoalveolar
Undifferentiated
   Large cell type
   Intermediate lymphomatoid
   Small cell type (oat cell)
   Giant cell
Bronchial gland
   Carcinoid
   Mucoepidermoid
   Adenoid cystic

* Material obtained at fine needle aspiration.

Small cell undifferentiated carcinomas make up 20% of all bronchogenic carcinomas.[16] They arise in a submucosal site, producing extensive compression of a bronchus. Endobronchial presentation and exfoliation may occur later. They are distinguished by early dissemination with extrathoracic metastases detected in 66% at diagnosis. Probably 90% are already metastatic. They are no longer considered surgical lesions because less than 0.5% survive for 5 years.[33] They are radiosensitive, but more important is the recent success reported with combined chemotherapy.[31,53] Therefore, poor-risk patients may be suitable targets for aspiration. Oat cell, fusiform, polygonal, and intermediate cell undifferentiated carcinomas may all respond to therapy,[27] and it is therefore useful to identify them.

Cytologically, the small cells may simulate lymphoma cells and the intermediate types must be distinguished from poorly differentiated cells of squamous or adenocarcinomatous origin (Fig. 5-20). Finding electron-dense secretory granules on electron microscopy (EM) is decisive. EM can be carried out on smears. Other clinical data, including fairly typical findings on sputum cytologic studies and increased levels of ectopic hormones (ACTH, SIADH), may provide sufficient support for a diagnosis of small cell undifferentiated tumor to allow immediate initiation of chemotherapy.

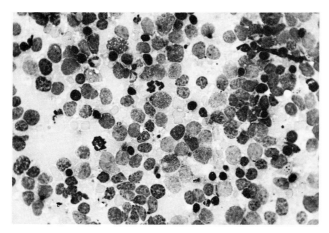

FIGURE 5-20: Dispersed, poorly differentiated cells simulate
lymphoma. Electron microscopy might distinguish them
from cells with squamous or adenocarcinoma origin.

Extensive staging including bronchoscopy, multiple scans, and bone
marrow biopsy is important for patients entered into clinical trial.[12] However, the simplicity of direct puncture, diagnosis, and treatment with chemotherapy in the usual clinical setting saves enormous amounts of time
and expense in a disease that is known to be systemic in such a high
percentage of cases.

Squamous carcinoma also is readily identified cytologically. Of importance is cavitary carcinoma, usually of squamous origin, in which the
central portion will consist of unidentifiable necrotic debris. Repeat puncture of the periphery of the abscess should be performed to obtain cellular
material. Carcinomatous abscess must be differentiated from an inflammatory abscess in which the material extracted will consist of sheets of
intact granulocytes.

Well-differentiated adenocarcinoma and bronchoalveolar carcinoma
are readily identified as adenocarcinoma, but are not easily distinguishable
cytologically from metastatic tumors. Clinical context is important, but it
may not be decisive.[37]

Large cell undifferentiated tumors are fairly characteristic cytologically.
However, poorly differentiated nasopharyngeal and prostatic cancers may
simulate a lung tumor cytologically. In an older male patient with a history
of smoking, chronic pulmonary disease, and a large solitary hilar mass, the
cytology is diagnostic. An appropriate report might state that the cytology
is diagnostic of large cell undifferentiated bronchogenic carcinoma "in the
clinical context stated."

One or more peripheral masses in a less characteristic patient should
prompt study of the prostate and nasopharynx because undifferentiated
large cell cytologic specimens are difficult to subclassify.

Giant cell tumors are quite dramatic cytologically. Glioblastoma multiforme, which does not metastasize, osteogenic sarcoma, and pancreatic and anaplastic thyroid carcinoma, among others, are sources of giant cells that are morphologically similar to giant cell tumors of the lung. Diagnostic difficulties that may arise are illustrated in the following case.

Case 5-10

The patient was a 63-year-old man complaining of pain and a limp in his right leg. X-ray films revealed periosteal alteration in the distal third of the femur. A mass was evident in the lower lobe of the right lung. On examination, a well-defined tender area was noted in the same region as the alteration of the femur seen on the x-ray films. At the bedside, a fine needle aspiration was carried out with a 22-gauge needle. No attempt was made to penetrate the bony cortex. Giant cells with massive polymorphous nuclei and phagocytosed neutrophils were obtained. Osteogenic sarcoma with metastasis to the lung was considered. The same cells were found on aspiration of the pulmonary mass (Fig. 5-21). The clinical course established that the origin of this tumor was the lung.

Tumors of bronchial gland origin may be suggested by exclusion and may require greater expertise in cytologic diagnosis.

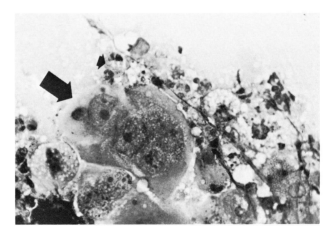

FIGURE 5-21: Giant cells with multiple nuclei (*large arrow*) are seen. Note the contrast with polymorphonuclear leukocyte (*small arrow*). Aspirate was obtained from giant cell tumor of the lung.

HOW DOES CYTOLOGIC IDENTIFICATION HELP THE CLINICIAN IN DIAGNOSIS AND MANAGEMENT?

The identification of oat cell carcinoma preoperatively has become an important procedure, as noted previously. Hamartoma is a benign lesion that may be identified cytologically.[28] In an early series by Dahlgren, 19 hamartomas were discovered in 693 patients in a health screening program.[11] Similarly, preoperative identification of carcinoid tumors will guide the surgeon to a more limited resection.

With increased experience and technical precision, very small lesions can be reached with a fine needle, clarifying small infiltrations that might have been neglected or in which diagnostic measures might have been postponed.

The following case illustrates a puzzling problem that might have been clarified by fine needle aspiration.

Case 5-11

The patient was a 49-year-old man complaining of difficulty swallowing and weight loss. He had been under the care of a gastroenterologist who had diagnosed an esophageal motility problem. The patient had smoked for many years, and a stellate "fibrotic" area, considered inflammatory in origin and measuring 1 cm by 1.8 cm, was seen on chest radiograph in his right upper lobe. He continued to lose weight. Esophagoscopy failed to disclose any mucosal lesion. Two weeks before his death, a small hard node was palpated behind the right clavicle. Fine needle aspiration yielded adenocarcinoma. At autopsy, a large retroesophageal mass of metastatic nodes was found. Adenocarcinoma was present in the stellate pulmonary lesion (scar carcinoma).

Many inflammatory lesions have been diagnosed by aspiration cytology. Such lesions may simulate tumors on radiograpic studies. Pneumonia,[6] abscess (see Case 5-1), and mycotic lesions[15] are all potential targets for fine needle aspiration. Clinical context is important, and anticipation in preparation for microbiologic studies should be part of the methodology. Aspiration of liquid or semiliquid material will yield numerous smears, some for biologic stains. The needle may be capped and the syringe submitted for culture.

Metastatic Tumors

Identification of solitary or multiple pulmonary lesions as metastatic has obvious clinical utility, particularly for guiding therapy. Breast, endometrial, and prostate cancers, where cytologically identified, may be treated with hormones. Thyroid carcinoma responds to radioactive iodine therapy, embryonal cancer to chemotherapy, and others (colon, melanoma, hypernephroma) potentially may be cured by resection. Specific cytologic diagnoses of these tumors and others has been defined.[24]

Because the lung is a common site for metastatic lesions with undetected primary,[5] the clinician must be alert to this possibility and must carefully review possible primary lesions before initiating a biopsy procedure. At the minimum, after reviewing history of tumors, the clinician should carefully examine the head and neck, breasts, abdomen, rectum, and prostate. The decision to search for a primary with imaging techniques before approaching the pulmonary lesion depends on the clinical context, including data on smoking or nonsmoking, and also depends on whether the radiograph reveals a single lung nodule or multiple lung nodules.

Diffuse or Extensive Regional Lung Disease

The dyspneic patient, usually hypoxic by oxygen measurement, often fails to yield diagnostic data by noninvasive methods.

Oncologic patients may have a diffuse lymphangitic pattern that appears insidiously on x-ray films. Initial films may be negative or merely suggestive. A high index of suspicion usually is nourished by fever, history of primary tumors (both intrathoracic and extrathoracic), and background for opportunistic infection (immunosuppression). Whole lung tomography and computed tomography may reveal lesions not evident on chest radiographs.[34,39] However, most patients are seen after the appearance of changes on routine x-ray studies. History of tumors with or without radiation, chemotherapy, and steroid therapy will provide useful data. Surgical history should be sought, including a review of small, often forgotten, lesions such as melanoma.

Examination of the sputum is, of course, the initial study. The limitations of sputum examination have been noted,[4] and apply equally to diffuse pattern disease. The positive yield is likely to be sparse because the lesions under consideration are not endobronchial, but interstitial and lymphangitic. However, alveolar carcinoma will often yield abundant tumor cells in sputum.

Bronchoscopic examination with endobroncheal biopsy will produce a low yield, particularly because lesions are extrabronchial. Transbronchial biopsies in an effort to sample parenchymal tissue have yielded significant numbers of positive diagnoses only by selected physicians.[2,13]

The clinician faced with a problem of diffuse parenchymal disease should be aware that reported statistics citing the value, yield, ease, and safety of a procedure such as transbronchial biopsy often are published by individuals and groups with extensive experience.[14,42,43] (See above.) It is not a procedure to be undertaken in a community hospital by less experienced operators with the expectation of similar statistical results.[18] In a series of 450 cases, pneumothorax occurred in 14%, which is in the range of such complications occurring with transthoracic fine needle aspiration. There was one death.[2]

Random puncture of an area of diffuse disease demonstrated on x-ray films may be a useful procedure. Potential yield already has been published.[24] As with many aspiration procedures, it has been considered the last thing to do in obtaining a diagnosis, but ultimately may become the initial step. Major advantages include ease of accomplishment without scheduling fluoroscopy or reserving an operating suite. Random puncture may be carried out at the bedside.

Complete opacification of one hemithorax, particularly with a pleural effusion on the contralateral side, is associated with dyspnea and hypoxia. Relief of hypoxia is sought by thoracentesis. If fluid is not obtained, the procedure usually is discontinued. In our experience, fine needle aspiration of the opacified lung by random puncture utilizing a 1.5-in, 22-gauge needle may easily yield cancer cells when the lung is heavily infiltrated with tumor.

The Lymphoid Smear

Aspiration of discrete pulmonary lesions, diffuse infiltrations, hilar masses, mediastinal masses, and pleural thickening may yield lymphoid smears.

Patients with extrathoracic proven Hodgkin's and non-Hodgkin's lymphoma may have pulmonary lesions. The differential diagnosis includes pulmonary or pleural lymphoma, pseudolymphoma, non-lymphoid neoplasm, drug-induced pneumonitis, and other inflammatory disorders.[1,29,45] In Case A-11 the expectation of lymphoid smears in a patient with known Hodgkin's disease was not realized.

Diagnosis may be sought by fiberoptic bronchoscopy and transbronchial biopsy (see above), by open biopsy, and by fine needle aspiration.

If fine needle aspiration yields a monomorphic smear (see Chap. 8), with a cell type similar to the extrathoracic lymphoma, the diagnosis is confirmed.

In the absence of a known diagnosis of lymphoma, reliance should be placed on cytologic variability in deciding the origin of the lymphoid cells. Pseudolymphomas should present smears similar to those of reactive lymph nodes (see Chap. 8).[21,29] However, some pseudolymphomas are monomorphic, and a positive diagnosis cannot be made with assurance cytologically or histologically in the absence of extrathoracic lymphoma.[21] When monomorphic smears are composed of large, immature lymphoid or cleaved cells, the diagnosis of lymphoma is likely. The content of the smears should be discussed with the pathologist.

Small mature lymphocytes may be extracted from lymphoid pneumonia, indolent thymomas that have extended to pleura and pericardium (see Case 5-5), and hilar lymph nodes. Mixtures of inflammatory cells—neutrophils, eosinophils, monocytes, and histiocytes containing carbon pigment and hemosiderin—should direct the diagnosis to an inflammatory etiology.

It must be kept in mind that lymphoid smears produced by fine needle aspiration in the absence of a clear-cut and specific diagnosis of lymphoma or non-lymphoid neoplasm are distinctly useful as clinical guides to be evaluated with all the other clinical data.[45] No attempt must be made to identify definitively what may be a complex histopathologic picture. However, the cytologic condition is a step beyond the radiographic picture in establishing a diagnosis.

Summary

Fine needle aspiration of the lung and thorax is a valuable addition to the clinician's diagnostic methods. The discovery of a pulmonary abnormality on examination or x-ray films will usually trigger a series of studies.[40] They involve collecting sputa, which requires a high level of compliance with cytologic screening and review by a pathologist. Endoscopies, CT scans, and tomography, which require scheduling, waiting for reports, repeat studies, further screening of lung cytology, preparation of histopathology, and the pathologist's report will all follow.

Pneumothorax, which has been the major limiting factor, is now considered a normal accompaniment of the puncture rather than a complication. Less concern with pneumothorax and increasing ease of its management allow fine needle aspiration to become a primary resource for the practicing physician. Suspicious chest abnormalities in many if not most clinical contexts should call for fine needle aspiration as an initial procedure. With diagnostic sensitivity as high as 99%[32] and allowing definitive therapy (surgery, radiation, chemotherapy) where clinically indicated, without further comfirmation, the litany of diagnostic measures can be cancelled immediately.

REFERENCES

1. Al-Saleem T, Peale AR: Lymphocytic tumors and pseudotumors of the lung. Am Rev Respir Dis 99:767, 1969
2. Anderson HA, Fontana RS: Transbronchoscopic lung biopsy for diffuse pulmonary diseases: Technique and results in 450 cases. Chest 62:125, 1972
3. Batata MA, Martini N, Huvos A et al: Thymomas: Clinicopathologic features, therapy and prognosis. Cancer 34:389, 1974
4. Caya JG, Wollenberg NJ, Clowry LV: The significance of "positive" respiratory cytology determinators in a series of 327 patients. Am J Pathol 82:155, 1984
5. Clary CF, Michel RP, Wang N-S et al: Metastatic carcinoma: The lung as the site of the clinically undiagnosed primary. Cancer 51:362, 1983
6. Covell JL, Feldman PS: Fine needle aspiration diagnosis of aspiration pneumonia (phytopneumonitis). Acta Cytol 28:77, 1984
7. Dahlgren SE, Nordenström B: Transthoracic Needle Biopsy. Stockholm, Almqvist and Wiksell, 1966
8. Dahlgren SE, Lind B: Comparison between diagnostic results obtained by

transthoracic needle biopsy and by sputum cytology. Acta Cytol 16:53, 1972

9. Dahlgren SE, Lind B: Transthoracic needle biopsy or bronchoscopic biopsy? Scand J Respir Dis 50:265, 1969

10. Dahlgren S, Sandstedt B, Sundström C: Fine needle aspiration cytology of thymic tumors. Acta Cytol 27:1, 1983

11. Dahlgren S: Needle biopsy on intrapulmonary harmartoma. Scand J Respir Dis 47:187, 1966

12. Dillman RO, Taetle R, Seagren S et al: Extensive disease small cell carcinoma of the lung. Cancer 49:2003, 1982

13. Ellis JH: Transbronchial lung biopsy via the fiberoptic bronchoscope: Experience with 107 consecutive cases and comparison with bronchial brushing. Chest 64:524, 1975

14. Feldman NT, Pennington JE, Ehrie MG: Transbronchial lung biopsy in the compromised host. JAMA 238:1377, 1977

15. Gleason TH, Hammar SP, Barthqs M et al: Cytological diagnosis of pulmonary cryptococcosis. Arch Pathol Lab Med 104:384, 1980

16. Greco FA, Oldham RK: Current concepts in cancer: Small-cell lung cancer. N Engl J Med 301:335, 1979

17. Gupta RK: Value of sputum cytology in the diagnosis and typing of bronchogenic carcinomas, excluding adenocarcinomas. Acta Cytol 26:645, 1982

18. Jenkins R, Myerowitz RL, Kavic T et al: Diagnostic yield of transbronchoscopic biopsies. Am J Clin Pathol 72:926, 1979

19. Kaminsky D: Aspiration Biopsy for the Community Hospital. New York, Masson, 1981

20. King EG, Bachynski JE, Mielke B: Percutaneous trefine lung biopsy. Evolving role. Chest 70:212, 1976

21. Koss MN, Hochholzer L, Nichols PW et al: Primary non-Hodgkins lymphoma and pseudolymphoma of lung. Hum Pathol 14:1024, 1983

22. Lalli AF, McCormick LJ, Zeich M et al: Aspiration biopsies of chest lesions. Radiology 127:35, 1978

23. Legha SS, Muggia FM: Pleural mesothelioma: Clinical features and therapeutic implications. Ann Intern Med 87:613, 1977

24. Linsk JA, Franzen S: Clinical Aspiration Cytology. Philadelphia, JB Lippincott, 1983

25. Linsk JA, Franzen S: Aspiration cytology of metastatic hypernephroma. Acta Cytol 28:250, 1984

26. Linsk JA, Salzman AL: Diagnosis of intrathoracic tumors by thin needle cytologic aspiration. Am J Med Sci 263:181, 1972

27. Livingston RB: Small cell carcinoma of the lung. Blood 56:575, 1980

28. Ludwig ME, Otis RD, Cole SR et al: Fine needle cytology of pulmonary hamartomas. Acta Cytol 26:671, 1982

29. Marchevsky A, Padilla M, Mamoru K et al: Localized lymphoid nodules of lung: A reappraisal of the lymphoma versus pseudolymphoma dilemma. Cancer 51:2070, 1983

30. Meyer JE, Ferrucci JT, Janower ML: Fatal complications of percutaneous lung biopsy: Review of the literature and report of one case. Radiology 96:47, 1970

31. Minna JD, Higgins GA, Glatstein EJ: Cancer of the lung. In DeVita VT Jr, Hellman S, Rosenberg SA: Cancer: Principles and Practice of Oncology, pp 396–474. Philadelphia, JB Lippincott, 1982
32. Mitchell ML, King DE, Bonfiglio TA et al: Pulmonary fine needle aspiration cytopathology. Acta Cytol 28:72, 1984
33. Mountain CF: Clinical biology of small cell carcinoma: Relationship to surgical therapy. Semin Oncol 5:272, 1978
34. Muhm JR, Brown LR, Crowe JK: Use of computed tomography in the detection of pulmonary nodules. Mayo Clin Proc 52:345, 1977
35. Nordenström B: New instruments for biopsy. Radiology 117:474, 1975
36. Pilotti S, Rilke F, Gribaudi G et al: Sputum cytology for the diagnosis of carcinoma of the lung. Acta Cytol 26:649, 1982
37. Pilotti S, Rilke F, Gribaudi G et al: Fine needle aspiration biopsy cytology of primary and metastatic pulmonary tumors. Acta Cytol 26:661, 1982
38. Pilotti S, Rilke F, Gribaudi G et al: Cytologic diagnosis of pulmonary carcinomas in bronchoscopic brushing material. Acta Cytol 26:655, 1982
39. Polga JP, Watnick M: Whole lung tomography in metastatic disease. Clin Radiol 27:53, 1976
40. Rosenow EC III, Carr DT: Bronchogenic carcinoma. CA 29:233, 1979
41. Sajjad SM, Lukeman JM, Llamas L: Needle biopsy diagnosis of thymoma. Acta Cytol 26:503, 1982
42. Scheinhorn DJ, Jagner LR, Whitcomb ME: Transbronchial forceps lung biopsy through the fiberoptic bronchoscope in pneumocystis carinii pneumoniae. Chest 66:294, 1974
43. Schoenbaum SW, Koerner SK, Ramakushna B et al: Transbronchial biopsy of peripheral lesions with fiberscopic guidance: Use of the fiberoptic bronchoscope. J Can Assoc Radiol 25:39, 1974
44. Schomberg PJ, Evans RG, Baules PM et al: Second malignant lesions after therapy for Hodgkin's disease. Mayo Clin Proc 59:493, 1984
45. Scully RE, Mark EJ, McNeely BU: Case records of the Massachusetts General Hospital. N Engl J Med 306:469, 1982
46. Silverman NA, Sabeston DC Jr: Primary tumors and cysts of the mediastinum. In Current Problems in Cancer Vol 2. Chicago, Year Book Medical Publishers, 1977
47. Sinner WN: Primary neoplasms diagnosed with transthoracic needle biopsy. Cancer 43:1533, 1979
48. Sinner WN: Transthoracic needle biopsy of small peripheral malignant lung lesions. Invest Radiol 8:305, 1973
49. Toomes H, Delphendahl A, Manke H-G et al: The coin lesion of the lung: A review of 955 resected coin lesions. Cancer 51:534, 1983
50. Turner-Warwick MEH: The responses of the lung to inhaled particles. In Weatherall DJ, Ledingham JGG, Warrell DA (eds): Oxford Textbook of Medicine. Oxford, Oxford University Press, 1983
51. Wallace RJ, Cohen A, Awe RJ et al: Carcinomatous lung abscess. JAMA 242:521, 1979
52. Walts AE: Localized pulmonary cryptococcosis: Diagnosis by fine needle aspiration. Acta Cytol 27:457, 1983
53. Weiss RB: Small-cell carcinoma of the lung: Therapeutic management. Ann Intern Med 88:522, 1978

54. Wolinsky H, Lischner MW: Needle track implantation of tumor after percutaneous lung biopsy. Ann Intern Med 71:359, 1969

55. Yesner R, Gerstt B, Auerbach O: Application of the World Health Organization classification of lung carcinomas to biopsy material. Ann Thorac Surg 1:33, 1965

56. Zavala DC: Diagnostic fiberoptic bronchoscopy: Techniques and results of biopsy in 600 patients. Chest 68:12, 1975

57. Zornoza J: Percutaneous Needle Biopsy. Baltimore, Williams & Wilkins, 1981

6   Palpable and Nonpalpable Abdominal Targets

The abdomen includes the body wall from the costal margins to the symphysis pubis including the flanks, and the abdominal and pelvic contents. Lesions in the pelvis reached by transrectal and transvaginal aspirations and occasional transabdominal puncture are considered in Chapter 7.

Intra-abdominal tissue pathology can be divided into intraluminal and extraluminal groups.

Intraluminal Tumors

The gastrointestinal tract makes up a large volume of the abdominal contents. Except for metastasis to the intestine,[1] lymphoma,[49] and unusual nonepithelial tumors, neoplastic change occurs in the mucosa. The earliest lesions may require careful endoscopic study. Ulcerating and polypoid cancers are detectable by barium studies and endoscopy. Such lesions are not initially targets for fine needle aspiration. However, it is not uncommon for patients to visit the clinic or office with abdominal symptoms, often pain, and a palpable mass. Large primary tumors of the gastrointestinal (GI) tract may become targets for fine needle aspiration. Colon carcinoma may give a fairly characteristic cytologic picture.[25,51] Other adenocarcinomas of the GI tract may be indistinguishable from one another, but the cytologic diagnosis of adenocarcinoma will point toward further studies (imaging studies and endoscopy).

Whether to carry out an immediate fine needle aspiration or to refer the patient for a barium enema, ultrasonography, or computed tomography is a matter of clinical judgment. Clinical judgment is guided by the patterns of clinical practice in the local area. In the absence of interest or expertise in the technique of fine needle aspiration and reading of slides on the part of the managing physicians, the patient ordinarily will undergo fiberoptic sigmoidoscopy, barium enema, upper GI and small bowel x-rays or colonoscopy, and panendoscopy of the upper GI tract, ultrasonography, computed tomography, and finally laparotomy, depending on the obscurity and urgency of the lesion. If a mass is palpable, fine needle aspiration when done initially will direct the diagnostic pattern and eliminate much of the above (see Fig. 6-1). This is illustrated in the following case.

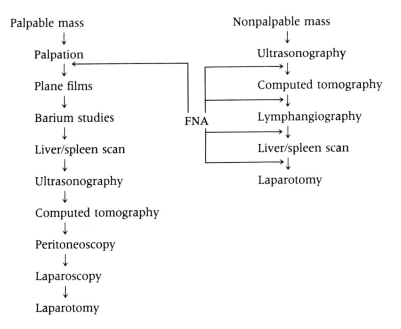

Palpable mass

↓

Palpation

↓

Plane films

↓

Barium studies   FNA

↓

Liver/spleen scan

↓

Ultrasonography

↓

Computed tomography

↓

Peritoneoscopy

↓

Laparoscopy

↓

Laparotomy

Nonpalpable mass

↓

Ultrasonography

↓

Computed tomography

↓

Lymphangiography

↓

Liver/spleen scan

↓

Laparotomy

Comment: FNA is carried out at once on palpable lesions and may eliminate a large number of studies, as well as forestall surgery.

FNA may be introduced after any of the visualizing procedures, and it may eliminate further study.

FIGURE 6-1: Diagnostic schema for abdominal masses.

Case 6-1

The patient was a 71-year-old man admitted to a gastroenterology service after appearing in the emergency room with weakness, anemia, and weight loss. The major finding was a massively enlarged liver.

Pertinent initial laboratory studies were as follows: hemoglobin, 8.6 g/dL; mean corpuscular volume (MCV), 69 μm^3; alkaline phosphatase, 138 U/L; gamma glutamyl transpeptidase, 210 U/L; and bilirubin, 2.6 mg/dL.

The initial study on admission was a liver scan followed by an upper GI series. The liver scan (Fig. 6-2) revealed multiple defects practically replacing the liver.

Oncologic consultation was requested, and fine needle aspiration of the liver yielded smears diagnostic of mucinous carcinoma. Barium enema was recommended because of the cytologic findings and hypochromic anemia.

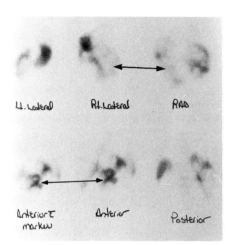

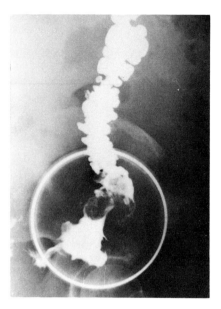

FIGURE 6-2: Liver scan with multiple gross defects (*arrows*).

FIGURE 6-3: A constricting lesion of the colon was revealed by the barium used in the upper GI series.

Meanwhile, a constricting lesion of the colon was already identified by the barium used in the upper GI series (Fig. 6-3).

COMMENT A patient with symptoms of systemic disease, hypochromic anemia, and a massive liver can be diagnosed most efficiently by immediate transabdominal puncture of the liver in an outpatient setting. The cytologic findings often will guide further studies, if any. Liver scan will most often be superfluous. The primary tumor in this patient was intraluminal, to which attention was directed by sampling an extraluminal mass.

Extraluminal Tumors

The major undiagnosed intra-abdominal targets for fine needle aspiration are extraluminal.

The bulk of fine needle targets seen in oncologic practice are solid tumors. In contrast, the majority of lesions punctured by radiologists may be cystic,[35] depending on referral patterns. Many of the cysts are renal. Sonographic guidance provided a correct diagnosis of cysts in almost 100% of cases.[35]

All aspects of body wall masses and intra-abdominal masses are considered below.

Clinical Presentation of Abdominal Targets

Unlike tumors of the head and neck, thyroid, salivary glands, breast, and thoracic wall, it is unusual for the patient to become aware of abdominal masses, some of which may be quite massive. For example, a massive spleen may announce itself by stomach compression and early satiety. The patient may have an advanced intra-abdominal mass because of recurrent cancer that remains unrecognized even though the patient is quite aware that he had a primary cancer previously treated. It is not uncommon for the patient to fail to recognize that the entire upper half of his abdomen is occupied by a smooth or even nodular tumor. Unless there is an accompanying systemic syndrome, the patient may fail to seek counsel until late in the course.

Unexpected late tumor is described in Case A-13 (see Appendix).

The main symptoms prompting abdominal examination are pain and varieties of dyspepsia. The major causes are benign and usually nonpalpable disorders (peptic disease, irritable colon, cholelithiasis). Of greater significance are anorexia and weight loss, because neoplasm is a leading consideration. Careful regional and deep palpation with the patient in a relaxed state is essential. The usual setting for this is the office or clinic. We have seen this sequence repeatedly. It eliminates innumerable studies and hospitalizations, as shown in Fig. 6-1. The diagnostic sequence in the symptomatic patient can be summarized as follows: Symptoms (anorexia, weight loss) → palpation → aspiration → diagnosis.

The Asymptomatic Patient

Asymptomatic patients present for examination in two settings. Most significant is the follow-up examination of the patient who has had a prior malignancy. An abdominal mass also may be observed during a physical examination done as part of the evaluation of a patient with an unrelated disorder (*e.g.,* a cardiac problem). Many persons who are not ill, and therefore are not patients, request routine annual physical examinations. Finding a palpable abdominal abnormality in an asymptomatic patient is a rare event. Regional palpable disease is summarized in Table 6-1.

Clinical Evaluation of the Palpable Abdominal Mass

The cardinal rule in all diagnostic problems is to be a clinician first and use special procedures, including x-rays and biopsies, for confirmation. The interpretation of cytologic smears is strongly influenced by the clinical history and physical presentation of the target. The attempt to interpret smears without clinical data is a form of gamesmanship that may be quite successful in skilled hands, but is not recommended. Of course, relying on

TABLE 6-1: Palpable Findings in Abdominal Tumors

Primary Site	Palpable Mass
Colon	Liver (right upper quadrant mass)
	Site of resection
	Pelvis, including presacral (requires transrectal palpation)
Stomach	Liver (right upper quadrant mass)
	Epigastrium
Kidney	Flank (nephrectomy site)
	Implantation tumor
	Left upper quadrant mass
	Right upper quadrant mass
Pancreas	Epigastric mass
	Left upper quadrant mass
	Liver (right upper quadrant mass)
Liver	Liver (right upper quadrant mass)
	Epigastric mass
	Left upper quadrant mass
Spleen	Left upper quadrant
	Left lower quadrant

clinical findings without satisfactory attention to morphologic details also is to be discouraged.

Therefore, it is important to formulate a clinical impression rapidly from the data at hand, but it is also important to remain rooted in microscopic criteria. This is illustrated in the following case.

Case 6-2

The patient was a pleasant and cooperative 66-year-old woman seen initially after colon resection. The colon carcinoma was a Duke C. Adjuvant chemotherapy using fluorouracil (5-FU) was recommended, and was administered for 6 months. Carcinoembryonic antigen (CEA) studies were not available at the time. The patient was free of disease for 1 year. On routine follow-up examination, a globular mass was palpated abdominally rising out of the pelvis. Pre-puncture diagnosis by the attending clinician and the consulting gynecologist was cystic ovarian mass, which carried a better prognosis than recurrent colon carcinoma.

Fine needle aspiration failed to yield fluid, but yielded semisolid, partially necrotic material. At the periphery of the smears there were clusters of columnar epithelium characteristic of colon carcinoma. On further study, the mass was deemed inoperable.

More often, however, clinical impression will predict or guide the cytologic diagnosis accurately.

The Right Upper Quadrant Mass

The dominant mass in the right upper quadrant is the liver. In the non-jaundiced patient, the initial impression is obtained by physical examination, primarily palpation, to delineate the lower edge and separate the organ from contiguous masses. An occasional error is failure to palpate the lower edge, in which case a massively enlarged smooth liver may be missed entirely. At this point, a review of the history may disclose cirrhosis (alcoholism, prior hepatitis), previous primary cancer (breast, lung, GI tract, kidney), a reticuloendothelial disorder (lymphoma, schistosomiasis) or a metabolic disorder (diabetes).

Potential findings are illustrated in the following case.

Case 6-3

The patient was a 52-year-old menopausal, jovial, but anxious obese women seen for adjuvant chemotherapy shortly after right mastectomy. The pathology report indicated invasive ductal carcinoma with 2 of 17 nodes positive for a metastatic carcinoma. A 9-month course of chemotherapy using fluorouracil, methotrexate, and cyclophosphamide (Cytoxan) was initiated. At the start of therapy, her hematologic status was normal. In the chemistry profile, the following values were noted: alkaline phosphatase (AP), 110 U/L; gamma glutamyl transpeptidase (GGT), 78 U/L; and fasting blood sugar (FBS), 155 mg/dL. She stated that she had mild diabetes that she controlled with diet. Her appearance did not indicate rigid dieting. Her liver edge was distinctly palpable at 3 cm below the right costal margin. On examination during the sixth month of therapy, the liver was palpated clearly at 6 cm. The edge was smooth. On liver/spleen scan, the spleen was normal in size, and the liver was enlarged and mottled. The following values were reported: AP, 120 U/L; GGT, 92 U/L; and FBS, 160 mg/dL. The patient's weight had increased. Fine needle aspiration with three separate punctures yielded fat and fat-laden hepatocytes. The diagnosis was fatty liver secondary to poorly controlled diabetes, possibly complicated by methotrexate. The patient was well at 3-year follow up.

The irregular or nodular liver surface and edge is highly suggestive, of course, of metastases, particularly in an oncologic patient with previous known carcinoma. Geographic pathology plays a role. For example, in South Africa over 60% of patients with enlarged, firm, nodular livers will have primary carcinoma of the liver.[13] (See below.)

Liver texture is important. Hard masses are highly suspicious. Again, history will be revealing. For example, cirrhosis often must be considered in unobtrusive drinkers who have consumed one or two six-packs of beer, or two to three martinis with lunch and dinner, for a number of years without episodic drinking bouts. Other physical evidence, including spider angiomata and ascites, may suggest cirrhosis in a patient who does not exhibit the wasting expected with advanced carcinoma.

The question arises at this point about reliance on the liver scan, both isotopic and with computed tomography. The isotopic scan is singularly unreliable in separating metastatic and benign diffuse liver disease.[8,18] Where it clearly demonstrates multiple discrete, classic defects of metastases, the liver almost invariably will be enlarged, irregular, and readily palpable—an excellent target for fine needle aspiration. As with thyroid scans (see Chap. 3), the liver scan is most often ordered as a reflex diagnostic measure. Retrospective evaluation in our experience demonstrates limited contribution of the procedure in the presence of palpable disease. This is illustrated in Case 6-4, which presents an important observation about the enlarged liver.

Case 6-4

The patient was a 32-year-old woman (see Chap. 4, Case 4-1) who developed carcinoma of the breast during pregnancy, who was seen 3 years after mastectomy (8 nodes positive) and adjuvant chemotherapy. She complained of back pain. Bone scan was normal. At this time the liver was palpable 5 cm below the right costal margin. In search of retroperitoneal nodes to explain the back pain, a CT scan was obtained. Several defects were noted in a rather massively enlarged liver (Fig. 6-4). On discussion with the radiologist, it was evi-

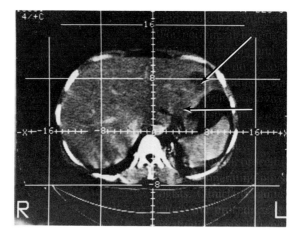

FIGURE 6-4: CT scan reveals discrete defects (*arrows*) in a rather massively enlarged liver. The enlargement was due to diffuse infiltration with cancer cells.

dent that the discrete defects noted on scan did not explain the massive liver enlargement. Random fine needle aspiration was carried out, yielding poorly differentiated carcinoma consistent with the original primary lesion. It was apparent that cancer diffusely infiltrated the liver or produced multiple small nodules not visible on scan in addition to the large defects noted.

COMMENT The CT scan failed to reveal a cause for the back pain. It did demonstrate the massive liver with defects. This palpable mass could have been diagnosed at the bedside at least 10 days before the CT scan finally was obtained. It must be noted that delay in scheduling, breakdown of the instrument, and travel to regional hospitals that have the instruments often prolong hospitalization and anxiety and often can be circumvented by prompt aspiration.

In the search for liver metastases, biochemical liver tests always should precede liver scan to improve the yield. With normal liver studies, the liver scan is quite insensitive.[45]

THE JAUNDICED PATIENT

The jaundiced patient with enlarged liver presents a different set of problems. History is extremely important, and biopsy procedures must be undertaken with some caution. Jaundice occurring with a palpable liver during the progression of a known intra-abdominal carcinoma (such as carcinoma of the gall bladder, bile duct, ampulla, pancreas, and stomach) should provide sufficient clinical evidence to forestall further invasive diagnostic testing. Puncture of the liver to demonstrate intrahepatic metastasis will add nothing to clinical management in this stage of progressive disease.

In the jaundiced patient with a palpable liver occurring without previous malignancy, liver function studies provide guidance. Obstructive jaundice requires imaging techniques (ultrasonography, computed tomography), which may lead to fine needle aspiration of an obstructing tumor (see below).

In the absence of extrahepatic obstruction, intrahepatic lesions must be sought. Liver scan may demonstrate one or more discrete lesions worthy of aspiration. Such lesions may be seen initially on the CT scan designed to demonstrate the presumed extrahepatic obstruction (see Nonpalpable Liver Targets).

Most malignant intrahepatic tumors in North America and Europe are metastatic even in the absence of an obvious primary. The liver is a potential site of metastasis for the most common tumors (tumors of the colon, stomach, breast, lung). However, 9000 cases of primary hepatocellular carcinoma occur annually in the United States, and cause approximately 5000 deaths each year.[7,12]

The relationship to cirrhosis is medically important. It is clear that nutritional or alcoholic cirrhosis does not ordinarily predispose to carcinoma.[12,29] Postnecrotic or posthepatitic cirrhoses are the types demonstrating correlation with primary carcinoma of the liver.[31] Therefore, screening for hepatitis antigens and antibodies is useful. Tumor in the presence of postnecrotic cirrhosis can be presumed to be hepatocellular carcinoma, which has a fairly distinctive cytologic pattern.[16,25,44] Cholangiocarcinoma does not engraft on cirrhosis. Its cytology would be indistinguishable from a variety of metastatic adenocarcinomas.

Although core biopsy may be done with limited morbidity,[27] the ease of fine needle aspiration as an office procedure should be emphasized. Finding carcinoma in association with elevated alpha fetoprotein[9] and the presence of hepatitis B surface antigen[50] is diagnostic.

Clinical criteria that help distinguish metastatic and primary tumors are listed in Table 6-2.

NONPALPABLE LIVER TARGETS

Finally, defects may be found, often unexpectedly, within nonpalpable livers, both jaundiced and nonjaundiced, as a result of liver scans, sonograms, or CT studies done for a variety of reasons. In the absence of any history or evidence of extrahepatic malignancy, such defects most often indicate benign disease, but did not in Fig. 6-5.

Current standard clinical practice on failure to diagnose any of the above clinical syndromes by examination, laboratory, or noninvasive imaging techniques usually will mandate an endoscopic procedure, a core biopsy, peritoneoscopy, or laparotomy.

TABLE 6-2: Liver Tumors

	Metastatic	Primary
Existence of cirrhosis	Uncommon	Cirrhosis present in 50% in North America[12,31]
Right upper quadrant pain	Late disease	May be useful sign earlier
Palpable mass, masses, or diffuse hepatomegaly	Nonspecific	Nonspecific
Routine laboratory studies	Nonspecific	Nonspecific
Alpha fetoprotein elevation	Occasional	75% to 90% positive;[9] levels over 4000 ng/mL highly suggestive[47]
Radionucleide scan	Filling defects	Filling defects
Angiography	Increased vascularity unusual	Increased vascularity characteristic[34]
HbsAG	Negative	Present in 80%[50]

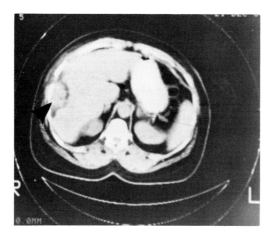

FIGURE 6-5: CT scan highlighting the liver reveals a discrete defect (*arrow*) that did not enlarge the liver, but proved to be a metastatic deposit.

THE APPLICATION OF FINE NEEDLE ASPIRATION TO PALPABLE AND NONPALPABLE LIVER DISEASE

Jaundice, enlarged liver, typical history of hepatitis, and confirmatory liver chemistry studies are usually sufficient for diagnosis of non-neoplastic liver disorders. However, fine needle aspiration has been used with satisfactory results in selected cases.[25,26,36,43] Where fine needle aspiration is revealing, core biopsy, which sometimes continues to produce potentially serious morbidity, can be eliminated from the work up. Evaluation of tissue structure is, of course, required at times.

The needle puncture may be random in the diffusely involved liver (see Case 6-4). A single puncture should yield adequate material. All jaundiced patients should have a satisfactory prothrombin time before puncture.

Neoplastic involvement of the liver by primary or metastatic tumors is unusual in the absence of abnormal liver function studies or palpable enlargement. Liver scan produces a low yield in their absence.[45] However, with the profusion of technologic imaging procedures now in vogue,[4] an inappropriate liver scan occasionally may demonstrate liver defects. In the absence of a known primary, such defects are almost always benign cysts. Suspicion must be aroused when a prior or concomitant primary carcinoma is known. Therapy may be totally dependent on diagnosis of the liver defects.

Puncture of liver defects is carried out rather simply under ultrasonographic or computed tomographic guidance.[3,7,36] Twenty-two gauge needles of varying lengths are used and the approach may be subcostal (anterior) or intercostal (anterior, lateral, or posterior). Where there are multiple discrete defects characteristic of liver metastases in a nonpalpable liver (this is unusual), material usually can be secured without guidance with multiple random passes of the needle.[16,26] An attempt to obtain a core biopsy using a large needle may obtain positive tissue, but it not infrequently yields benign tissue because the needle has missed tumor nodules. Multiple passes from multiple sites using a thick needle are impractical and hazardous.

The overutilization of imaging techniques is illustrated in Case A-14 of the Appendix.

Scan may demonstrate a diffuse infiltrative pattern in a liver that is not enlarged or is minimally so. Although a non-neoplastic diffuse process, such as hepatitis, cirrhosis, or granulomatous inflammation, is usually present and is ordinarily best demonstrated by histologic examination of a core biopsy specimen, fine needle aspiration may unexpectedly yield carcinoma. Granulomatous alteration also may be identified easily by this method.[43]

A mottled diffuse pattern may be due to multiple metastatic nodules. The size threshold for identifying metastatic nodules on liver scan is 2 cm.

In summary, the random puncture may yield intra- and extracellular fat (fatty liver, cirrhosis [see Case 6-3]); hepatocytes with intranuclear inclusions (diabetes, hepatitis); increased lymphocytic, monocytic, or granulocytic cells (lymphoma or leukemia [see Case 6-8]); Gaucher's cells (storage disease); and malignant cells (metastatic or primary hepatocellular carcinoma).

Puncture of liver parenchyma in the presence of obstructive jaundice carries with it the hazard, albeit slight, of bile leak and bile peritonitis. Sudden pain and muscle guarding immediately after the puncture is suspicious for this eventuality. With supportive therapy, fluids, and antibiotics, the outcome should be benign.

TECHNIQUE OF PUNCTURE

Where the palpable irregularity is readily detected and the abdominal wall is thin, a 3.8-cm (1.5-in), 22-gauge needle is quite satisfactory. The needle is passed through the skin, with or without local anesthesia, and is poised over the target. Then, with the patient in inspiratory apnea, it is passed into the liver and material is extracted in the usual manner (see Chap. 1).

A hard liver edge may be felt just below the rib margin, in which case the needle may be passed tangentially cephalad into the edge while the patient is in inspiratory apnea.

Targets above the costal margin are reached by an intercostal approach. The length of the needle is determined by the depth of the lesion. The choice of anterior, lateral, or posterior approach is based on radiographic guidance.

CYTOLOGY

Liver cells are fairly distinctive, and they are easy to distinguish from carcinoma cells, particularly when seen in juxtaposition. Adenoma or well-differentiated hepatoma may pose a problem. The specific cytologic diagnosis of hepatocellular carcinoma has been reported in several studies.[17,26]

Necrosis is common in smears obtained from larger masses. Tumor cells may be seen in faded groups near the periphery. However, necrosis alone in the clinical context of a metastatic tumor is virtually diagnostic. Multiple liver abscesses may simulate tumor (see Case A-14), but the yield will be granulocytes. The major yield is usually smears with abundant tumor cells, often specifically unclassifiable as to origin (but see Case A-11).

Bile stains black with Romanowsky's stain. This intracellular black pigment may simulate melanin in the clinical context of suspected metastatic melanoma.

Intranuclear inclusion may occur in hepatoma (Fig. 6-6), melanoma,[25] and hypernephroma,[24] in addition to the benign disorders noted above. Discrimination of these cytologic details requires much experience on the part of the cytopathologist, but, as always, he should be guided by clinical information.

Additional palpable right upper quadrant masses include upper pole of the right kidney, hepatic flexure carcinoma, gall bladder, metastatic masses, and lymphoma. It is evident that the most direct method of distinguishing these lesions is fine needle aspiration. Again, clinical context is important, but it may be deceptive, as illustrated in the following cases.

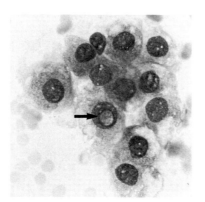

FIGURE 6-6: Hepatoma, aspiration biopsy. There is an intranuclear inclusion (*arrow*) also seen in hypernephroma and melanoma. Clinical correlation is important.

Case 6-5

The patient was a 74-year-old woman seen initially for left axillary adenopathy. Nodes measured up to 3 cm, and were rubbery and discrete. On fine needle aspiration, a mixed pattern of equal numbers of large and small lymphocytes were present. A diagnosis of non-Hodgkin's lymphoma, mixed lymphocytic/histiocytic, was made. Surgical biopsy was carried out and the histopathology was non-Hodgkin's lymphoma, mixed lymphocytic/histiocytic nodular. Bone marrow smears contained sheets of intermediate lymphocytes. General physical examination was otherwise negative. In particular, the liver and spleen were not palpable. After chemotherapy with six cycles of COP (Cytoxan/Oncovin/prednisone), all nodes disappeared and the marrow picture improved. The patient was seen at 3 months, and then neglected to return for 7 months, at which time she complained of mild anorexia and dyspepsia. On examination, a right upper quadrant mass was palpated easily. The patient was referred for radiotherapy (computed tomography and ultrasonography were not available). Adequate radiation failed to reduce the mass. Transabdominal fine needle aspiration yielded typical cytologic findings of colon carcinoma confirmed by barium enema.

Case 6-6

An 84-year-old woman was seen in the office for follow-up examination after recent lumpectomy for carcinoma of the left breast. She had declined mastectomy. Estrogen receptors were positive. On examination, a right upper quadrant mass not detected previously was palpated. It was rather hard and globular, and was palpable on deep pressure through a lax abdomen. Fine needle aspiration was carried out in the office, and yielded 3 mL of brown bile. The patient experienced minimal discomfort with no residual effects. There were no gall bladder symptoms. The patient was kept under surveillance while receiving tamoxifen with no tumor recurrence or biliary problems at 2 years. The gall bladder remained palpable. A similar case was reported by Pelaez.[32]

Finding adenocarcinoma on aspiration of a nonhepatic right upper quadrant mass may not identify the target. Gastrointestinal neoplasms (including colonic, gastric, and biliary neoplasms) may be difficult to distinguish cytologically. Other clinical diagnostic measures, including the usual imaging techniques, may be required. The identification of renal tumors is considered later in this chapter.

The Left Upper Quadrant Mass

The most common palpable left upper quadrant mass is the spleen. Spleno-megaly almost invariably is detected by a physician. The spleen may be enlarged as part of a variety of readily identifiable clinical syndromes or for no apparent reason. Potential causes are listed in Table 6-3.

Perhaps the largest published experience with fine needle aspiration of the spleen is that of Söderström.[39,40,41] He stressed that the presumed dangers of splenic puncture are minimized when the fine needle and the one-hand syringe are used in one continuous action to puncture and aspirate simultaneously, release the plunger, and withdraw, all in seconds.

For enlarged spleens, the puncture is made in the midportion of the spleen below the ribs with the patient in inspiratory apnea. For the non-palpable spleen, the puncture is made between the middle and anterior axillary lines through the ninth or tenth interspace in expiratory apnea after several breaths.

Before the puncture, routine coagulation studies (prothrombin time, partial thromboplastin time, platelets) should be obtained.

It is best to enter the subcutaneous compartment first with the needle, before thrusting into the spleen. Local anesthesia may be used. Although Söderström recommends needles 9 cm in length, it is certainly possible to obtain satisfactory specimens utilizing 3-cm needles in patients with spleens easily palpable beneath a fat-depleted abdominal wall. Shorter needles also require a shorter time for the complete maneuver. Splenic tissue structure is uniform throughout. Clinical judgment should determine the needle length. The finer the needle, the less the possibility of trauma to the splenic capsule. We have found 22-gauge needles to be a reasonable compromise.

The spleen mirrors multiple systemic processes. A question has been posed concerning puncture of the normal-sized spleen to obtain useful clinical data.[40,41] Certainly, a normal-sized spleen may be a repository of granulomatous disease and Hodgkin's disease (see below). If that area remains in doubt, there should be no doubt about the importance of puncturing an enlarged spleen even where the clinical context would ap-pear to make the puncture superfluous. Spleen puncture should be carried out in particular when a clinical syndrome is puzzling or fails to conform to the expected evolution of a disease process. This is illustrated in the following cases.

Case 6-7

The patient was a 72-year-old man admitted with disorientation, vomiting, and dehydration. History revealed rather longstanding chronic lymphocytic leukemia (CLL) treated previously with chlor-ambucil, prednisone, and subsequently vincristine (Oncovin). During much of the preceding 3 months, he had been hospitalized in an-

TABLE 6-3: **Splenomegaly**

Associated Disorders*	Initial Finding in Unrecognized Syndrome	Chronic Inflammatory Disorders	Diagnosis Known by Hematologic and Serologic Studies	Studies Required Prior to Splenic Puncture
Chronic leukemia	Lymphoma (may be the only site)	Cirrhosis with portal hypertension	Agnogenic myeloid metaplasia	Bone marrow
Lymphoma	Sarcoidosis	Malaria	Hemolytic anemia	Lymphoma
Acute inflammatory disorder	Hypersplenism	Other tropical parasites	Congenital	Hematologic disorders
Infectious mononucleosis	Splenic vein thrombosis		Acquired	Gaucher's disease
Enteric infections	Gaucher's disease		Systemic lupus erythematosus	CT scan of abdomen
Subacute bacterial endocarditis			Leukemia	Lymphoma
				Serologic studies
				SLE
				Hemolytic anemias

*Known or suspected at time of examination.

other institution because of anemia, weakness, fever, and general deterioration. His spleen, described as massive, had been treated with radiation.

On admission, the patient was dry, wasted, and disoriented. Temperature was 100.3 °F. There was regular sinus tachycardia. The lungs were clear. There were no enlarged lymph nodes. The liver was not palpable. Spleen was irregularly enlarged with a prominent lower bulge. The edge was 10 cm below the left costal margin. Laboratory studies were as follows: hemoglobin, 10 g/dL; WBC, 4300/μL with 50% polys, 5% bands, 43% lymphocytes, and 2% monocytes. Platelets were 103,000 mm³; albumin/globulin (AG), 4.3/2.1; and calcium, 15 mg/dL. Chest x-ray was unremarkable. Bone marrow smears contained focal aggregates of fairly mature lymphocytes sufficient to identify lymphoproliferative disorder in an otherwise normal marrow.

The patient was treated with fluids and diuretics, with lowering of his calcium and partial recovery of normal mental status. He indicated that his spleen was painful and tender. Ten days were spent lowering his calcium and carrying out studies to explain his downhill course in the face of so little gross or hematologic evidence of CLL.

Spleen punctures yielded smears consisting entirely of blast cells, interpreted either as extramedullary acute lymphocytic leukemia or poorly differentiated lymphoma. Transformation of chronic lymphocytic leukemia to an acute phase, while unusual, must be considered. After suitable preparation, a splenectomy was performed.

The following case illustrates the importance of careful examination.

Case 6-8

The patient was an alert, thin, 69-year-old retired dancer who lived alone. She was seen in consultation in the hospital. She had lost 30 lb in a period of 3 months, and had been examined and studied for 1 month by her family doctor. A massive liver enlargement extending across the upper abdomen was interpreted as metastatic in origin. There was no history of drinking or of any primary tumor. The breasts were negative to palpation. A barium enema and upper GI had been done and were reported as negative.

On examination, the liver was not only palpable, it was visible through the thin abdominal wall. It extended below the umbilicus with an irregular edge that could be palpated over to the left upper quadrant.

Fine needle aspiration yielded hepatocytes extensively intermixed with atypical lymphoid cells, some with enlarged irregular nuclei and nucleoli. At this point, the patient was reexamined, and it was determined that the left upper abdominal extension of the liver could be distinguished from a moderately enlarged, firm spleen. Fine needle aspiration of the spleen yielded sheets of large immature lymphoid cells, some of which could be characterized as Sternberg–Reed cells. There were occasional scattered eosinophils. No normal or well-differentiated lymphocytes were present.

The diagnosis was Hodgkin's disease involving liver and spleen.

The patient was treated promptly with cyclophosphamide (Cytoxan), vincristine (Oncovin), procarbazine, and prednisone without any further study. There was dramatic shrinkage of the liver and spleen with clinical improvement.

COMMENT This patient again illustrates the importance of careful physical examination. Palpation required methodical fingertip separation of liver and spleen, done best when the examiner is sitting by the patient. Pursuit of the assumption that the liver enlargement and downhill course were due to metastatic disease would have led to early death of the patient.

Although the unexpected may be produced by aspiration, as in the above cases, more often the clinical hematologic status of the patient will suggest the likely cytologic yield. All such information must be presented along with the smears to obtain the most accurate readings. The most common splenic "tumor" is the congested spleen or the spleen of hypersplenism often caused by portal or splenic vein obstruction. Although the typical cytology has been presented clearly by Söderström, diagnostic smears are not always obtained. However, by exclusion a diagnosis can be entertained. Such a "negative" smear will largely exclude the obvious pathologic entities such as lymphoma, leukemia, myeloid metaplasia, sarcoidosis, and storage diseases discussed below.

It may be difficult at times to distinguish a left upper quadrant mass of lymphomatous nodes (see below) from splenic lymphoma. The cytologic smears will be identical. Imaging techniques often, but not always, will settle the issue. Primary lymphoma confined to the spleen may be a surgical target, and identification is important where possible.

Granulomatous involvement of the spleen by sarcoidosis, tuberculosis, and other inflammatory disorders may be identified cytologically.[37,43] Hodgkin's disease may yield granulomatous alterations (epithelioid and giant cells) without clearly identifiable Sternberg–Reed cells. However, such changes are highly suspicious in a patient with splenomegaly and known nodal Hodgkin's disease. On the other hand, not all splenomegaly in Hodgkin's disease is due to invasion by the disease. In addition to hypersplenism, Söderström has described useful cytologic patterns for lymphoma.[25] Such disorders as agnogenic myeloid metaplasia and Gaucher's disease yield fairly self-evident smears.

On occasion, carcinomas may invade the spleen and produce spleno-megaly. A palpable spleen in this setting usually raises the suspicion of a double primary (carcinoma and lymphoma), or of splenic vein thrombosis secondary to carcinoma. A puncture is usually decisive.

However, all left upper quadrant masses are not of splenic origin.[40] Clinically, a mass may closely simulate a spleen, but may arise from a strikingly different source. This is illustrated in Case A-17 in the Appendix. It must be noted in reviewing this case, which predates the era of ultra-sonography and computed tomography, that this instrumentation is not uniformly available throughout the world, and that even in the western countries, such instrumentation is regionalized in many areas and it is sometimes difficult and inconvenient for patients to travel distances.

Renal tumors, particularly Wilms', may be mistaken for a spleen. Neu-roblastomas, adult adrenal masses, retroperitoneal sarcomas, and less likely, primary and metastatic epithelial carcinomas also must be considered. Con-fusion may arise as illustrated in the following case of left upper quadrant retroperitoneal sarcoma.

Case 6-9

A 62-year-old man returned to a community hospital from a major medical center with a left upper quadrant mass. He had been referred to the medical center with a history of fever, microscopic hematuria, heart murmur, weight loss, and congestive heart failure, in addition to the mass. Admitting diagnosis was subacute bacterial endocarditis. Studies at the medical center included: repeated blood cultures, neg-ative; liver/spleen scan, no splenomegaly; sonogram, left upper quad-rant mass, which was palpable; IVP, poor function of left kidney (nondiagnostic); CT scan of abdomen, left upper quadrant mass; and bone marrow, reactive.

Laparotomy was considered, but it was excluded because of the patient's medical status. Discharge diagnosis was probable lym-phoma. Time in hospital was 4 weeks.

A transabdominal fine needle aspiration of the palpable mass yielded a cytologic diagnosis of fibrosarcoma.

Treatment was initiated with radiotherapy.

COMMENT A diagnosis of subacute bacterial endocarditis was reason-able on the assumption that the mass was spleen. Other aspects in-cluding hematuria and fever raised the question of hypernephroma. The mass was palpable and fine needle aspiration was diagnostic. Diagnosis could have been made on the first day of admission, and further studies could have been limited to those necessary to define the mass for radiotherapy.

Patients with palpable abdominal masses of unknown origin who are studied at large, particularly academic, medical centers, are more likely to have extensive duplicative, repetitive, often highly technological, and time-consuming studies. In part, this is due to the multiple consultation system in which each consultant applies his own expertise, skills, and procedures. Fine needle aspiration performed in the office or clinic usually will intercept or shorten this proceeding. We have found that procedures and hospitalizations can be avoided. This is illustrated in the next section.

Midabdominal Masses

A midabdominal mass may be a surprise finding during a routine abdominal examination. In older patients, the mass may be pulsatile and may be recognized by the physician as an abdominal aneurysm. It is self-evident that pulsatile masses should not be punctured. In patients who have vegetative gastrointestinal symptoms without localization, palpation of the liver in search of diffuse liver disease and metastases rarely is omitted. The midabdomen may not receive the same searching scrutiny. Absolute relaxation of the abdominal wall is essential and may require patience and time. In young children, abdominal palpation sometimes is done successfully with the patient in a warm tub. Unfortunately, palpation has lost its priority since the advent of computed tomography, which encourages physicians to rush through the physical examination.

In our experience, palpable extraluminal midabdominal masses are metastatic or recurrent carcinomas and lymphomas. Less commonly, primary intraluminal, pancreatic, adrenal, renal, and pelvic primary tumors and retroperitoneal sarcomas may present as midabdominal masses. Case 6-10 illustrates the interesting evolution of a diagnosis.

Case 6-10

The patient was a 73-year-old man admitted to the hospital with weakness, weight loss, and migratory skeletal pains. Initial laboratory studies yielded the following values: hemoglobin, 8.8 g/dL; MCV, 90 μm^3; urinary protein, 100 mg/dL; and creatinine of 2.3 mg/dL.

Initial physical examination was negative for lymph nodes and masses. Enlargement of the liver and spleen was not detected. Gastrointestinal and skeletal x-rays were done. The left hip, a major pain source, revealed a lytic defect in the left femur (Fig. 6-7). A presumptive diagnosis of multiple myeloma was made, and protein studies, including electrophoresis, were ordered.

Hematologic consultation was requested with particular attention to aspiration of the lytic lesion. Review of the films before examining the patient suggested that penetration of the femur would not be accomplished easily because the cortex was intact.

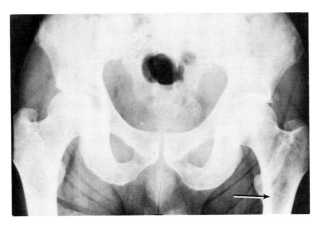

FIGURE 6-7: Radiograph of pelvis and hips. There is a lytic defect in the left femur (*arrow*) suggesting a diagnosis of myeloma. Final diagnosis was metastatic prostate carcinoma.

On physical examination, a pulsating aorta was easily palpable through a lax abdominal wall. A para-aortic mass could be detected. Immediate fine needle aspiration yielded an epithelial tumor cytologically consistent with prostate carcinoma. At this point, palpation of the prostate revealed an indurated area. Prostate aspiration was requested, confirming a diagnosis of prostatic carcinoma.

COMMENT The patient had a 12-day hospitalization before a diagnosis was established, primarily because of an incomplete physical examination. The prostate was clearly abnormal but rectal examination had not been performed. The midabdominal mass was evident on careful examination. Although lytic lesions are not usual in metastatic prostate disease, they do occur.

History of prior or concurrent tumors, particularly colonic, gastric, pancreatic, and ovarian, is most important in evaluating midabdominal masses of unknown origin. GI metastases from bronchogenic carcinoma are not rare, but cases reported fail to describe physical findings.[1] Metastases to abdominal nodes from oat cell carcinoma producing palpable masses occasionally have been seen in our experience. Intra-abdominal metastases to the omentum from pancreatic, gastric, colonic, and ovarian carcinoma are readily palpable and easily aspirated. Mesenteric and nodal masses may require deeper palpation unless they are quite bulky. Then the diagnosis is usually apparent clinically and biopsy confirmation is not necessary. This is particularly true of ovarian masses, which may fill the abdomen in a patient otherwise free of remote metastases. Such a patient may be ambulatory, in contrast with a patient with advanced bulky gastrointestinal or pancreatic carcinoma, who is usually debilitated by intrahepatic and remote metastases. In such patients, fine needle aspiration contributes little to clinical management.

Local recurrence of resected tumors of the stomach and colon may become palpable targets. In the routine follow up of resected intraluminal tumor, hematological, stool, and endoscopic examination usually will reveal local recurrence before a mass is palpated. CEA determination may be even more sensitive. Palpation should not be neglected, however, and the discovery of local intra-abdominal induration at the site of surgery should be followed by fine needle aspiration, which will readily yield carcinoma cells, if present.

Local tumor induration is simulated by the effects of radiation. This is similar to the irradiated breast (see Chap. 4), and may require periodic aspiration to exclude local tumor infiltration, particularly in the symptomatic patient. (Another source of local induration is illustrated in Case 7-3.)

Metastatic deposits subperitoneally or in the abdominal wall are useful targets with and without prior radiation or known primary. This is illustrated in the following case.

Case 6-11

The patient was a 55-year-old moderately retarded woman with a history of colon resection (Duke C) at age 52 years. She lived alone with minimal supervision, and finally was brought to the clinic by a friend. She complained of a "dragging sensation" in her lower abdomen. On examination, the left lower abdominal wall was densely infiltrated, thickened, and dusky. The edges of the infiltrated area were delimited rather easily (Fig. 6-8). The healed incision of the colon resection ran through the middle of the area. A clinical diagnosis of recurrent infiltrated colon carcinoma (implantation tumor) was made. However, fine needle aspiration yielded cellular smears composed of somewhat pleomorphic and fragile immature lymphoid cells. The final diagnosis was non-Hodgkin's lymphoma, poorly differentiated and diffuse—a second primary.

Abdominal puncture occasionally will yield fluid indicating a cystic structure. Pancreatic cysts may present in the midabdomen and the left side (see Case A-17 in Appendix). Where suspected, the fluid, often brownish, should be submitted for amylase determination.

Mesenteric cysts yield clear yellow fluid. In endemic regions, care must be taken to avoid puncturing an *Echinococcus* cyst. Similarly, presumed ovarian cysts palpated in the lower midabdomen should be aspirated with

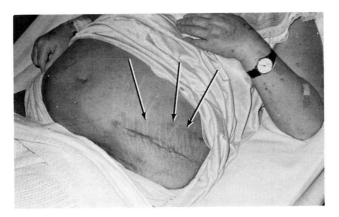

FIGURE 6-8: There is dense, visible, and palpable infiltration of the abdominal wall adjacent to an abdominal incision. When it is due to tumor infiltration, fine needle aspiration almost invariably will be diagnostic.

care to avoid spillage of carcinoma (see Chap. 7), or aspiration should be omitted.

The midabdomen also may be the site of extension of an enlarged liver, kidney, or adrenal gland, usually recognized as such but sometimes not diagnosed without imaging techniques. Puncture may yield surprise findings. (Unusual abdominal findings are presented in Case A-13 of the Appendix.)

Nonpalpable pancreatic, renal, adrenal, and lymph node masses are considered in a later section.

Intra-abdominal Lymphoma

Gastrointestinal lymphoma is an intraluminal tumor presenting with signs and symptoms indistinguishable from carcinoma. 104 cases were collected at Memorial Hospital in New York City during the period 1949–1978. The lesions ranged in size from 1 cm to 20 cm (surgical specimen). How many were clinically palpable is not stated.[49] One may assume that some of the larger masses were palpable and therefore suitable targets for aspiration.

It may be difficult clinically to distinguish a palpable primary GI lymphoma from an extraluminal tumor arising in lymph nodes (see below). In practical terms, such a mass rarely becomes a target for aspiration before GI studies have been done. Such studies are prompted by gastrointestinal symptoms (*e.g.,* nausea, vomiting, cramps, bleeding).

The major intra-abdominal palpable lymphoma is extraluminal, involving lymph nodes. Lymphomas arising in the retroperitoneal nodes and presenting as palpable abdominal masses are firm, fixed, smooth, or irregular masses. In contrast, primary gastrointestinal tumors are more likely to be vague in outline and moveable.

Direct diagnosis of extraluminal palpable intra-abdominal lymphoma is accomplished easily with direct transabdominal puncture. The yield will consist of well, moderately, and poorly differentiated lymphoid smears consistent with non-Hodgkin's lymphoma. Peripheral nodes, spleen, and liver may be nonpalpable. Bone marrow may be normal. Having diagnosed retroperitoneal lymphoma cytologically and confirmed the presence of retroperitoneal nodes by CT scan, decision must be made concerning histopathological diagnosis requiring laparotomy. Clinical context is important (Table 6-4).

The relationship of cytology to the histopathology of lymphomas and to clinical analysis is considered in Chapter 8.

Puncture of Nonpalpable Lesions of the Abdomen

The instrumentation and details for locating nonpalpable lesions of the abdomen and carrying out the biopsy have been presented most knowledgeably in reports by radiologists who have developed the technique and are often the first to advocate the methods of fine needle aspiration in many institutions.[19,28,52]

There is a tendency for the clinician to remain outside of this diagnostic arena. However, it is important to remember that the attending physician assumes responsibility and it is both his duty and option to select the appropriate diagnostic studies. Therefore, it is in the patient's interest that he remain involved. This begins with consideration of which imaging pro-

TABLE 6-4: Procedural Steps in Dealing with a Lymphoid Smear Extracted from the Abdomen (Guidelines)

Known Lymphoma	DeNovo Finding		
↓	↓		
Reclassify stage	Consider age and clinical status		
↓	↓	↓	↓
CT scan (optional)	Elderly or debilitated		Young and vigorous
	(Symptomatic vs. asymptomatic)		
Treat (clinical decision)	No treatment depending on cytology and symptoms	Well differentiated (treat or observe)	Poorly differentiated (consider laparotomy for tissue structure)
	Well differentiated	Poorly differentiated	
	Observe	Consider treatment	

cedure to use when retroperitoneal disease is suspected. Rather than order
a series of studies, he will be better advised to discuss the contemplated
studies with the radiologist. Much depends in each institution on the
experience of the radiologist in obtaining material, and that of the pathologist in interpreting aspiration biopsy smears. As important as experience,
after the aspiration and before the slides are read, well-prepared smears
must be available (see Chap. 1). The clinician may be able to make such
smears after instruction and practice. It will be rewarding to be present at
the puncture to discuss possible pathologic findings with the radiologist,
make the kind of smears satisfactory to the pathologist, and at the same
time, make his presence known to his patient.

Ultrasonography, computed tomography, and image intensifying fluoroscopy are the major tools required. Many punctures were done successfully using single plane fluoroscopy before the advent of ultrasonography
and computed tomography. Various marker systems including skeletal landmarks, introduction of barium, angiography,[46] ERCP,[15] and lymphangiography[14] have provided satisfactory technical and topographical aides
in locating the lesion and guiding the needle direction.

Bipedal lymphangiography to opacify nodes has provided a useful
marker for transabdominal puncture. The technique is used to stage carcinomas including those of the cervix, ovary, testicle, bladder, and prostate.[33,48] Opacification of lymphomatous nodes allows aspiration after therapy to determine residual disease.

The use of ultrasonography with a transducer allows visualization of
the needle within the target. Computed tomography provides even greater
technical refinement, reveals extremely small lesions, and allows visualization of the needle within the target. However, it is time consuming and
expensive, and it increases radiation exposure.[32]

Having located the lesion, biopsy is done in a fairly uniform manner
regardless of the type of target. The patient should be reassured, and rarely
requires any sedation. An opaque marker is placed on the abdominal wall
over the site of the target. The skin and subcutaneous tissue are anesthetized
with xylocaine 1%. The needle (22 gauge) and stylet are introduced vertically through the skin. A small incision may be necessary. The needle is
advanced, and may elicit minimal pain on traversing the peritoneum. If
the target is small and it is anticipated that several passes may be necessary
with some deviation of direction each time, then a guide needle (18 gauge)
may be left within the abdominal wall. The needle is advanced slowly
through the abdominal contents, stomach, and so forth, meeting no resistance until it enters the lesion, retroperitoneal tissues, pancreas, and so
forth. The direction is guided by fluoroscopy. Aspiration is accomplished in
the usual manner by oscillating the needle in one tract with full suction
applied. If the target is missed, the needle is withdrawn and reinserted with
a directional change.

For the usual palpable abdominal lesion, gloves are not necessary for sterility. However, in using a long needle that may require stabilization at the skin level, gloves are mandatory. With many years of experience and repeated punctures of viscera, we have not seen infection introduced or released from the bowel even in immunosuppressed patients.[25] A representative lesion is seen in Figure 3-14.

The Pancreas

The diagnosis of pancreatic carcinoma is very often obscure and as a result is late, rendering the tumor incurable in 90% of cases.[30] Early symptoms are vague, often ignored by the patient and misinterpreted by the physician. It is agreed that the noninvasive, although expensive, modalities (*e.g.,* ultrasonography, CT scanning) should be employed first in the search for pancreatic carcinoma.[3,30] However, they are not screening measures and the exercise of clinical judgment is important.

Upper abdominal symptoms together with anorexia and weight loss provide some focus. Obstructive jaundice, history of pancreatitis, and recent diabetes should further encourage prompt investigation.[23]

There are technical reasons for utilizing ultrasonography as the initial study in children and elderly or emaciated patients with reduced retroperitoneal fat.[30] However, there are technical problems in general that require an adequate level of expertise to assure reliability.[3] For the clinician who needs a clinical decision in a particular patient, it is prudent to discuss the specific diagnostic potential of ultrasonography with the physicians responsible for imaging in the particular institution. General rules and expectations cannot be relied upon. The specific question must be asked, "Can you demonstrate a lesion that can be reached with a transabdominal fine needle puncture?" Computed tomography offers the best possibility of detecting small lesions.

Having localized a pancreatic mass, puncture ordinarily can be done accurately and the cytologic diagnosis can be obtained in a high percentage of cases.[2,28,32] Immediate examination of the smears is suggested; therefore, prearranged collaboration between clinician or radiologist and cytopathologist is important. Failure to obtain satisfactory material should prompt repeat puncture.

The cytology of adencarcinoma can be distinguished rather easily from that of islet cell or carcinoid (small cell) tumors.[25] Lymphoma is also distinctive (see Chap. 8). Therefore, the method of fine needle aspiration has specificity as well as sensitivity.

Peripancreatic lymph node enlargement often is noted in CT scan studies. Fine needle aspiration of a lymph node yielding metastatic adenocarcinoma in a patient with clinical and x-ray evidence of pancreatic carcinoma should be decisive.

Peroperative fine needle aspiration of metastatic nodes and primary tumors is a useful procedure.[25] Such slides may be submitted for immediate reading, similar to a frozen section.

The Renal Puncture

The kidneys and adrenals provide significant extraluminal targets, both palpable and nonpalpable. Puncture is particularly useful because of the distinctive cytology.[24] The most common tumor is hypernephroma, which produces widespread pathophysiological alterations of great interest to internists and a variety of subspecialists.

Pathophysiological alterations include fever,[6] hypercalcemia,[10,11] hepatic dysfunction,[42] anemia,[10,11] polycythemia,[5] and amyloidosis.[11] A clinical syndrome encompassing one or more of these paraneoplastic findings should prompt immediate focus on the kidneys. Although the majority of renal tumors are detected on IVP, which is done to investigate microscopic hematuria, obstruction, infection, or disturbance in renal function, careful palpation in a relaxed state should be the first diagnostic maneuver. Forty-five percent of 309 nephrectomized patients had a palpable mass.[38] A palpable mass coupled with hematuria and one or more of the paraneoplastic disorders noted above narrows the diagnostic focus and should point immediately to the prospect of fine needle aspiration. Urinalysis should precede the puncture to avoid factitious hematuria, and even though the mass is palpable and suitable for direct puncture, IV urogram or ultrasonography ordinarily are indicated before aspiration, as discussed below.

DIFFERENTIAL DIAGNOSIS

Other left upper and right upper quadrant masses (see above) raise questions of differential diagnosis. The standard approach to identification of the tumor as of renal origin includes nephrotomography, intravenous pyelography, arteriography, ultrasonography, and computed tomography. Any or all of these techniques may be employed. At what point should fine needle aspiration be considered (Fig. 6-9), and is it indicated or justified?

The most common renal mass is the benign cyst.[21,22] It is not usually palpable and is discovered on IVP. Identification and puncture with the aid of ultrasonography is the usual sequence, and almost invariably yields benign fluid. Cysts ordinarily are not important clinical problems for the clinician. Puncture is done by radiologists.

The most common tumor, as indicated above, is renal cell carcinoma (hypernephroma). The cytology is highly specific, and therefore an early attempt to obtain cells for study is reasonable.[25] The cytology of transitional cell carcinoma of the kidney is also fairly characteristic.[25] It can be distinguished from liver and spleen cytology as well as a variety of adenocarcinomas within the abdomen.

THE CLINICAL APPLICATION OF FINE NEEDLE
ASPIRATION TO RENAL LESIONS

In our experience, the palpable flank mass should be punctured immediately after urinalysis and IVP. It is an outpatient procedure. CT scan

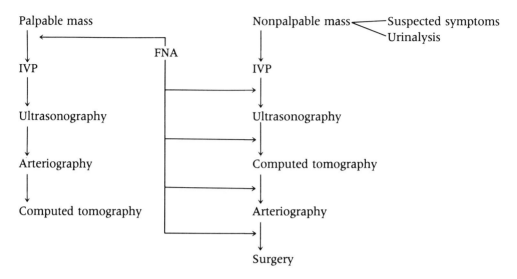

Comment: Palpable renal mass should be diagnosed immediately with FNA, eliminating imaging procedures. Puncture of nonpalpable mass requires imaging procedures (Case 6-12).

FIGURE 6-9: Diagnostic schema for renal masses.

and arteriography are not necessary for identification of the tumor, but may be clinically indicated for staging and presurgical evaluation.

Suspicion of a renal tumor based on symptoms (see above) should immediately prompt careful palpation of the renal sites with the patient in a relaxed state. Failure to detect a mass raises questions of a nonpalpable renal tumor, and detection requires imaging techniques. Earlier attempts at renal puncture and tumor identification utilized IVP[51] and then arteriography.[51] Ultrasonography and CT scanning (see Fig. 6-9) may have replaced them as adjuvant techniques for renal puncture.[35] Puncture of small lesions is accomplished easily.

The clinically relevant yield from palpable and nonpalpable tumors includes identification of renal cell carcinoma, transitional cell, Wilms' tumor, angiolipoma, and metastatic masses. Metastasis to the kidney is illustrated in the following case.

Case 6-12

The patient was a 57-year-old man with a dull left flank pain, microscopic hematuria, and an abnormal IVP. A definite mass could not be palpated. The findings were reviewed by a urologic surgeon and the patient was explored by a flank incision. Mobilization of the kidney was difficult, requiring interruption of the procedure. Further study demonstrated a colon carcinoma that had invaded the kidney and distorted the renal calyces.

Renal cell carcinoma and colonic carcinoma cytology usually are distinguished easily, and preoperative puncture would have guided the surgeon appropriately.

Pretherapeutic identification of the tumor is valuable for several other reasons.

1. Cytologic classification of renal cell carcinomas into well-, moderately, and poorly differentiated tumors has been found useful at Radiumhemmet. All poorly differentiated tumors are preferentially treated with radiotherapy.
2. Before infarction therapy by arterial occlusion, it is necessary to have a definitive morphologic diagnosis.[20]
3. Identification of benign lesions may forestall nephrectomy.

In this area, as in all others in the body, where a technique is available to atraumatically provide pretreatment information for the clinician, only sophistry and the imperative of vested interest can raise any objections.

Postoperative follow up should include careful palpation of the flank or abdominal incision. Implantation tumors may be detected quite early, and fine needle aspiration of the implantation site may yield a prompt diagnosis. Recurrent tumor in the flank is illustrated in the following case.

Case 6-13

The patient was a 58-year-old woman seen in the emergency room in a stuporous state. Two months previously, left nephrectomy was done for staghorn calculus that had been present for 15 years. The pathologic report was squamous carcinoma of the kidney. Studies revealed serum calcium to be 15 mg/dL. The patient was treated with intravenous isotonic saline and furosemide with gradual improvement. On examination and deep palpation of the left flank, an ill-defined palpable mass could be detected. Fine needle aspiration utilizing a 22-gauge, 7-cm needle with stylet was done, and squamous carcinoma was extracted. Radiation therapy maintained a normal calcium level after it controlled the tumor.

Summary

The primary physician will find that the abdomen and its contents are a fruitful source of diagnostic data. The critical issue is that of clinical rather than technological diagnosis. This is achieved by careful history and searching physical examination, which will often reveal a target for fine needle aspiration. Having discovered the target, immediate sampling should be done or the patient should be referred for the procedure before ordering x-rays, sonograms, and scans. Overcoming inhibitions to the direct puncture of the abdominal wall may require some instruction and a good deal of patience together with sound clinical judgment.

All nonpalpable masses revealed by a variety of imaging techniques can be punctured as easily as palpable masses. For the most part, the radiologist must be relied upon to carry out the procedure or to direct the clinician. Modern imaging techniques markedly reduce the expected difficulties in reaching a remote lesion.

REFERENCES

1. Antler AS, Ough Y, Pitchumoni CS et al: Gastrointestinal metastasis from malignant tumors of the lung. Cancer 49:170, 1982
2. Beazley RM: Needle biopsy diagnosis of pancreatic cancer. Cancer 47:1685, 1981
3. Bernardino ME, Barnes PA: Imaging the pancreatic neoplasm. Cancer 50:2681, 1982
4. Bernardino ME, Lewis E: Imaging hepatic neoplasms. Cancer 51:2666, 1982
5. Berger L, Sinkoff MW: Systemic manifestations of hypernephroma. Am J Med 22:791, 1957
6. Bottinger LE: Fever in carcinoma of the kidney. Acta Med Scand 156:477, 1958
7. Cancer statistics, 1980. CA 30:24, 1980
8. Cedermark BJ et al: The value of liver scan in the follow-up of patients with adenocarcinoma of the colon and rectum. Surg Gynecol Obstet 144:745, 1977
9. Chen DS, Jung JL: Serum alpha-feto protein in hepatocellular carcinoma. Cancer 40:779, 1977
10. Chisholm GD: Nephrogenic ridge tumors and their syndromes. Ann NY Acad Sci 230:403, 1974
11. Chisholm GD: Paraneoplastic syndromes: Introduction. In Küss R, Murphy GP, Khoury S et al (eds): Renal Tumors, pp 277–282. Paris, Alan R Liss, 1981
12. Chlebowski RT, Tong M, Weissman J et al: Hepatocellular carcinoma: Diagnostic and prognostic features in North American patients. Cancer 53:2701, 1984
13. Geddes EW, Faulkson G: Differential diagnosis of primary malignant hepatoma in 569 Bantu mineworkers. Cancer 31:1216, 1973
14. Göthlin JH: Post-lymphographic percutaneous fine needle biopsy of lymph nodes guided by fluoroscopy. Radiology 120:205, 1976
15. Ho CS, McLaughlin MJ, McHattie J et al: Percutaneous fine needle aspiration of the pancreas following endoscopic retrograde cholangiopancreatography. Radiology 125:351, 1977
16. Ho CS, McLaughlin MJ, Tao LC et al: Guided percutaneous fine-needle aspiration biopsy of the liver. Cancer 47:1781, 1981

17. Johansen P, Svedsen K: Scan guided fine needle aspiration biopsy in malignant hepatic disease. Acta Cytol 22:292, 1978

18. Johnson PM, Sweeney WA: The false positive hepatic scan. J Nucl Med 8:451, 1967

19. Katz RL, Shobhana P, Machary B et al: Fine needle aspiration cytology of the adrenal gland. Acta Cytol 28:260, 1984

20. Lalli AF, Peterson N, Bookstein JJ: Roentgen-guided infarction of kidney and lungs. Radiology 93:434, 1969

21. Lang FK: Roentgenographic assessment of asymptomatic renal lesions. Radiology 109:257, 1973

22. Laucks SP Jr, McLachlin MSF: Aging and simple cysts of the kidney. Br J Radiol 54:12, 1981

23. Lee Y, Tatter D: Carcinoma of the pancreas and periampullary structure. Arch Pathol Lab Med 108:584, 1984

24. Linsk JA, Franzen S: Aspiration cytology of metastatic hypernephroma. Acta Cytol 28:250, 1984

25. Linsk JA, Franzen S: Clinical Aspiration Cytology. Philadelphia, JB Lippincott, 1983

26. Lundquist A: Fine needle aspiration biopsy of the liver. Acta Med Scand (Suppl 520), 1971

27. Menghini G: One second biopsy of the liver: Problem of its clinical application. N Engl J Med 283:582, 1970

28. Mitty HA, Efremedis SC, Yeh H-C: Impact of fine-needle biopsy on management of patients with carcinoma of the pancreas. AJR 137:1119, 1981

29. Moertel CG: The liver. In Holland JF, Frei E III (eds): Cancer Medicine, pp 1541–1547. Philadelphia, Lea & Febiger, 1973

30. Moosa AR: Pancreatic cancer: Approach to diagnosis, selection for surgery and choice of operation. Cancer 50:2689, 1982

31. Mori W: Cirrhosis and primary cancer of the liver. Cancer 20:627, 1967

32. Pelaez JC, Hill MC, Dach JL et al: Abdominal aspiration biopsies with sonographic and computed tomographic guidance. JAMA 250:2663, 1983

33. Prando A, Wallace S, Von Eschenbuch AC et al: Lymphoangiography in staging carcinoma of the prostate. Radiology 131:641, 1979

34. Reuter SR: The current status of angiography in the evaluation of cancer patients. Cancer 37:532, 1976

35. Rosenblatt KR: The role of ultrasonography in the diagnosis of the renal mass and impaired renal function. JAMA 251:2561, 1984

36. Schwerk WB, Schmita-Moorman P: Ultrasonically guided fine-needle biopsies in neoplastic liver disease. Cancer 48:1469, 1981

37. Selroos O: Fine-needle aspiration biopsy of the spleen in diagnosis of sarcoidosis. Ann NY Acad Sci 278:517, 1976

38. Skinner DG, Calvin RB, Vermillan CD et al: Diagnosis and management of renal cell carcinoma. Cancer 28:1165, 1971

39. Söderström N: Fine-Needle Aspiration Biopsy. New York, Grune and Stratton, 1966

40. Söderström N: How to use cytodiagnostic spleen puncture. Acta Med Scand 199:1, 1976

41. Söderström N: Spleen. II. Cytology of infradiaphragmatic organs. In Weid GL (ed): Monographs in Clinical Cytology. Basel, S Karger, 1979

42. Stauffer MH: Nephrogenic hepatosplenomegaly (abstr). Gastroenterology 40:694, 1961
43. Stormby N, Akerman M: Aspiration cytology in the diagnosis of granulomatous liver lesions. Acta Cytol 17:200, 1973
44. Tao LC, Ho CS, McLaughlin MG et al: Cytologic diagnosis of hepatocellular carcinoma by fine-needle aspiration biopsy. Cancer 53:547, 1984
45. Tempero MA, Peterson RJ, Zetterman RK et al: Detection of metastatic liver disease. JAMA 284:1329, 1982
46. Tylen U, Arnesjö B, Lindberg LG et al: Percutaneous biopsy of carcinoma of the pancreas guided by angiography. Surg Gynecol Obstet 142:737, 1976
47. Waldman TA, McIntire KR: The use of a radioimmunoassay for alpha-feto protein in the diagnosis of malignancy. Cancer 34:1510, 1974
48. Wallace S, Jing B, Zornoza J: Lymphangiography in the detection of the extent of metastatic carcinoma. Cancer 39:706, 1977
49. Wermgrad DN, DeCosse JJ, Sherlock P et al: Primary gastrointestinal lymphoma. Cancer 49:1258, 1982
50. World Health Organization: Groups on prevention and control of hepatocellular carcinoma, Zuckerman AJ, chairman. Lancet 1:463, 1983
51. Zajicek J: Aspiration Biopsy Cytology. Cytology of Infradiaphragmatic Organs. Basel, S Karger, 1979
52. Zornoza J: Abdomen. In Zornoza J (ed): Percutaneous Needle Biopsy. Baltimore, Williams & Wilkins, 1981

Lesions of the Pelvis: Transrectal and Transvaginal Aspirations 7

The small pelvis can be visualized as a bony cylinder, the entrance of which is bounded by the pubic and ischial bones and the sacrum and coccyx. The iliac bones complete the cylinder. The organs within the cylinder open caudally by means of the rectum and anus in men and women and the vagina in women. With the patient in a relaxed position, preferably lying supine, with legs up and the sacrum flattened against the table, it is possible to palpate in a sweeping manner far laterally, posteriorly in the sacral hollow, and anteriorly to include the prostate in men and the anterior vaginal wall and bladder in women. The cervix is palpable vaginally. Rectally it may be mistaken for a tumor. Where the finger can distinctly palpate a nodular or indurated area, a specific target for fine needle aspiration becomes apparent. This is illustrated in case 7-1.

Case 7-1

This patient was a 73-year-old woman seen for the first time 6 months after an abdominoperineal resection, complaining of gradual onset of burning pain in the perineum.

On examination, the liver was not enlarged and no abdominal masses were palpable. Her colostomy was functioning well with no evident local induration or palpable mass on intrastomal palpation. Attention was then directed to the perineum. There were no external nodules and no masses could be palpated on deep pressure into the perineal tissues.

Deep transvaginal examination revealed a palpable mass fixed in the right presacral space. Transvaginal aspiration was carried out (Fig. 7-1) utilizing a one-handed syringe and a Franzen needle guide. Smears diagnostic of adenocarcinoma were obtained. The patient underwent radiation, with symptomatic relief.

COMMENT This case stresses the importance of focused physical examination in solving a clinical problem. Clinical judgment indicates persuasively where the pathology must be. Persistent physical examination—often by more than one observer—should be done before turning to technologic aids (see Case 7-7).

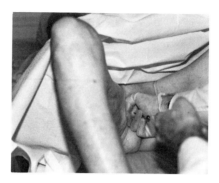

FIGURE 7-1: The palpable target is initially located; then the needle guide is fitted, and the index finger is placed as high on the mass as possible. The syringe with the needle attached is then inserted and the aspiration is done. (See Chap. 1.)

Diffuse or somewhat vague induration which may be present postoperatively or postirradiation is sampled by a series of fanlike aspirations, as described by Sevin[19] (see below).

The pelvic and rectal examination is or should be part of any general examination. In an informal study of patients examined in a community hospital, it was noted that more than 90% of patients (excluding those admitted by proctologists and gynecologists) did not have rectal and pelvic examinations as part of the initial evaluation. Some patients had been examined before admission, but it was quite apparent that many patients were not examined fully. The ready availability of fine needle aspiration as a tool might encourage clinicians to pursue routine examination of the pelvic contents more diligently.

The Examination

History

History of disease in the pelvis or of malignancy in an extrapelvic site should be reviewed. Disorders that indicate potential pelvic masses are summarized in Table 7-1. If the clinician notes the historic factors listed in Table 7-1, he will perform a more searching examination of the perineum, pelvis, and rectum.

Inspection and Palpation

Examination of the pelvis and its contents, as with all portions of the body, begins with inspection. In patients with abdominoperineal resection, the anal crease, perineum, and buttocks are examined for local scar infiltration

TABLE 7-1: Disorders Predisposing to or Indicating Potential Pelvic Masses

Disorder	Potential Pelvic Mass
Breast carcinoma	Ovarian metastases
Gastric carcinoma	Krukenberg tumor
Extrapelvic Hodgkin's and non-Hodgkin's lymphoma	Nodal masses
Colon carcinoma	Pelvic mass
	Krukenberg tumor
	Presacral mass
Abdominoperineal resection	Incisional or perineal recurrence
Bladder carcinoma	Primary tumor mass
	Recurrent tumor mass
	Postirradiation induration
Endometrial carcinoma	
Pretreatment	Primary tumor mass
Posthysterectomy	Presacral mass
Bright rectal bleeding	Anal or rectal mass
Urinary obstruction	Prostatic and cervical carcinoma
Dysmenorrhea and dyspareunia	Endometriosis
Abnormal vaginal bleeding	Uterine and ovarian mass
Constant back or leg pains	Prostate carcinoma
Hypercalcemia	Ovarian, prostate, or cervical carcinoma

or asymmetric bulges. Similarly, enlargement of one labia may be noted. The inguinal region (which also is dealt with in Chapter 8) may reveal hernias, lymph nodes, and aneurysms. Aspiration, of course, must be applied judiciously with reliance on clinical judgment.

Palpation of all scars is important. Running the tips of the fingers along a linear scar will detect small early elevations. Suture granulomas or unresolved thickening at the site of sutures may be confused with implanted tumor. Fine needle aspiration easily distinguishes the two possibilities. This is illustrated in the following case.

Case 7-2

The patient was a 62-year-old man treated for rectal carcinoma by abdominoperineal (AP) resection 9 months before he was seen in the oncology clinic. Deep sacral pain occurred 5 months after surgery, and a mass that was eroding the sacrum was detected radiographically. Pain was relieved by radiation. He now was having difficulty sitting. On examination, two nodules were palpated in the anal crease. Fine needle aspiration of the anterior nodule yielded chronic granulomatous material consistent with a suture granuloma. However, aspiration of the posterior nodule yielded adenocarcinoma.

Both nodules were excised for palliative relief, and the patient remained under observation.

COMMENT Although surgical biopsy would have been done to solve this problem, preoperative diagnosis in this and other cases helps guide the surgeon in the extent of his procedure.

Pelvic recurrences after abdominoperineal resection have been reported in over 50% of cases[21] and are often announced by onset of deep aching perineal pain, as in Cases 7-1 and 7-2. In contrast to the above, recurrence may be detected by palpation of smooth, deep, usually tender perineal induration.

The labia, particularly if one is enlarged, should be palpated. Bartholin's gland abscess or cyst should be distinguished from tumor[5] preoperatively to allow proper therapy. This is accomplished with fine needle aspiration.

After irradiation, there may be induration of the suprapubic tissues, sometimes with a suspicious firm ledge. In patients with irradiated endometrial or bladder cancer, the ledge cannot be distinguished from carcinoma invading the body wall. Radiation after surgery for colon carcinoma that was found to have extended to the body wall may also result in deceptive induration. This is illustrated in Case 7-3.

Case 7-3

The patient was a 58-year-old auditor who was referrred for chemotherapy of metastatic colon carcinoma. He was well up to 6 months before when he developed cramping accompanied by intermittent constipation. Barium enema revealed a constricting lesion in the sigmoid colon. Resection was performed to palliate the symptoms even though extensive tumor was invading the mesentery. Pathologic examination revealed infiltration of the tumor through the wall of the bowel extending into the root of the mesentery, a wedge of which was removed. Four nodes were positive. Following surgery, radiation (4000 rads) was delivered to the tumor site. Three months after irradiation, the patient complained of persistent discomfort and occasional pain at the surgical and radiation site. Computed tomography (CT) scan (Fig. 7-2) revealed a mass involving the abdominal wall. A radiologic diagnosis of "tumor invading the lower anterior wall" was rendered and confirmed in discussion with the radiologist.

On examination, there was densely infiltrated tissue running parallel to the surgical scar. The edges could be defined clearly and the mass was in clear contrast to the surrounding soft abdominal wall tissue.

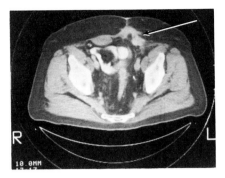

FIGURE 7-2: Note the smooth contour of the cross section of the rectus muscle on the right (*R*) compared to the distorted muscle on the left (*L; arrow*). This change was secondary to radiation and surgery.

Fine needle aspiration was done in several sites. The tissue was dense and the cytologic yield consisted of tissue fluid and a few fibrocytes. The cytologic diagnosis was "scar tissue secondary to surgery and radiation."

Two months later, the patient was admitted for a small bowel obstruction. At surgery, there were adhesions and one focus of carcinoma involving the serosa of the appendix. Generous biopsies of the pelvic abdominal wall revealed only dense collagenized tissue without tumor cells.

COMMENT The CT scan was a false-positive.

Intrapelvic palpable masses may become targets for transabdominal wall puncture in the same manner as other abdominal masses. Deep palpation above the inguinal ligament, along the path of the iliac vessels, and within the pelvic brim may yield palpable targets. However, muscle bundles palpable within the pelvic brim may simulate tumor. Asymmetry is an important differential feature.

The Anus and Rectum

The anal verge should be palpated carefully to detect early carcinoma or basaloid tumors that can be mistaken for external hemorrhoids or fibrotic nodules. The anal canal should be palpated for areas of induration. Basaloid (small cell) tumors made up 35% of a series of anal carcinomas.[1] This is a highly malignant tumor with frequent systemic metastases, and early diagnosis is useful.

On digitally entering the rectum, the most neglected region is the posterior wall and presacral space. Sarcoma, lymphoma, chordoma, and recurrent carcinoma, particularly colonic, may present with a smooth, easily missed bulge.

Figure 7-3 illustrates an x-ray film in which the definitive diagnosis was presacral mass displacing the rectum forward in a patient with known prior colon carcinoma. However, on careful palpation the posterior rectal wall could easily be pressed against the sacrum. No mass was palpated. At subsequent laparotomy (see Case 7-3) no tumor was present in the pelvis. This is a false-positive x-ray diagnosis.

In contrast, digital examination of the rectum failed to palpate a large presacral mass (Fig. 7-4) because attention was focused on the prostate and anterior rectal wall. The mass, which was fairly soft, was subsequently aspirated. The smears contained several large, primitive, unidentified tumor cells with extensive surrounding necrosis. The surgical pathology was anaplastic chordoma.[10]

Gross nodular enlargement should be detected easily. Induration of the rectal wall is often present postirradiation, and poses the familiar problem of distinguishing tumor and fibrous tissue. Fine needle aspiration is usually decisive.

Carcinoma of the anus is illustrated in Case 7-4.

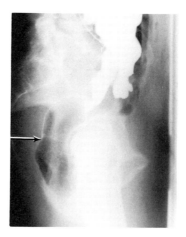

FIGURE 7-3: The air-filled rectum is placed forward suggesting a retrorectal mass (*arrow*). The area was normal to palpation and no mass was present at surgery.

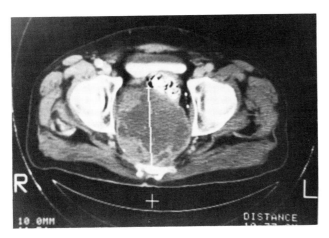

FIGURE 7-4: There is a huge, soft presacral mass (AP diameter indicated by vertical marker) that was not noticed on digital examination of the rectum. Transrectal aspiration yielded necrosis, and puncture yielded tumor cells. The histologic finding was anaplastic chordoma.

Case 7-4

The patient was a 63-year-old woman treated for an anal fissure and hemorrhoids with local applications for several months. She then medicated herself for 2 more months. She had persistently rejected surgery.

On examination, a cauliflower, superficially necrotic mass could be visualized easily (Fig. 7-5). On palpation, the mass was found to extend under intact skin. Fine needle aspiration was done through intact skin, yielding smears with abundant cellularity diagnostic of squamous carcinoma (Fig. 7-6). Confronted with the diagnosis, the patient then consented to definitive therapy.

Transrectal palpation of Blumer's shelf is an extremely important maneuver in that it demonstrates pelvic metastases from a suspected primary site, often in the upper abdomen (stomach, pancreas). Transrectal fine needle aspiration will confirm the diagnosis (see Case 7-6).

Gynecologic Disorders

It is fairly apparent that a gynecologic specialist would have little difficulty detecting vaginal and pelvic abnormalities. However, for the general clinician awareness of potential palpable disease and the possibility of immediate diagnosis with fine needle aspiration is useful.

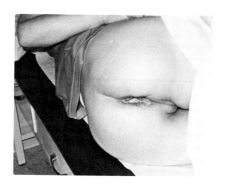

FIGURE 7-5: Infiltrated granular tissue is visible at the anal verge.

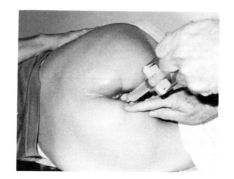

FIGURE 7-6: To avoid the necrotic portion of the tumor, the needle is inserted into intact skin where tumor has infiltrated. An abundant cell yield was obtained. The cytologic finding was carcinoma.

The cervix may be confused with tumor, particularly where examination of the pelvic organs has not been carried out routinely (see above). Historic factors are important. Where a patient reports hysterectomy in the past, the date may be useful. Before 1950, supracervical hysterectomy was a common procedure, leaving the cervix as a potentially confusing rectal mass. Where a mass is palpated through the anterior rectal wall after total abdominal hysterectomy, of course, tumor must be suspected. The first question then must be concerned with the reason for the hysterectomy—for example, fibroids versus endometrial carcinoma versus ovarian carcinoma. Such historic factors are not always readily available, depending on the patient population.

In the pelvic examination, vaginal nodules and subvaginal masses may be missed if they are not sought. Palpation of the vaginal wall after total abdominal hysterectomy may reveal asymmetries, which can be clarified by judicious fine needle aspiration. Exfoliation of cancer cells with resulting positive Papanicolaou smears requires permeation and penetration of the epithelial layer. Submucosal tumor cannot be detected by exfoliative studies. Hypernephroma metastatic to the vaginal wall has been diagnosed by fine needle aspiration.[13]

Again, historic factors must be considered, including symptoms of endometriosis, prior pelvic organ carcinoma, and genitourinary or rectal carcinoma.

The bimanual examination requires that the patient be relaxed and cooperative. Examination under anesthesia is not unusual in gynecologic departments. From the standpoint of fine needle aspiration, gross identification of an enlarged uterus, which is most often due to leiomyomas, is not the main goal. Similarly, cystic masses confirmed by ultrasonography require immediate surgery, and fine needle aspiration usually is contraindicated. In the relaxed patient, induration may be palpated, often laterally, and such palpable targets may yield useful cytology. The clinical context is often that of a postoperative or postirradiation status[19] (see above).

Bladder Palpation

Transvaginal and transrectal bimanual examination is also important in evaluating bladder lesions, both before and after surgery or radiation. Cystoscopic biopsy may yield superficial tissues with inflammatory or radiation alterations, and may miss the penetration of the vesical wall by tumor. Anterior palpation may define induration, which can be reached by fine needle aspiration. Clinical staging, associated with a 50% error, can only be improved with the use of fine needle aspiration.[17]

Enlargement of One Leg

Enlarged nodes in the inguinal and femoral region are considered in Chapter 8. However, a common problem encountered by the oncologist as well as the general physician is enlargement of one or both legs with unknown cause. Careful lateral transvaginal and transrectal palpation may detect enlarged, often indurated, nodes capable of producing pressure on venous or lymphatic channels. Direct invasion of a vein by a pelvic primary or metastatic tumor, resulting in clot formation and stasis, also occurs. Such tumor masses may be detectable by palpation. Failure to detect an obstructive lesion on initial examination should be followed by venogram, which can indicate whether the blockage is intraluminal or extraluminal. Following this examination, palpation should again be attempted to find a possible target for fine needle aspiration. Where an intraluminal venous blockage is detected and anticoagulation is contemplated, invasive procedures should be done first. Palpation of the prostate is discussed later in the chapter.

Fine Needle Aspiration of Pelvic Targets

External Targets

All palpable external pelvic targets can be reached by a fine needle, and most will yield a definitive diagnosis. This eliminates the need for surgical biopsy, or guides the surgeon in his approach both to biopsy and excisional therapy.

Nodules within scars or in subcutaneous or exposed submucosal sites (introitus, anal verge) are aspirated in the routine fashion ultilizing 22-gauge or 25-gauge, 1-cm or 2-cm needles. Both Romanowsky's and Papanicolaou's stains are important to define lymphoid, renal, squamous, and other cytologic variants, which are best evaluated with one of these stains.

Identifiable lesions that are reached easily by a short (1-cm to 3-cm) needle are listed.

Pelvic Lesions Reached by Short Needles

Anal carcinoma
   Squamous (see Case 7-4)
   Basaloid
Labial and proximal vaginal masses
   Metastatic invasion[13,15]
   Primary squamous carcinoma
   Tumors of labial glands[5]
   Endometriotic nodules
Scar nodules
   Squamous carcinoma
   Adenocarcinoma (see Case 7-2)
   Poorly differentiated carcinoma
Suprapubic induration
   Tumor invasion
   Radiation (see Fig. 7-2 and Case 7-3)

Invasion of the pelvic walls, perineum, and buttocks may be reached with longer needles. Satisfactory results can be obtained with 5-cm to 9-cm, 22-gauge needles.

The onset of deep perineal pain with intrapelvic recurrence (see above) may prompt surgical biopsy with its associated morbidity. Puncture will yield excellent material, often mucinous carcinoma arising from colon carcinoma, in our experience.

Less common is asymmetry of the buttocks because of deep tumor proliferation. Metastatic masses are rare, but the buttocks may be the site of primary sarcoma of muscle and nerve tissue. Sacral chordoma also may enlarge a buttock. Puncture with a long needle may yield diagnostic material. Chordoma in particular is recognized easily by smears stained with Romanowsky. Buttock lesions may be surprisingly deep—for example, neurofibrosarcoma arising from deep nerve trunks and displacing normal muscle bundles. Use of computed tomography now should make it easy to reach such lesions.

Destructive lesions of the pelvic skeleton are dealt with in Chapter 10. However, tumors do break out of the bony structure to involve soft tissue and present as soft tissue masses. Palpation of masses above the inguinal ligaments, suprapubically along the iliac vessels, and within the pelvic brim are approached with 5-cm to 9-cm, 22-gauge needles containing a stylet. Palpation and puncture of such targets are made more difficult by an excess of body fat.

Intrapelvic Masses

Potential intrapelvic targets are palpable primary pelvic tumors arising in uterus, ovaries, fallopian tubes, and bladder (Table 7-2).[19] Transvaginal aspirations are discussed later. Metastatic and lymphomatous lymph nodes and subperitoneal deposits may become targets.

Lesions reached by longer (5-cm to 9-cm) needles are listed.

Lesions Reached by Longer Needles

Intraperineal targets
   Metastatic carcinoma
Buttock asymmetries and masses
   Sarcomas, chordoma
Intrapelvic masses (externally palpable)
   Metastatic nodes, primary tumors

OVARIAN MASSES

Concern has been expressed about puncture diagnosis of ovarian masses that unexpectedly turn out to be cystic.[3,7] Such a puncture potentially could disseminate cancer cells, although there are no data on this point. Nevertheless, all possible ovarian masses should be screened for fluid content by ultrasonography.

TABLE 7-2: Intrapelvic Targets

Gynecologic Targets	Nongynecologic Targets
BENIGN	Enlarged nodes
Leiomyomas—uterus	Metastatic carcinoma
Theocomas—ovaries	Lymphoma
Dermoid cyst—ovaries	Postlymphangiographic enlarged
Serous and mucinous cystadenomas—ovaries	nodes
	Gastrointestinal tumors
MALIGNANT	Primary sigmoid carcinoma
Carcinomas	Metastatic masses (see Table 7-1)
Cervical	Genitourinary tumors
Endometrial	Bladder carcinoma and sarcoma
Ovarian	
Serous and mucinous cystadenocarcinomas	
Uterine sarcomas	
Leiomyosarcoma	
Malignant mixed mesodermal tumor	
Endometrial stromal tumor	
Special ovarian tumors	
Germ cell tumors	
Granulosa cell tumors	

Solid masses are excellent targerts for puncture, but they should always be considered within a clinical context. Pre-existing or concurrent tumors that may produce ovarian masses simulating primary tumors include gastric, colonic, and breast carcinomas, carcinoid, and lymphomas.[15,20,22,23] Ovarian metastases were present in 8% of Willis' autopsy series of women with malignant disease.[23] The ovaries were the most common site of metastases to the female genital tract in a study by Mazur.[15] Knowledge of the primary neoplasm simplifies the cytologic interpretation.

The most common pelvic enlargement is the fibroid uterus. Careful gynecologic examination will identify this disorder in the appropriate clinical context (age, abnormal bleeding, no malignancy history) in almost all cases. However, problem cases do occur in which the gynecologist cannot identify the mass with assurance. This is illustrated in the following case.

Case 7-5

The patient was a 72-year-old woman presenting initially with a left pleural effusion and an obvious carcinoma that had distorted her left breast and invaded the axilla. The pleural fluid contained malignant cells. Fine needle aspiration of the breast that appeared to be permeated with tumor yielded characteristic ductal carcinoma. A wedge biopsy was done for estrogen receptors, which were strongly positive. The pleural effusion was treated with tube thoracostomy and tetracycline. The patient was treated with tamoxifen and combined chemotherapy utilizing cyclophosphamide, methotrexate and fluorouracil. The breast shrank progressively, with a virtual automastectomy (Fig. 7-7). The axillary tumor disappeared, leaving residual induration.

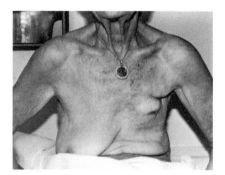

Figure 7-7: There is marked shrinkage of the breast. The nipple is still visible. The patient did not have a mastectomy. No tumor was present on aspiration of residual breast tissue.

One year later, there appeared to be no local tumor recurrence. Chemotherapy had been discontinued at 9 months. The patient was losing weight. On examination, a mass not previously noted could be palpated through a thin lower abdominal wall suprapubically. No mass had been noted during the initial examination 1 year previously. On bimanual examination, the mass had some physical characteristics of a fibroid uterus, but had atypical features. The strong presumption was that pelvic metastasis had occurred in a patient with initially far advanced local tumor. Fine needle aspiration was done transabdominally. The needle entered dense tissue with difficulty and extracted benign appearing fusiform muscle cells consistent with leiomyoma. The recent onset of diabetes accounted for the weight loss. The patient remained under observation with no further chemotherapy, but continued to receive tamoxifen.

COMMENT The usefulness of fine needle aspiration here is self-evident. The patient's diabetes was an important clinical clue.

Patients with ovarian carcinoma often are referred to major cancer centers for oncologic surgery after a laparotomy has been performed at a community hospital. Gynecologists may not be trained in oncologic surgery, which may require major debulking. A pelvic mass may be discovered by examination and defined in part by imaging techniques. Nevertheless, the separation not only of a uterine tumor but also of a colonic carcinoma from an ovarian mass may be difficult or impossible. Fine needle aspiration can often identify ovarian carcinoma, and then allow a rational choice of surgery depending on clinical factors such as size of the mass. Future management then may be discussed with the patient. Case 7-6 illustrates the problems of relying on indirect data.

Case 7-6

A 73-year-old woman complained of a cramping lower abdominal pain. Examination detected a pelvic mass, and a barium enema was requested. This demonstrated persistent narrowing of the sigmoid colon, which was interpreted as a primary infiltrating colon carcinoma. At surgery, the surgeon found the left colon entering into and bound down by a large mass that appeared to be an extensive locally invasive colon carcinoma. The area was deemed inoperable, but thickened omentum was detected and a portion was submitted for frozen section. Metastatic adenocarcinoma was diagnosed.

The surgeon told the patient that her disorder was incurable but that she possibly could benefit from chemotherapy. The oncologist reviewed the films from the barium enema with the radiologist. They concluded that the narrowing could be extraluminal. The pathologic findings then were reviewed, and the pathologist agreed that the omental metastases easily could have arisen from the ovary.

With ultrasonic guidance, a transabdominal puncture of the pelvic mass was done. It yielded smears consistent with ovarian carcinoma. The patient was referred to a gynecologic oncologist, who performed a major debulking procedure. At the initial procedure, preoperative or perioperative fine needle aspiration would have been appropriate.

The patient was placed in a chemotherapy program with good results.

COMMENT Although preoperative aspiration cytology will not always allow a distinction to be made between an ovarian and a gastrointestinal neoplasm, such differential diagnoses are often possible. From a clinical standpoint, it is more important to obtain as much preoperative data as possible than to speculate about the merits of the procedure. In the area of pelvic tumors, as illustrated in this case, and in all other areas, aspiration should be one of the initial diagnostic procedures.

Transvaginal Aspirations

Transvaginal aspiration is done utilizing the Franzen needle guide originally designed for prostate aspiration (see Fig. 7-1). The needle point can emerge from the guide as much as 2 cm (see Fig. 1-4). Following careful palpation, the needle can be introduced into lesions of the vaginal wall and the cervix. Cervical lesions, of course, usually are sampled by Pap-stained exfoliative smears, followed by surgical biopsy with or without colposcopy. Fine needle aspiration of the cervix has been done under two circumstances. A patient with a coagulation disorder (von Willebrand's disease) could not have a biopsy done surgically because of excessive bleeding. The cervix was markedly enlarged and appeared to be permeated by an invasive endocervical carcinoma, which could not be visualized. A fine needle was passed easily directly through the mucosa of the exocervix deep into the cervical tissue, and poorly differentiated squamous carcinoma was extracted.

An elderly woman with vaginal bleeding could be examined only with difficulty because of vaginal atrophy and synechiae. An irregular cervix could be palpated with one finger, and a more extensive examination would have required anesthesia. Exfoliative smears were unsatisfactory. Aspiration was done using the needle guide, and fairly well-differentiated squamous carcinoma was extracted.

Palpation beyond the vaginal canal may detect the targets listed previously in Table 7-2.

Experienced observers usually can distinguish these tumors cytologically,[6,19] but as always, cytologic diagnosis is rendered in conjunction with clinical considerations including the history, findings on physical examination, and the texture of the tumor as determined by the "feel" of the needle as it penetrates the mass.

The intravaginal palpating finger should press the vaginal wall against the potential target. The sigmoid colon drapes into the pelvis and is easy to puncture inadvertently. Obtaining fecal material on puncture appears to result in no ill effects. However, Sevin recommends prophylactic antibiotics.[19]

A major clinical problem is the evaluation of the postirradiation pelvis. Ill-defined indurated tissues may harbor infiltrating carcinoma. The problem is similar to that of the postirradiation breast (see Chap. 4). Sevin has approached this problem by carrying out a series of fanlike punctures under anesthesia.[19]

Transrectal Aspirations

Primary carcinoma of the rectum within reach of digital examination usually is diagnosed by direct visualization followed by surgical biopsy. Fine needle aspiration occasionally has been useful when an obvious tumor is necrotic and surgical biopsy fails to obtain satisfactory specimens. Deep penetration of the needle often will obtain diagnostic smears, and radiation therapy can proceed at once.

An unusual circumstance is penetration of a prostate carcinoma through Denonvilliers' fascia producing an exophytic, sometimes fungating, intrarectal tumor that is mistaken for a primary rectal carcinoma. The cytology is rather distinctive, and where there is any doubt fine needle aspiration should be done. We have seen two such cases, in one of which a surgeon was attempting an AP resection until he realized his error.

Transrectal aspiration of palpable intrapelvic masses is done in the same manner as transvaginal aspirations. The choice depends on the ease of reaching the mass.

Solution of a systemic clinical problem by transrectal aspiration is illustrated in Case 7-7.

Case 7-7

The patient was a 68-year-old man referred for evaluation of anemia and mild anorexia. He had lost 5 pounds in 2 months. Prior to the referral, complete blood count, chemistry profile, barium enema, and upper GI series had been reported normal and negative except for normochromic anemia with hemoglobin value of 10 g/dL and MCV of $92\mu m^3$. The red cells on smear were unremarkable. The negative studies suggested an extraluminal problem (see Chap. 6). No enlargement of the liver had been detected. A digital rectal examination was reported to show mild enlargement of the prostate and no rectal lesions.

Repeat examination was carried out. An extraluminal mass could be detected impinging on the high posterior rectal wall.

With the patient in a flexed position on his side, transrectal fine needle aspiration was done using the Franzen needle. Smears were obtained diagnostic of signet ring cell carcinoma metastatic to the retrorectal tissues. At this point, upper GI endoscopy was recommended. A fairly circumscribed superficial spreading carcinoma was detected, and a biopsy was done.

COMMENT This case stresses the importance of a searching reexamination of a patient who obviously has an undefined organic syndrome. Failure to palpate the mass would have resulted in a CT scan, which may well have failed to detect a small pelvic mass.

Failure to reach above the prostate in a patient with bright red rectal bleeding may miss a palpable exophytic tumor. Patients who have bright red bleeding deserve at least a deep digital rectal examination before referral to a subspecialist for endoscopic studies.

The Prostate

One of the major and still underutilized clinical diagnostic advances in medicine has been fine needle aspiration of the prostate gland. The significance of this advance is underscored by the following observations.

1.   With increasing life expectancy in the male, the incidence of carcinoma of the prostate will continue to rise. At present, unlike restriction of smoking in lung cancer or high-fiber diet in colon cancer, there is no evident prophylactic measure to be undertaken.

2.   Although many prostate cancers are incidental findings and many are indolent, it is now the third major cause of cancer death in males. Apart from that, the morbidity, discomfort, incapacitation, and expense caused by advanced disease is incalculable.

3.   Prostate cancer shares with breast carcinoma ready access to the lesion in large numbers of cases. In both cancers, a major failure is neglecting the examination during routine patient evaluation. Since the large majority of prostate cancers are in the putative posterior lobe, they are within easy reach of the digital examination. Any nodular alteration that can be palpated on simple digital examination can be aspirated and diagnosed.

4.   The cause of palpable findings in the prostate can only be surmised. The degree of accuracy in evaluating prostate induration varies from 50%

to 80% among skilled urologists.[4,9] Reliance on digital findings by the general clinician is a potentially serious error. Indurated highly suspicious glands can easily be due to chronic prostatitis. On the other hand, isolated nodules referred for aspiration on suspicion of cancer often have been found benign on several annual examinations and repeat aspirations.

5. Early localized prostate cancer will be detected only if patients are screened and if they consent to biopsy. Consent for fine needle aspiration is obtained readily, whereas urologists and patients are reluctant to proceed to core biopsy in borderline cases.[2] This is illustrated by the following case.

Case 7-8

A 45-year-old man was examined by an experienced urologist who palpated an indurated gland. He diagnosed chronic prostatitis, partially because of the patient's age, prescribed for it, and suggested a return visit but did not document the recommendation. The patient did not return. Six months later, the patient had a hernia repair, and a lymph node was removed from the inguinal region. The node was reported to contain adenocarcinoma of unkown origin. After 2 months of further investigation, he was seen by a second urologist who diagnosed prostatic cancer with a core biopsy. By this time, he had a positive bone scan. A large legal action was brought against the first urologist.

Several issues are raised by this case. Was it reasonable to assume that an indurated prostate in a 45-year-old man with burning urination was chronic prostatitis to be treated with antibiotics? If there was any suspicion at all, shouldn't a follow-up appointment have been documented? Should all patients with clinical chronic prostatitis have a biopsy to rule out cancer? Why didn't the general surgeon who did the hernia repair palpate and identify an abnormal prostate as part of his routine presurgical examination? Why wasn't the prostate promptly investigated on finding the metastatic inguinal node?

Fine needle aspiration, which is a rapid, inexpensive, outpatient procedure, answers several of these questions. Where the biopsy is conveniently available, as at the Karolinska and other hospitals in the Stockholm area, it is done frequently and a significant number of benign aspirates are obtained. Where the biopsy is done infrequently, cases are usually selected and only those suspicious for cancer are referred for biopsy. This method is clearly not a screening technique, but it is probably valid that patients with a low level of clinical suspicion of cancer are better biopsied than observed. As with all aspects of the aspiration biopsy method, clinical judgment is paramount and it improves with experience. The judgment of the urologist in Case 7-8 has been altered by experience. It has been recommended that patients in the older age group with palpably normal prostates should undergo biopsy because of the rising incidence of the disease.[25] This is an unsettled question. A 45-year-old man with an indurated, nontender prostate falls into the group with low suspicion of cancer. Clinical judgment must dictate how decisively a follow-up appointment should be arranged. However, it must be stressed that when the prostate is tender or exhibits other evidence of acute inflammation, needle biopsy is contraindicated because of the possibility of sepsis.

On the question of failure of the general surgeon to examine the prostate prior to a hernia repair, it unfortunately may represent a norm in modern practice that must be corrected. Basic examinations clearly have been downgraded in the face of demands on time and the attractions of technology.

Metastatic inguinal nodes rarely originate in the prostate gland unless the case is well advanced. The normal pathway of the prostate lymphatic drainage is to the iliac nodes. Blockage of these pathways will result in spread to inguinal nodes.

Nine patients with prostatic carcinoma presenting as metastatic cancer of unknown origin have been reported.[24] None of the metastases was in inguinal nodes. Prostate enlargement was detected in five of the nine patients. None of the patients had prostatic biopsies (tissue biopsies) until after extensive workup, including lymph node and lung biopsies with acid phosphatase stains. Based on current experience, it is reasonable to suggest that all nine patients should have had a fine needle biopsy of the prostate as one of the initial studies. It would have afforded a high likelihood of establishing an early diagnosis and forestalling many expensive, uncomfortable, and time-consuming studies. It may be added that the metastatic lesions also could have been sampled with a fine needle.

THE CLINICAL APPLICATION OF
FINE NEEDLE ASPIRATION OF THE PROSTATE

Patients become subjects for fine needle aspiration of the prostate after discovery of a suspicious lesion or in the presence of metastatic disease of unknown origin, as discussed above.

The patient is apprised of the possibility of aspiration, and the procedure is explained and questions are answered. The potentialities of a positive diagnosis also may be discussed. In office practice, it is useful to demonstrate the needle guide and show that the long needle emerges only 1 cm or 1.5 cm from the end of the guide (see Fig 1-4).

Two approaches have been used to carry out the procedure. In office practice, the patient drops his trousers and underwear, stands on a small stool, flexes his body over the examining table, and rests on his elbows. The procedure then is done as discussed below as a routine digital rectal examination. In office practice, this has the virtue of minimal preparation and, for the most part, no need of assistants. In a busy practice, it may take 5 minutes to do the puncture and make the smears.

The other approach occurs in clinic practice (Karolinska Hospital). The patient lies on his back with his legs up in stirrups (Fig. 7-8). Either the patient or an assistant elevates the external genitalia, and the puncture is carried out as illustrated.

Some clinical hints are useful. Ample lubricant must be used. The fingertip should extend beyond the proposed point of puncture,[12] since the needle emerges behind the fingertip and enters the target about 0.5 cm proximal to the fingertip.

An attempt should be made to introduce the needle precisely into the nodule or indurated area. Several repeat aspirations may be necessary. Where both lobes are indurated, they both should be punctured.

Occasionally, the prostate is massive and rounded, and the needle may enter it tangentially and yield rectal mucosa. If the needle extends too high laterally, it may puncture the seminal vesicles, yielding a fairly characteristic smear that less experienced cytologists may mistake for malignancy.

In office practice, it is useful to stain and review the smears at once, if possible, to be sure the needle has been placed satisfactorily and adequate smears made as well as to advise the patient of the diagnosis where that is appropriate.

In the original reports of the fine needle method, Romanowsky's stain was used. Papanicolaou's stain should be prepared also if enough material is available.

As a rule, patients do not complain about repeat punctures, but they may.

The major complication is sepsis, which is rare. It is avoided for the most part if acute prostatitis is not punctured. Rarely, urethral bleeding

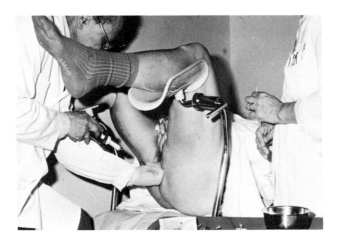

FIGURE 7-8: Transrectal aspiration of the prostate. The patient's legs are in firm stirrups, and he holds his genitalia. The operator has excellent control.

may occur. It may be an indication of increased vascularity, and the surgeon should be alerted.

Prophylactic antibiotics have not been necessary in our experience, although there are some who use them. It may be an important concern in the immunocompromised patient.

The instrumentation and method of use have been described else-where,[12] but will be repeated here. The instruments consist of a one-hand syringe and needle guide and a long, 22-gauge needle (see Fig. 1-2). The needle guide is placed over the gloved finger (see Fig. 1-3), and then is fixed in place by a finger cot.

Normally, the target has been palpated previously. However, we have found that when referral has been made by an experienced observer, and particularly if the referral is accompanied, as it should be, by a note with a small drawing, then a preliminary digital examination is not necessary. This reduces the annoyance that the patient must endure.

The finger and needle guide are inserted, and the target area is iden-tified. The finger should extend beyond the palpable lesion, allowing the needle to enter it. Figure 7-9 schematically illustrates the puncture.

The needle, first checked for patency while attached to a one-hand syringe, is inserted through the guide. The lesion is penetrated, full suction is applied, the needle tip is oscillated briefly, suction is released, and the needle and the guide are withdrawn.

To avoid drying, the needle is separated immediately and the material is expelled on a glass slide before taking time to remove the guide and glove. Alternatively, a trained assistant may make the smears. There may not be sufficient material for both Romanowsky and Papanicolaou smears,

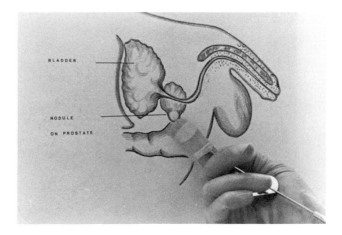

FIGURE 7-9: Schematic diagram of prostate aspiration. The fingertip should extend above the nodule to allow the un-derlying needle to enter the target.

and the choice may be left to the cytologist. The advantage of the Diff-Quik (Romanowsky's) stain is a 20-second preparation, which allows immediate examination and repeat aspiration if necessary. This depends on the ability of the aspirating physician to read the smears. A variety of arrangements can be made with the cytopathologist and the patient with respect to microscopic diagnosis and speed of reporting. As with the breast and other areas, the procedure generates a fair amount of anxiety, and patients are extremely grateful for prompt reporting.

PITFALLS IN THE FINE NEEDLE ASPIRATION METHOD

1. The prostate for purposes of aspiration biopsy cytology is divided schematically into five lobes.[8,14] The posterior lobe, which backs up intimately against the rectal mucosa (separated by Denonvilliers' fascia; see above), is the repository of the great majority of carcinomas. Suprapubic prostatectomy leaves this fertile source of neoplastic change. Palpable nodules and localized or generalized induration usually mean disease in the posterior lobe. However, a definite number of carcinomas are found in the lateral and anterior portions (lobes) of the gland and may be missed by the needle.
2. The palpating finger may cover the localized target and the needle will enter a surrounding benign area.
3. Lateral placement of the needle may result in puncture of the seminal vesicle, producing atypical smears.
4. The cytologist may overread an atypical hyperplasia as cancer.
5. The cytologist may fail to distinguish transitional carcinoma (arising from the urethra or bladder and penetrating the gland or arising in the gland) from prostatic carcinoma, and hormonal manipulation may inappropriately follow.
6. The cytologist may fail to recognize metastatic invasion of the prostate.
7. The report may convey a benign diagnosis with finality, rather than indicating the possibility that cancer could have been missed by the needle.

These pitfalls are corrected by increasing the experience of the aspirator and the cytologist. However, most important is the application of clinical data, clinical judgments, and good clinical habits (see Case 7-8), without which the entire method fails.[11]

The diagnostic schema for prostatic nodules, masses, and indurations is presented in Figure 7-10.

Nonpalpable Targets

The major nonpalpable targets are enlarged lymph nodes, which most usually are metastatic from the cervix or the prostate, but potentially from any pelvic organ. Such nodes may be impalpable but can be demonstrated

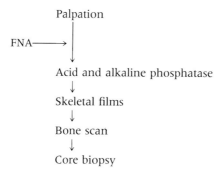

Comment: Prompt diagnosis by FNA eliminates core biopsy. Other ancillary studies are related to staging, but are sometimes done before the diagnosis of prostatic carcinoma is established in an effort to obtain indirect evidence. Computed tomography and lymphangiography may be used for staging, after primary diagnosis is established, and may provide further targets for FNA.

FIGURE 7-10: Diagnostic schema for prostatic nodules or masses.

by lymphangiography,[16,18] CT scan, and ultrasonography. Nodes opacified by lymphangiography are aspirated easily under fluoroscopy where the advancing needle is seen. In addition, lymphomatous nodes in the pelvis, although illuminated by lymphangiography, may not provide a sufficiently characteristic x-ray pattern to allow restaging. For example, clinical stage I Hodgkin's disease may be converted to stage III by the x-ray pattern of a lymphangiogram. On the other hand, fine needle aspiration may be necessary to confirm an inconclusive x-ray picture.

The technique of ultrasonography allows identification of many pelvic masses that may not be palpable on routine examination. Some of these masses may become palpable if the examination is done by an experienced gynecologist or possibly under anesthesia. Nevertheless, suspicious masses seen on a sonogram may be punctured with guidance by the ultrasonographer. Gynecologists, oncologists, or radiologists may become skilled in carrying out this procedure. The pelvic skeleton is dealt with in Chapter 10.

Summary

The concept of the generic "tumor" (see Chap. 1) applies strongly to the pelvis, which is a crossroads for primary and metastatic tumors. This is emphasized by the diversity of tissue types, including epithelial and mesenchymal, and the number of systems that are present, including gastrointestinal, urinary, and genital. As a result, definitive diagnosis by purely clinical techniques is difficult. Reliance cannot be placed on indirect data.

Fine needle aspiration, while not providing 100% sensitivity or specificity, is more than a useful adjuvant method in defining the pathology with no loss of time, little expense, and virtually no morbidity.

REFERENCES

1. Bowman BM, Moertel CG, O'Connell MJ et al: Carcinoma of the anal canal. Cancer 54:114, 1974
2. Chodak GW, Schoenberg, HW: Early detection of prostate cancer by routine screening. JAMA 252:3261, 1984
3. Christoferson WW: Cytologic detection and diagnosis of cancer: Its contributions and limitations. Cancer 51:1201, 1983
4. Esposti PL: Aspiration Biopsy Cytology in the Diagnosis and Management of Prostate Carcinoma. Stockholm, Stahl, Accidens, Tryck, 1974
5. Frable WJ, Goplerud DR: Adenoid cystic carcinoma of Bartholin's gland: Diagnosis by aspiration biopsy. Acta Cytol 19:152, 1975
6. Ganjei P, Nadji M: Aspiration cytology of ovarian neoplasms: A review. Acta Cytol 28:329, 1984
7. Hadju SI, Melamed MR: Limitations of aspiration cytology in the diagnosis of primary neoplasms. Acta Cytol 28:237, 1984
8. Ham AW, Cormack DH: Histology, 8th ed. Philadelphia, JB Lippincott, 1979
9. Jewett AJ: Significance of the palpable prostatic nodule. JAMA 160:838, 1956
10. Kaiser TE, Pritchard DJ, Krishnau KU: Clinicopathologic study of sacrococcygeal chordoma. Cancer 54:2574, 1984
11. Linsk JA, Axilrod HD, Solyn R et al: Transrectal cytologic aspiration in the diagnosis of prostatic carcinoma. J Urol 108:455, 1972
12. Linsk JA, Franzen S: Aspiration biopsy cytology of the prostate gland. In Linsk JA, Franzen S (eds): Clinical Aspiration Cytology, pp 243–266. Philadelphia, JB Lippincott, 1983
13. Linsk JA, Franzen S: Aspiration cytology of metastatic hypernephroma. Acta Cytol 28:250, 1984
14. Lowsley OS: The development of the human prostate gland with reference to the development of other structures of the neck of the urinary bladder. Am J Anat 13:299, 1972
15. Mazur MT, Hsueh J, Gersell D: Metastasis to the female genital tract. Cancer 53:1978, 1984
16. Mennemeyer R, Bartha M, Kidd CR: Diagnostic cytology and electron microscopy of fine needle aspirates of retroperitoneal lymph nodes in the diagnosis of metastatic pelvic neoplasms. Acta Cytol 23:370, 1979
17. Paulson DF, Perez CA, Anderson T: Genito-urinary malignancies. In DeVita VT Jr, Hellman S, Rosenberg SA (eds): Cancer: Principles and Practice of Oncology, pp 732–787. Philadelphia, JB Lippincott, 1982
18. Prando A, Wallace S, Van Eschenbush AC et al: A lymphangiography in staging carcinoma of the prostate. Radiology 131:641, 1979
19. Sevin B-U, Nadji M: Pelvic fine-needle aspiration cytology in gynecology. In Linsk JA, Franzen S (eds): Clinical Aspiration Cytology, pp 221–242. Philadelphia, JB Lippincott Co, 1983

20. Ulbright TM, Roth LM, Stehman FB: Secondary ovarian neoplasia: A clinicopathologic study of 35 cases. Cancer 53:1164, 1984

21. Villalon AH, Green D: The use of radiotherapy for pelvic recurrence following abdominoperineal resection for carcinoma of the rectum: A 10 year experience. Aust NZ J Surg 51:149, 1981

22. Warren S, Macomber WB: Tumor metastasis. VI: Ovarian metastasis of carcinoma. Arch Pathol 19:75, 1935

23. Willis RA: The Spread of Tumours in the Human Body, 3rd ed. Sevenoaks, England, Butterworths, 1973

24. Yam LT, Winkler CF, Janckila BS et al: Prostatic cancer presenting as metastatic carcinoma of undetermined origin: Immunodiagnosis by prostatic acid phosphatase. Cancer 51:283, 1983

25. Zinke H, Campbell JT, Utz DC et al: Confidence in the negative transrectal needle biopsy. Surg Gynecol Obstet 136:78, 1973

The Enlarged Lymph Node   8

Lymph node enlargement is one of the cardinal objective findings in the broad spectrum of medical and surgical disease. Primary central nervous system lesions and vascular, degenerative, and metabolic disorders ordinarily will not produce lymph node enlargement. Almost all other inflammatory and neoplastic diseases carry the potential for regional, distant, or multicentric lymph node enlargement. Although nodes may be involved without associated enlargement (*e.g.*, subcapsular lymph node metastases in mastectomy axillary specimens), they do not ordinarily become targets for fine needle aspiration because they are not palpable. This is one of the limitations of the method.

The enlarged node is a prime target for fine needle aspiration (Fig. 8-1). Clinical evaluation precedes a puncture and very often will predict the cytologic yield. The importance of clinical context is illustrated in the following examples.

1. Enlarged, hard, fixed axillary nodes draining a breast carcinoma should yield carcinoma cells on aspiration.
2. Bilateral palpable posterior cervical nodes in a patient with scalp inflammation should provide a picture of reactive lymphadenitis.
3. Large, rubbery, confluent femoral nodes in a patient with biopsy-proven Hodgkin's disease above the diaphragm can be expected to yield a typical cytological picture of Hodgkin's, resulting in stage III.
4. Firm-to-hard discrete right inguinal nodes in a patient with a prior excision of a level III pigmented melanoma below the knee of the right leg should yield pigmented tumor cells.
5. Supraclavicular nodes in a patient with bilateral hilar infiltrations can be expected to yield granulomatous smears (sarcoid).[11]
6. Left supraclavicular nodes in a young man with a testicular mass can be expected to yield a germinal smear (see Testis, Chap. 3). With no testicular mass, occult tumors must be considered. (See Case A-7 in Appendix.)
7. Enlarged, firm anterior cervical nodes in a patient with a firm ulcerated lesion of the tongue should yield squamous cells.

The above expectations are most often fulfilled, but the clinician must retain his searching and imaginative faculties in the event of an unexpected finding.

Concern has been expressed about the difficulty, and therefore the danger, of interpreting lymph node aspirations in the diagnosis of lym-

Palpation

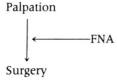

Surgery

Comments on smears
  If squamous: Detailed head and neck examination
  If nonsquamous: Judicious search for primary below the clavicle
  If lymphoid: Mixed, well differentiated
                   Search for focal infection
                   Viral studies
                   In children—observe for several weeks
                   Biopsy if no regression or diagnosis
              Monomorphic and/or poorly differentiated, or with
              Sternberg–Reed cells
                   Bone marrow
                   Chest x-ray
                   Surgical biopsy

Surgical violation of the neck for diagnosis of metastatic disease
is contraindicated.

FIGURE 8-1: Diagnostic schema for enlarged cervical nodes.

phoma.[7,13] In spite of the frequency of lymph node enlargement and the
ready availability of nodes as targets for fine needle aspiration, there is a
scarcity of papers published on the subject.[16,20] This is noted particularly in
comparison with transthoracic and transabdominal (retroperitoneal) punctures, about which perhaps hundreds of papers have been published, and
which are associated with fairly extensive technology, and with hazards.

   This concern deals entirely with the feasibility of making a definitive
diagnosis of lymphoma based on the cytology of smear preparations. It will
tend to extend to all lymph node enlargements, and therefore will inhibit
the utilization of an extremely valuable clinical procedure. The following
pathologic nodes all may yield useful and often definitive data in diagnosis.

   Suppurative nodes
   Reactive (hyperplasia/lymphadenitis)
   Toxoplasmic lymphadenitis[6]
   Cat-scratch lymphadenitis
   Infectious mononucleosis lymphadenopathy
   Postvaccinal lymphadenitis
   Post-lymphangiography lymphadenopathy
   Anticonvulsant lymphadenopathy

Non-Hodgkin's lymphoma
  Well differentiated
  Intermediate differentiated
  Poorly differentiated
Hodgkin's lymphoma
Plasma cell myeloma (see Case 2-2, Chap. 2)
Eosinophilic granuloma
Metastatic carcinoma and sarcoma

All clinicians dealing with the broad spectrum of clinical disorders during their workweek will easily recognize disorders in the above list that may be seen weekly, monthly, or even once or twice a year. The practical usefulness of immediate puncture and referral of slides for prompt diagnosis, or exclusion of a diagnosis such as metastasis, is immediately apparent. The aspiration is part of an overall clinical evaluation as considered below.

The Clinical Evaluation of Lymph Node Enlargement

The interpretation of smears from any of the nodal enlargements listed previously must be preceded by clinical evaluation or accompanied by clinical data. In perhaps no other area of fine needle aspiration is the clinical component of the diagnosis more important. Clinically, patients can be divided into two groups: those with a known antecedent malignancy, and those without. Metastatic lymph nodes with unknown primary will be considered below. As with all aspects of clinical aspiration, history and focused physical examination are fundamental.

Lymph node enlargements are seen for evaluation because of referral from another physician, discovery by the patient, or discovery during a routine examination or an examination for some other purpose, for example, a cardiac or pulmonary problem. In pursuit of the diagnosis, the following questions are raised:

"Did you have prior surgery?"
"Was the surgery for a malignant tumor?"
"Did you ever have a mole or skin bump removed?"
"Were you ever treated for a lymphoma?"
"Do you know what kind of treatment and what kind of lymphoma?"
"Have you had any localized infections?"
"Have you had a generalized febrile illness?"
"Do you have any pets?"
"Are they dogs or cats?"
"Are the cats young?"
"Do you take any medication for seizures?"

"Have you had a recent vaccination?"
"Do you have a venereal disease or any lesion on your genitalia?"
"What is your sexual preference?"

To obtain this history, it is important to keep in mind late recurrence of both carcinoma and lymphoma. The original tumor may date back many years, with disease-free intervals of up to 30 years.[27]

The physical examination includes review of all node-bearing areas regardless of the presenting enlargement. This includes scalp, facial lymphoid deposits, preauricular, anterior, lateral and posterior cervical, suboccipital, submandibular, intraparotid angle of jaw, axillary, epitrochlear, inguinal, and femoral nodes (Fig. 8-2).

There are several important aspects of lymph node examination. Scalp examination (see Fig. 9-12) with the flat hand may detect an unusual lymphoid mass. Suboccipital nodes often are ignored when the patient is sitting in confrontational position. This applies also to angle of the jaw, preauricular, and submandibular nodes (Fig. 8-3). The axillae require deep palpation with the patient's arm hanging loosely flexed and resting on the examiner's arm or shoulder (Fig. 8-4). (Aspiration is illustrated in Fig. 4-10.) Experience with fine needle aspiration heightens skills in physical examination, particularly in delineating small nodal masses for puncture.

If the nodes are in the superficial axillary tissue, they may be grasped when the arm is extended (Fig. 8-5). Puncture is accomplished easily if the nodes can be fixed with one hand. Epitrochlear adenopathy is rarely included in the routine examination. In addition to disseminated inflammatory disorders, such as infectious mononucleosis and syphilis, nodular lym-

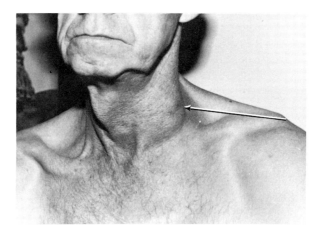

FIGURE 8-2: Enlarged lymph nodes (*arrow*) in this patient's neck were detected initially on routine physical examination. Further examination revealed a primary carcinoma of the lung.

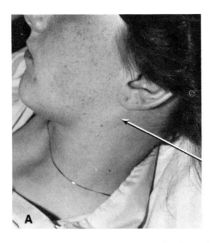 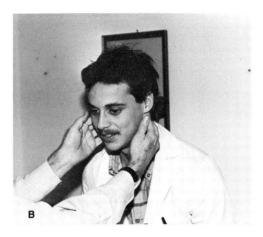

FIGURE 8-3: (*A*) This patient had a subtle mass (*arrow*) at the angle of the jaw. (*B*) Palpation below the ear directly behind the jaw angle may reveal an important hard fixed node.

phoma as well as Hodgkin's disease may involve the epitrochlear nodes. An unusual case is presented later in the chapter (see Case 8-6).

Physical Characteristics

The physical characteristics of the node are often nonspecific. However, some clues to identity may be noted. Enlarged tender nodes occur primarily as a result of an acute suppurative process. Nodes forming conglomerate

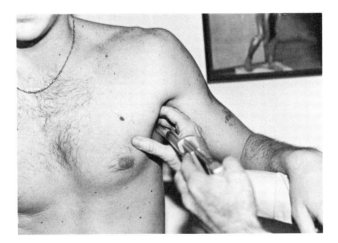

FIGURE 8-4: The arm must be relaxed to palpate deep into the axilla. Nodes are brought down and pinioned against ribs.

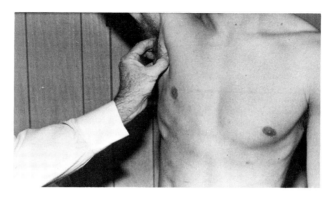

Figure 8-5: Lymph nodes here are grasped with the arm in extension.

masses, particularly if the overlying skin appears to be infiltrated, are seen in Hodgkin's disease. However, in the same case an isolated node that also may be involved with Hodgkin's disease may be palpated in a remote region. In addition, Hodgkin's disease may be heralded by a single, mobile, rubbery node (see Case 2-8). Nontender, enlarged, mushy nodes may be caseated. Discrete rubbery nodes, in groups or singly, suggest non-Hodgkin's lymphoma. Single, small, firm nodes may be exhibited by the patient for an opinion. Although benign neglect may not be hazardous even in patients subsequently proved to have non-Hodgkin's lymphoma, it is always reassuring to extract a smear characteristic of chronic inflammation.

Metastatic nodes vary considerably but in general tend to be hard compared to those of lymphoma. They may be rocky in texture. A solitary, fixed, hard node in the presence of concurrent or past known carcinoma is a sentinel sign. In the presence of a conglomerate mass of nodes it may be useful to aspirate a regional solitary node to avoid necrosis, which occurs in large masses (Fig. 8-6). The distinction of obviously pathological carcinomatous nodes from lymphomatous nodes cannot always be made clinically. History of the disorder is useful.

There are three types of nodal enlargement that enable the physician and cytopathologist to focus their attention and dispense to a large extent with the concern about feasibility of metastatic, reactive, or lymphomatous lymph node diagnosis (Table 8-1).

The management of enlarged nodes by the fine needle aspiration technique is simplified by attention to the following cardinal rules:

1. Normal nodes are not targets.
2. If enlargements are due to metastases, carcinoma cells will be extracted.
3. If no carcinoma cells are extracted from an enlarged node, the diagnosis will be reactive (acute, chronic, or granulomatous infection) or lymphoma.

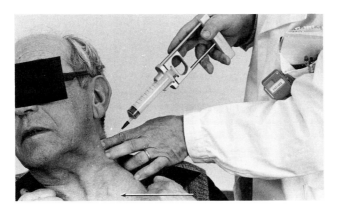

FIGURE 8-6: A conglomerate mass of nodes (*arrow*) is evident in the supraclavicular space. Aspiration of a solitary regional node was diagnostic.

4. If a monomorphic smear is obtained, consider non-Hodgkin's lymphoma.
5. If a mixed lymphoid smear is obtained, consider reactive nodes or Hodgkin's disease.
6. If there are equal numbers of large and small cells, consider "lymphocytic–histiocytic" non-Hodgkin's lymphoma.

Metastatic Nodes

Familiarity with a lymphoid smear[18] readily allows the identification of contrasting metastatic cytology. One of the areas of difficulty is undifferentiated carcinoma, oat cell and intermediate cell type. Clinical data and careful cytologic analysis ordinarily will solve this problem. In a patient with, for example, a known squamous cell primary, the findings of squamous cancer cells in the lymph node aspirate forestall surgery. On the other hand, an undifferentiated smear with no known primary may require

TABLE 8-1: Types of Nodal Enlargement

Metastatic nodes
Reactive nodes
    Acute suppurative
    Subacute suppurative
    Reactive hyperplasia
    Granulomatous
Lymphomatous nodes
    Hodgkin's disease
    Non-Hodgkin's disease

TABLE 8-2: Likely Primary Sites of Metastatic Regional Adenopathy

Cervical nodes	Lesions of the head and neck, 50%
	Primaries below the clavicles, 50%[9,28]
Occipital nodes	Scalp (squamous carcinoma and melanoma)
Intraparotid nodes	Scalp, face, and ears (squamous carcinoma and melanoma)
Submandibular and submental nodes	Lips, mouth, and tongue
Angle of jaw	Nasopharynx
Supraclavicular nodes	Lung, gastrointestinal tract, breast, germinal (in young men)
Axillary nodes	Breast, lung, melanoma
Inguinal nodes	Lower extremities, buttocks, external genitalia, melanoma

surgical excision for histologic evaluation. With histology, difficulties in distinguishing undifferentiated carcinoma and lymphoma also exist. Electron microscopy, cell markers, and monoclonal antibodies have been used to differentiate cell type and, in particular, to separate lymphoma from carcinoma.[12] Table 8-2 summarizes the potential points of origin of localized regional adenopathy. (Also see Chap. 2.)

NODE INVOLVEMENT IN ATYPICAL SITES

Lymphatic permeation by motile carcinoma cells in a centrifugal fashion is a recognized process. This accounts for the well-known skin implants occurring in the skin of the thorax and abdomen during postmastectomy recurrence. However, early lymph node involvement as secondary deposits occurs as a result of a lymphatic embolic process. The combined processes of permeation to a new site followed by embolic spread to an even more remote lymph node site may account for some of the unusual deposits. However, perhaps the main mechanism is retrograde lymphatic spread as a result of a blocked primary pathway. This leads to contralateral cervical nodal metastases in cancers of the head and neck, contralateral axillary metastases in cancer of the breast, and inguinal metastases in abdominal visceral carcinoma and prostate carcinoma.[27]

METASTATIC NODES WITH INAPPARENT PRIMARY

In oncologic practice, metastatic nodes with an inapparent primary are a common finding. An extensive literature on the subject of cryptogenic primary has been recorded.[3,4,8,10,15,26] There is general agreement that, as with so-called primary branchogenic carcinoma (see Chap. 2), exhaustive examination must be done in search of the primary. There is also general agreement that surgical biopsy of a suspicious cervical node to establish a diagnosis is contraindicated.[4] Such intervention will worsen the prognosis. Surgical biopsies in other regions, such as the axillae, may be appropriate.

However, it is precisely at this point that fine needle aspiration has one of its most important applications.

If fine needle aspiration is not done and surgery is contraindicated, the other approach is initiation of a search for a primary with physical examination, x-ray, and laboratory studies. Without knowing the nature of the metastasis, this may be a time-consuming and expensive process. It must be remembered that half of the metastatic cervical nodes may originate below the clavicle.[9,28] Information yielded by fine needle aspiration will have extremely valuable applications, depending on the experience and skill of the cytopathologist.

The initial yield will be the usual determination that the tumor is squamous or adenocarcinoma. Other, less common, broad groups including melanoma, germinal tumors, and sarcomas also may be readily definable. This information immediately guides the diagnostic work up and shortens the time immeasurably. Detailed study and review by Willis confirms that the metastasis is highly representative of the primary.[27] In spite of the search, the primary is not found in a significant number of patients. Treatment of metastatic cervical nodes even without finding the primary will salvage up to 30% for a 5-year period.[8]

Case 8-1 illustrates metastatic nodes with unknown primary.

Case 8-1

The patient was a 79-year-old woman reporting for an examination with a vague complaint of "not feeling well" (Fig. 8-7). She denied gastrointestinal or genitourinary symptoms and, in fact, her appetite

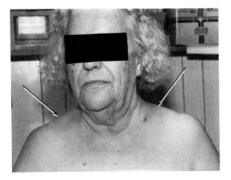

FIGURE 8-7: This patient had left supra-clavicular lymphadenopathy. The region bulged compared to the hollow on her right (*arrows*). Fine needle aspiration yielded adenocarcinoma.

and weight were well maintained. On inspection, it was evident that the supraclavicular hollow seen on her right was not evident on her left. Palpation confirmed the presence of a nodal mass, and fine needle aspiration yielded metastatic adenocarcinoma. The results of a complete physical examination, including breasts and pelvis, were negative. Chest x-ray and mammography were normal. The patient was considered to have metastatic carcinoma with unknown primary and was observed in follow-up rather than studied at that time with endoscopy and gastrointestinal x-rays.

Reactive Lymph Nodes

ACUTE SUPPURATIVE LYMPHADENITIS

Tender confluent nodes in the presence of an obvious pyogenic infection, such as acute pharyngitis, ordinarily will not require morphologic (cytologic or histologic) confirmation. The nodal mass is often fluctuant, and the overlying skin may exhibit changes of cellulitis. However, inadequately treated infection may result in soft to firm nontender nodal masses (often not recognized as nodes) that yield acute suppurative exudate (pus) on aspiration. A cervical mass, simulating a deeper proliferating tumefaction, sometimes may occur and the extraction of pus, somewhat thinner than in the acute case, will be a surprise finding. The focus of infection may be an infected tooth or tonsil that is relatively asymptomatic. In all cases it is worthwhile to submit the exudate for bacterial smear and culture. This may require a second puncture preceded by a povidone–iodine (Betadine) swab.

This is illustrated in the following cases.

Case 8-2

The patient was a 20-year-old woman referred for aspiration of a smooth, firm, rubbery submental mass (Fig. 8-8). She had been treated intensively with antibiotics by an otolaryngologist on the presumption that the mass was a collection of inflammatory nodes even though no primary site of infection could be detected. On examination, the mass was nontender, nonfluctuant, and poorly delimited. Apart from the relatively short history (6 weeks), it resembled a lymphomatous mass rather than an infection.

Fine needle aspiration yielded 1.5 mL of thick, yellow pus that yielded *Streptococcus* organisms on culture.

Residual lymphoid elements were not evident. It is conjectural whether we are dealing with abscess formation in cellulitis or a breakdown of suppurative nodes.

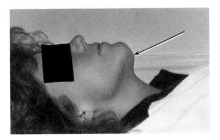

FIGURE 8-8: A smooth, rubbery, non-tender submental mass (*arrow*) is shown in a patient with negative intraoral examination. Aspiration yielded pus.

Case 8-3

The patient was a 27-year-old woman who had left inguinal adenopathy. She was asymptomatic, and the nodes had enlarged gradually over a period of 10 days.

On examination, an inguinal mass appeared to consist of confluent, soft to rubbery, nontender nodes (Fig. 8-9). There was no history or evidence of infection of the left extremity, buttock, perineum, or external genitalia.

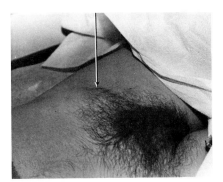

FIGURE 8-9: A conglomerate rubbery mass (*arrow*) is shown in the left inguinal region. It was clinically suspicious for lymphoma. There was no regional infection. Streptococcal pharyngitis had been treated 10 days previously. Fine needle aspiration yielded pus that was negative on Gram stain and culture.

The clinical diagnosis was "suspicion of lymphoma." Fine needle aspiration yielded purulent material consisting of granulocytes, histiocytes, and considerable cellular degeneration. Gram stain and culture were negative.

At this point, a history was elicited of acute streptococcal pharyngitis treated with penicillin 10 days earlier. Seeding of the inguinal nodes was presumed. No other source of infection was evident.

Case 8-4

There was a confluent mass involving the left side of the neck of a 67-year-old man. The mass had appeared fairly rapidly over a period of 3 weeks. There was no antecedent pharyngitis or history of local inflammation.

On examination, the mass was nontender and felt like a confluent nodal mass (Fig. 8-10). A thorough head and neck examination for a primary lesion was negative. The pre-aspiration diagnosis rendered by the referring otorhinolaryngologist was neoplasm of unknown origin.

Fine needle aspiration yielded 3 mL of pus, which was negative on culture. At this point, the patient said he had taken some antibiotic tablets 2 weeks earlier.

COMMENT In Cases 8-2, 8-3, and 8-4, the mass was suspicious for neoplasm, with lymphoma a major consideration. The masses were

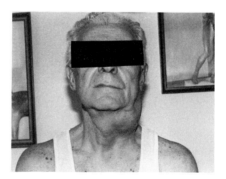

FIGURE 8-10: This 67-year-old man had a confluent nonfluctuant nodal mass. It had appeared rapidly without antecedent infection. Results of head and neck examination by an otorhinolaryngologist were normal. Fine needle aspiration yielded sterile pus. The patient then indicated he had medicated himself with antibiotic pills.

nontender and rubbery. Fine needle aspiration was decisive in rapidly establishing the diagnosis.

The finding of enlarged nodes on physical examination should prompt immediate clinical evaluation. Attention is directed to history and general physical findings that might be related, such as known prior neoplasm or enlarged spleen. Surgical biopsy is the last diagnostic measure to consider. Immediate fine needle aspiration (see Table 8-1) will shorten the workup. Cytologic diagnosis is influenced by clinical findings to the same degree that clinical diagnosis is established or guided by cytologic findings. It is quite important that the clinician remain in control of the patient, particularly in follow up when cytology is not done, or when cytology does not conform to the clinical impression.

SUBACUTE SUPPURATIVE LYMPHADENITIS

The presence of microabscesses on histologic study of lymph nodes indicates cat-scratch disease, lymphogranuloma venereum, and tularemia.[1] The largest experience that we have had is with cat-scratch disease, in which fine needle aspiration is a useful guide.

Unexplained lymphadenopathy in children is a major source of parental anxiety. The appearance of enlarged nodes is not an immediate cause for concern. It is their persistence for 2 weeks to 4 weeks that prompts the investigation. Our experience as referral physicians reveals the pattern of primary care. When first seen, patients usually have had one or more follow-up visits with the primary physician for throat and general examination. A blood count, mononucleosis test, and often throat culture already have been performed. Occasionally, chest x-ray has been ordered. Cervical nodes in the anterior chain are the usual sources of concern. Occipital, posterior cervical, supraclavicular, and axillary nodes are less common sites.

On physical examination at this point, the nodes are not distinctive. They are soft to firm, mobile, discrete, and nontender. Clinically, distinction from lymphomatous nodes cannot be made. Cat scratch disease may also simulate malignant lymphoma histologically.[19]

In children, the initial question concerns young cats belonging to the child or a neighbor. History of exposure (scratching may be denied) is ordinarily sufficient to guide the diagnosis. The smears are reactive with increased granulocytes. They may not, of course, be diagnostic but the history and polymorphonuclear leukocytes are sufficient to forestall surgical excision in most cases. Findings are illustrated in Case 8-5.

Case 8-5

The patient was a 5-year-old girl referred for evaluation of lymphadenopathy present for ten days. Lymph nodes were palpable in the right submandibular and right axillary regions (Fig. 8-11). The pa-

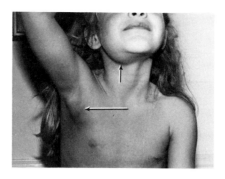

Figure 8-11: Reginal lymphadenopathy (*arrows*) is illustrated in a child with cat-scratch disease.

tient was afebrile and had no complaints. Workup including complete blood count, sedimentation rate, mononucleosis test, and chest x-ray was negative or normal. Further questions determined that there were no pets in the family. However, a neighboring child with whom the patient played did have a young cat.

Fine needle aspiration of the nodes yielded mixed lymphoid cells with foci of granulocytes, confirming a diagnosis of cat-scratch disease. The nodes regressed without treatment.

The next case illustrates the importance of clinical evaluation.

Case 8-6

The patient was a 16-year-old, healthy, muscular boy referred for evaluation and aspiration of massive bilateral epitrochlear nodes (Fig. 8-12). There was no history of fever, malaise, or any other acute or chronic disorder. There were no pets. A neighbor's home had a cat, and the patient had visited the home but had not handled the cat.

On physical examination, the nodes were firm, rubbery, mobile, and nontender, and each was 3 cm in diameter. They were visible and bulged the volar concavity of the upper arm. There were similar enlarged nodes in the left axilla. No other nodes were palpable. The liver and spleen were not palpable.

Fine needle aspiration of one epitrochlear node yielded smears with mixed lymphoid cells and increased numbers of atypical histiocytes, some with macronucleoli. There were occasional granulocytes and eosinophils. No definite Sternberg–Reed cells were seen.

The diagnosis rendered was atypical lymphoid smears, suspicious for Hodgkin's disease. Surgical biopsy was recommended.

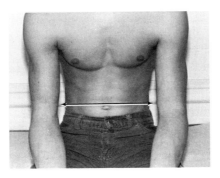

FIGURE 8-12: There is massive, bilateral, nontender epitrochlear adenopathy evident as visible bulges (*arrows*), and easily palpable. Each measured 3 cm in diameter.

The surgeon removed a large axillary node. The histopathologic diagnosis was cat-scratch disease. There were microabscesses and granulomatous changes. Follicles were well preserved with no evidence of lymphoma.

COMMENT Although the cytologic diagnosis was in error, final diagnosis is always guided and often modified by clinical findings. Perhaps acute suppurative changes or some other specific diagnosis might have forestalled surgery.

REACTIVE HYPERPLASIA
The most common lymphoid cytologic smear is reactive, nonspecific hyperplasia. There may or may not be a regional focus of infection. The reaction usually includes a mixed lymphoid population without the specificity of clusters of histiocytes, plasma cells, epithelioid cells, or granulocytes. In children, the usual recommendation should be to treat expectantly, possibly with an antibiotic, but for the most part to observe and not to do a biopsy surgically. Viral agents may be responsible for many of these nodes. It is precisely with this common cytologic pattern that the problem of differential diagnosis with non-Hodgkin's lymphoma arises.

The clinical presentation, as with all potential targets for aspiration, is diagnostically important. Slides should be accompanied by clinical description and clinical impression. The separation of attempted lymphoid smear interpretation from the clinical data increases the difficulty. Although the cytologist is better advised to request data and, of course, to expect satisfactory smears before attempting a diagnosis, in practical terms, many less than optimal studies are presented and interpreted. Cytologic clues such as possible Sternberg–Reed cells in a suboptimal smear may be useful in guiding the clinician to a diagnosis. Cytologic findings with clinical correlation are shown in Table 8-3.

Unless the clinician is interested in microscopy, the cytologic findings do not require detailed study. Nevertheless, the cytopathologist's report will be more meaningful if the cytologic details are correlated with the clinical findings.

The effects of aspiration on lymph node histology must be minimal, because correlation of cytology and histology is excellent. One study has been done on the effect of benign lymph node histology, and no problems reading the histology were found.[5]

TOXOPLASMIC LYMPHADENITIS

Toxoplasmic lymphadenitis, which is a specific type of adenitis, accounts for up to 15% of cases of unexplained lymphadenopathy in young adults.[6,17,22] The most common site is the cervical region. The nodes may be quite asymptomatic, of long standing, and may simulate lymphoma,

TABLE 8-3: Evaluation of Lymphoid Smears

Cytologic Findings	Likely diagnosis
NODAL	
Randomly scattered transformed cells	Reactive
Mixed lymphoid with reactive plasma cells, eosinophils, granulocytes, and histiocytes*	Reactive vs. Hodgkin's
Immature monomorphic lymphoid cells	Non-Hodgkin's lymphoma
Mature monomorphic lymphoid cells*	Non-Hodgkin's lymphoma
Sternberg–Reed cells	Hodgkin's
Increased granulocytes	Microabscesses
Caseation	Tuberculosis
Increased histiocytes	Toxoplasmosis; anticonvulsants; postvaccinial
EXTRANODAL	
Immature plasma cells	Plasmacytoma
Immature monomorphic lymphoid cells	Non-Hodgkin's lymphoma
Mixed mature and immature lymphoid cells in relatively equal numbers	Lymphocytic–histiocytic lymphoma
Sternberg–Reed cells	Hodgkin's
Mature monomorphic lymphoid cells	Non-Hodgkin's lymphoma vs. pseudolymphoma

* Problem areas.

accounting for the number that come to surgical biopsy. Important in the history is exposure to cats' feces (cleaning the litter box) or ingestion of nonpasteurized milk and partially cooked meat.

Serologic studies may be fairly diagnostic. However, an elevated titre, if not confirmed by serial rise in an appropriate clinical context, may leave a lingering doubt concerning the nature of the specific adenopathy in a specific patient. A large number of the world's population may have serologic elevations indicating prior infection. Therefore, patients with lymphoma may fortuitously still have a positive titre for toxoplasmosis.

Fine needle aspiration yields a characteristic, if not pathognomonic, cytologic pattern that with clinical data will strongly suggest the diagnosis and forestall lymph node biopsy.[6] In the natural history of the lymphadenopathy, spontaneous regression occurs. The typical cytologic feature that identifies the disease is the presence of aggregates of epithelioid cells. Toxoplasma cyst has been identified on fine needle aspiration.[2] This specific finding is quite unusual. It is also an unusual finding on histological examination.[25]

GRANULOMATOUS LYMPHADENITIS

The identification of granulomatous alteration in cytologic smears is fairly straightforward.[11,18,28] The prototype of noncaseating granulomas is sarcoidosis. Fine needle aspiration of peripheral lymphadenopathy is extremely useful.

A clinical diagnosis of sarcoidosis may be made in the presence of bilateral hilar adenopathy in the appropriate clinical context. Such patients may be kept under observation by experienced pulmonologists. More often, however, morphologic confirmation is sought. Procedures including mediastinoscopy, supraclavicular fat pad excision, and anterior diagnostic thoracotomy have been utilized. Failure to palpate supraclavicular nodes is associated with a poor surgical yield in fat pad diagnosis. Palpation of nodes, whether cervical, supraclavicular, or axillary, allows fine needle aspiration and the potential diagnosis of granulomatous lymphadenitis (sarcoid).

The clinical presentation is useful, but it is not always diagnostic, as illustrated in the following case.

Case 8-7

The patient was a 40-year-old black female admitted for investigation of an abnormal chest film. Radiographically, there was hilar adenopathy highly suggestive of sarcoidosis. On examination, the patient was afebrile. Left supraclavicular lymph nodes measuring up to 1.5 cm were palpable. Cervical, axillary, and inguinal adenopathy was insignificant. There were no findings on auscultation. Liver and spleen were not palpable.

Fine needle aspiration of the palpable node was done. It yielded caseous necrosis. Tuberculosis was identified by smear and culture. It is of interest that a tuberculin skin test was not done before the diagnosis.

Along related lines, 26 patients were admitted to a large cancer center for evaluation of physical and radiographic findings that had prompted a diagnosis of malignancy.[21] In none of the patients was a tuberculin test performed prior to admission, and it was done in only 9 patients after admission. Of the 26 patients, 8 had enlarged lymph nodes because of tuberculous lymphadenitis interpreted as malignant on physical examination. In all of them, and in a number of the other admissions, fine needle aspiration would have established or guided a diagnosis before admission. Symptoms of tuberculosis were uncommon in the entire group of 26 patients. To quote the commentary from the report, "An earlier diagnosis could have avoided the patient's anxiety related to the erroneous diagnosis of neoplasm and could have decreased the expensive, complicated workups."

INFECTIOUS MONONUCLEOSIS AND SYPHILIS

Systemic disorders usually associated with adenopathy, such as infectious mononucleosis, should provide sufficient clinical data to establish a firm diagnosis without any biopsy procedure. However, exceptions occur as illustrated in Case 8-8.

Case 8-8

A 22-year-old male had enlarged rubbery nodes, cervical, axillary, and inguinal. He had a persistent fever, unremarkable blood count, and negative titres for mononucleosis, toxoplasmosis, herpes, and cytomegaloviruses. A diagnosis of secondary lues emerged following fine needle aspiration that yielded richly reactive smears with groups of epithelioid cells. A VDRL test was strongly positive and was consistent with a subsequently obtained history of exposure.

COMMENT Clinical diagnosis failed because of bad clinical habits leading to errors of omission.

We have not had sufficient experience with the lymphadenopathy seen in homosexuals as well as that seen in patients with acquired immune deficiency diseases to characterize the clinical course and cytology. However, it is apparent that with appropriate study, this may be an area in which the fine needle aspiration method may give early clues.

GRANULOMATOUS CYTOLOGY

Some varieties of granulomatous cytology yielded by FNA with associated clinical disorders are listed.

Sarcoidosis—Epithelioid and giant cells
Tuberculosis—Epithelioid and giant cells, with caseation
Syphilis—Epithelioid and giant cells, with histiocytes
Hodgkin's disease—Epithelioid and Sternberg–Reed cells
Seminoma—Epithelioid and giant cells, and germinal tumor cells[23]

The clinician should be aware of the differential diagnosis, and should raise the following questions with the cytopathologist.

Could it be sarcoidosis or tuberculosis? The presence of Langhans' cells, giant cells, or caseation should be decisive (see Case 8-7).

Could it be cat-scratch disease or lymphogranuloma venereum (particularly if inguinal nodes are affected)? In both entities, together with tularemia, there are multiple nodal microabscesses that will be seen on smear as clusters of granulocytes.[1]

Could it be Hodgkin's disease or non-Hodgkin's lymphoma (Lennert's type)? This is a major differentiation, but the presence of Sternberg–Reed cells or the monomorphic pattern of non-Hodgkin's lymphoma (see below) should aid the differentiation.

For the clinician, in these as in all nodal diseases, the ambiguities ordinarily can be resolved by a lymph node biopsy. But this is contrary to judicious medicine. Particularly in children, surgical violation of the neck is unwarranted. First, the application of clinical judgment should include the linear history of the enlargement, the surrounding circumstances of exposure, the physical characteristics of the nodes, and finally, fine needle aspiration. Where the above do not yield absolute criteria of diagnosis, they will at least encourage a seasoned clinician to counsel a period of observation.

Lymphomatous Nodes

THE CLINICAL DISTINCTION OF REACTIVE
AND LYMPHOMA NODES

The clinical assessment of reactive and lymphoma nodes is summarized in Table 8-4. Age of the patient, history of the disorder, and location and physical character of the nodes can be assessed rapidly and are very often diagnostic.

Reactive nodes, particularly cervical nodes, are common findings in children. (See Chap. 2.) In contrast, Hodgkin's disease occurs in the second, third, and fourth decades and non-Hodgkin's lymphoma occurs in the fourth, fifth, and sixth decades. Although there is overlap, these distinctions are important. A cytologic picture suggestive of a lymphoma in a child (under 10 years of age) must be quite compelling before we recommend

TABLE 8-4: Guidelines to Clinical Assessment of Lymphoma
Versus Nonlymphoma Nodes

	Lymphoma*	Nonlymphoma
AGE	> 15 years	< 15 years
HISTORY OF ENLARGEMENT	Longstanding	Recent
RAPID ONSET	Lymphoblastic Pleomorphic Burkitt's	Associated with acute infection
INTERMITTENT ENLARGEMENT	Infrequent	Common
PRESENCE OF SYSTEMIC DISORDERS	Uncommon	Common
FOCAL INFECTION	Not seen	Common
VACCINATION	Not seen	Common
ANTICONVULSANTS	Hodgkin's reported (rare)	Common
HOMOSEXUALITY	Rare; common with AIDS†	Common as precursor of AIDS†

* Hodgkin's and non-Hodgkin's.
† Acquired immune deficiency syndrome.

surgical excision. Non-Hodgkin's lymphoma is the third most common malignancy in childhood after acute lymphoblastic leukemia and neuroblastoma. However, it is rare when compared to the number of patients with reactive adenopathy. Aspiration cytology may be decisive, as discussed below. Observation of the patient usually will resolve the issue. A cardinal rule in all of aspiration biopsy cytology, but particularly in the decision process regarding lymphoid nodes, is that clinical control of the patient must be maintained until the process is resolved. Total reliance on the cytologic impression is unwarranted. It represents one aspect of the diagnosis. However, where the cytologist is definitive and recommends excision, this decision should be followed.

In the older age group, the appearance of significant nodal enlargement yielding lymphoid smears is ominous. In the absence of focal infection, it is highly suspicious for lymphoma (usually non-Hodgkin's lymphoma) and frequently for chronic lymphocytic leukemia.

History of the nodal enlargement is essential information. Have the nodes been present for days, weeks, or months? How rapidly have they enlarged? Have they been recurring intermittently? Are they associated with a systemic disorder (such as infectious mononucleosis)? Is there a focus of infection producing regional adenopathy? Has there been a vaccination recently? Is the patient receiving anticonvulsants?

The attempt to diagnose lymph node cytology and histology without a history is hazardous. Twenty cases of postvaccinial lymphadenitis were submitted to the Armed Forces Institute of Pathology, of which nine were histologically diagnosed lymphoma. In 14 cases, the history of vaccination was overlooked. Enlarged reticular cells may simulate Sternberg–Reed cells. Similar changes occur with infectious mononucleosis, herpes zoster, and dermatopathic lymphadenitis.[14]

It is evident from this review that the clinical history is crucial. The primary clinician with access to detailed history and physical examination is undoubtedly in the best position to provide all the diagnostic data, including the smears.

The incidence of Hodgkin's disease in children can be appreciated by reviewing a collected series from a major referral cancer center (Roswell Park Memorial Institute). From 1921 to 1973, 106 cases were collected. Ages varied from 3.5 years to 7 years with a mean of 12.6 years.[24]

For the clinician, concern about the feasibility of cytologic diagnosis of lymphoma is lessened because of his appreciation of the clinical picture, which is not completely available to the cytopathologist and is not necessarily evident to the subspecialist.

This is illustrated in the following case.

Case 8-9

A 19-year-old athletic boy was seen by an otolaryngologist for evaluation of enlarged nodes in the lateral neck and extending up to the mastoid and retroauricular area. Results of a complete intraoral examination were negative. Before scheduling an excisional biopsy, the physician submitted two aspirated smears for cytologic diagnosis. The cytology was suspicious for mixed non-Hodgkin's lymphoma consisting of a mixture of small lymphocytes and numerous scattered histiocytic cells.

The cytopathologist requested to see the patient. Examination revealed large, rubbery, partially confluent nodes extending up to the mastoid, clinically very suggestive of lymphoma (Fig. 8-13). General examination revealed no other lymph node enlargement of hepatosplenomegaly. The patient appeared fairly vigorous, but on questioning, he noted that he had experienced some night sweats, which he had attributed to heavy exercise in the summer.

On complete blood count, a white count of 12,000/μL with 10% lymphocytes—a distinct lymphopenia—was found. The overall clinical picture was that of Hodgkin's disease.

A repeat aspiration yielded the same morphology, and no Sternberg–Reed cells were seen. Surgical biopsy led to an initial diagnosis of malignant lymphoma, probably mixed non-Hodgkin's type. Convincing Sternberg–Reed cells were not seen. Diagnosis rendered on consultation was Hodgkin's disease, mixed cell type, which conformed to the clinical diagnosis of Hodgkin's disease with B symptoms, staging to be determined.

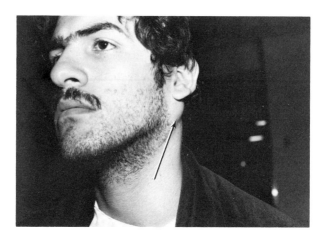

FIGURE 8-13: Large rubbery nodes (*arrow*) are visible in the mastoid region. On careful palpation, a chain of nodes was detected down to the clavicle, prompting surgical staging with laparotomy. The final stage was IV.

COMMENT This case demonstrates that the cytologic diagnosis of lymphoma should not stand nakedly without clinical support and histologic confirmation. This rule is valid, even though in experienced hands unequivocal cytologic diagnosis of Hodgkin's disease and poorly differentiated non-Hodgkin's lymphoma has been rendered repeatedly without error.

Nodes that have been enlarging slowly and progressively in the adult suggest lymphoma. However, some inflammatory nodes regress quite slowly and must be considered (see Cases 8-1, 8-2, and 8-3). Rapid enlargement of nodes ordinarily is diagnostic of an inflammatory process. Non-Hodgkin's lymphoma in children, including lymphoblastic lymphoma, pleomorphic lymphoma, and Burkitt's lymphoma, may appear and enlarge fairly explosively. Adult non-Hodgkin's lymphoma is ordinarily much more indolent.

Intermittent nodal enlargement ordinarily should put to rest concerns about malignancy. However, experience has shown that lymphoma may proceed in fits and starts with intermittent enlargement. In the pre-aspiration era, we saw a patient who had three successive lymph node biopsies at 6 month to 8 month intervals, which were interpreted as reactive nodes, atypical hyperplasia, and finally non-Hodgkin's lymphoma.

Location of the nodal enlargement is, of course, a guide to the diagnosis. Scalp and suboccipital nodes in the absence of focal infection are suspicious for lymphoma. In contrast, anterior cervical nodes in a patient with pharyngitis are largely self-explanatory. Axillary nodes are often palpable on deep palpation during routine examination. They share with inguinal nodes the frequency of regional hyperplasia in response to recurrent extremity infection. However, enlarged rubbery nodes in the absence of overt distal infection must be viewed with suspicion. Epitrochlear nodes may be the site of nodular lymphoma and Hodgkin's disease in addition to secondary lues and infectious mononucleosis. Cat-scratch disease as a cause is cited earlier in Case 8-6.

THE APPLICATION OF FINE NEEDLE ASPIRATION
TO THE DIAGNOSIS OF LYMPHOMATOUS NODES

The clinical and physical characteristics of nodal lymphoma are noted above. Fine needle aspiration allows the evaluation of palpable nodes of all sizes in all regions and in atypical locations. Nonpalpable nodes (intrathoracic and retroperitoneal) can be reached with the help of imaging techniques (see Chaps. 5 and 6). Where the alternatives are fine needle aspiration, continued observation, or surgical biopsy, the advantage of informed fine needle aspiration is apparent.

Hodgkin's disease lends itself to diagnosis by fine needle aspiration because of the distinctive cytology highlighted by the Sternberg–Reed cell (see Fig. 2-11). All positive cytologic diagnoses are accompanied by a recommendation for surgical excision to determine the tissue structure. Where the diagnosis has been established in one region, positive cytologic diagnoses of nodes in other regions do not require surgical follow up.

False-negative results may occur. Reactive nodes with eosinophils and increased numbers of histiocytes, or with epithelioid cells but no Sternberg–Reed cells, must be considered with suspicion. The decision for a surgical biopsy versus follow up remains with the clinican (see above).

The diagnosis of Hodgkin's disease has been made and confirmed by experienced cytopathologists in innumerable patients. It is our opinion that pathologists with no specific experience in fine needle aspiration interpretation can recognize Hodgkin's disease after moderate experience with these preparations.

Smears consisting of sheets of primitive, often poorly preserved, lymphoid cells obtained from enlarged nodes in both children and adults are recognized easily by hematologists and pathologists who have experience with bone marrow and peripheral blood preparations from patients with acute leukemia. The distinction among Burkitt's, pleomorphic, or poorly differentiated lymphocytic lymphoma is difficult and may be impossible. However, it is not important, since primary diagnosis will be followed by surgical biopsy to determine whether the structure is nodular or diffuse. As with Hodgkin's disease, establishment of a primary diagnosis in one region may be supplemented by cytologic diagnosis alone in other regions. In the pre-aspiration era, it was not uncommon to have repeated and multiregional surgical excisions to determine the content of enlarged nodes. An important consideration is the evaluation of inguinal nodes, known to enlarge regularly as the result of repeated lower extremity infections, in a patient with previously diagnosed and treated lymphoma above the diaphragm.

Well-differentiated non-Hodgkin's lymphoma and the uncommon lymphocyte-rich Hodgkin's disease will yield fairly uniform and mature lymphocytes. Experienced cytologic interpretation may suggest strongly that a monomorphic pattern of these cells points to lymphoma. At this point, the clinician must decide whether to rcommend excision, or to observe the patient. Clinical studies that may be useful include chest film, lactic dehydrogenase (LDH), complete blood count (CBC), Coombs' test (if there is any anemia), and serum protein electrophoresis (SPE). Positive findings in any of these would hasten the decision to excise. However, in children, a smear of mature lymphocytes is almost never seen in lymphoma.

Small, atypical, sometimes single nodes may yield useful diagnosis as illustrated in Case 2-8. Enlarged nodes also may yield plasma cells or plasmacytoid lymph cells with a resulting diagnosis of Waldenstrom's macroglobulinemia or multiple myeloma as illustrated in Case 2-2. Adjuvant studies include SPE, urine, immunoelectrophoresis for light chains, bone marrow, and appropriate films.

Summary

Critical understanding of the diagnosis of lymph node disease emerges clearly from an appreciation that enlarged nodes must yield foreign cells (carcinoma, sarcoma) or lymphoreticular cells on aspiration. Problems in identifying cancer cells are minimal. Problems in separating reactive from lymphomatous nodes remain formidable. Evaluation of nodal disease must be dominated by clinical data. The clinical picture will predict what the cytology will reveal in most cases. Where the clinical picture is obscure or nondirective, experienced reading of the slides will yield a diagnosis or guide the clinician in further study.

Surgical biopsy will be recommended to assess lymph node structure (diffuse or nodular lymphoma) or to make a diagnosis when the aspiration fails. Particularly in children, delay in node biopsy is encouraged by benign or equivocal findings on smears.

Carcinomatous nodes in the absence of a primary should be studied by the fine needle method and should not be subjected to excisional biopsy.

Optimum diagnostic results are obtained by correlating FNA with the clinical picture. Microscopic diagnosis in the absence of clinical data should be discouraged.

REFERENCES

1. Anderson WAD, Kissane JM: Pathology, 7th ed. St Louis, CV Mosby, 1977
2. Argyle JC, Schumann GB, Kjeldsberg CR et al: Identification of a toxoplasma cyst by fine-needle aspiration. Am J Clin Pathol 80:258, 1983

3. Barrie JR, Knapper WH, Strong EW: Cervical nodal metastasis of unknown origin. Am J Surg 120:466, 1970

4. Batsakis JG: Tumors of the Head and Neck. Baltimore, Williams & Wilkins, 1974

5. Behm FG, O'Dowd GJ, Frable WJ: Fine-needle aspiration effects on benign lymph node histology. Am J Clin Pathol 82:195, 1984

6. Christ ML, Feltes-Kennedy M: Fine needle aspiration cytology of toxoplasmic lymphoadenitis. Acta Cytol 26:425, 1982

7. Christopherson WW: Cytologic detection and diagnosis of cancer: Its contributions and limitations. Cancer 51:1201, 1983

8. Devine KD: Cancer in the neck without obvious source. Mayo Clin Proc 53:644, 1978

9. Engzell U, Jakobsson PA, Sigurdson A et al: Aspiration biopsy of metastatic carcinoma in lymph nodes of the neck. Acta Otolaryngol (Stockh) 72:138, 1971

10. Fitzpatrick PJ, Kotalik JF: Cervical metastasis from an unknown primary tumor. Radiology 110:659, 1974

11. Frable MA, Frable WJ: Fine needle aspiration biopsy in the diagnosis of sarcoid of the head and neck. Acta Cytol 28:175, 1984

12. Gatter KC, Alcock C, Heryet A et al: The differential diagnosis of routinely processed anaplastic tumors using monoclonal antibodies. Am J Clin Pathol 82:33, 1984

13. Hajdu SI, Melamed MR: Limitations of aspiration cytology in the diagnosis of primary neoplasms. Acta Cytol 28:337, 1984

14. Hartsock RJ: Postvaccinial lymphadenitis: Hyperplasia of lymphoid tissue that simulates malignant lymphomas. Cancer 21:632, 1968

15. Jesse RH, Perez CA, Fletcher GH: Cervical lymph node metastasis: Unknown primary cancer. Cancer 31:854, 1973

16. Kline TS, Kannan V, Kline IK: Lymphadenopathy and aspiration biopsy cytology. Cancer 54:1076, 1984

17. Krick JA, Remington JS: Current concepts in parasitology. Toxoplasmosis in the adult: An overview. N Engl J Med 298:550, 1978

18. Linsk JA, Franzen S: Clinical Aspiration Cytology. Philadelphia, JB Lippincott, 1983

19. Luddy RE, Sutherland JC, Levy BE et al: Cat scratch disease simulating malignant lymphoma. Cancer 50:584, 1982

20. Morrison M, Samwick AA, Rubenstein J et al: Lymph node aspirations: Clinical and hematologic observations in 101 patients. Am J Clin Pathol 22:255, 1952

21. Pitlik S, Fainstein V, Bodey GP: Tuberculosis mimicking cancer: A reminder. Am J Med 76:822, 1984

22. Remington JS: Toxoplasmosis in the adult. Bull NY Acad Med 50:211, 1974

23. Richter HJ, Leder LD: Lymph node metastasis with PAS-positive tumor cells and massive epithelial granulomatous reaction as a diagnostic clue to occult seminoma. Cancer 44:245, 1979

24. Shah NK, Freeman AI, Freedman M et al: Hodgkin's disease in children. Med Pediatr Oncol 2:87, 1976

25. Stansfield AG: The histological diagnosis of toxoplasmic lymphadenitis. J Clin Pathol 14:565, 1961

26. Ultman JE, Phillips TL: Management of the patient with cancer of unknown primary site. In DeVita VT Jr, Hellman S, Rosenberg SA (eds): Cancer: Principles and Practice of Onocology, pp 1518–1533. Philadelphia, JB Lippincott, 1982
27. Willis RA: The Spread of Tumours in the Human Body. London, Butterworth, 1973
28. Zajicek J: Aspiration Biopsy Cytology, Part 1. Basel, S Karger, 1974

The Diagnosis of Surface Lesions, Lumps, and Bumps 9

The body surface, which has abnormalities often taken for granted, presents an enormous terrain for the clinician. Discrete lesions that may become targets for fine needle aspiration most often are seen initially by primary care physicians, including internists. They then may choose to observe, or refer to a surgeon or possibly to a dermatologist. Discrete lesions may be epidermal, subcutaneous, or even deeper in origin, but all present with a change in surface texture, shape, or contour. Casual appraisal of a patient who has a specific problem (which may be an upper respiratory infection, cardiac disorder, abdominal cramps, or hemorrhoids) often will pass over a local alteration that may be quite significant. The patient shown in Figure 9-1 had a mild parotid swelling that he ignored and a resident physician missed. It was found to be a malignant tumor (mucoepidermoid) on fine needle aspiration. In contrast to observation of such a gross change in contour, minute scrutiny of small lesions, particularly keratotic facial lesions, may be aided by using the magnifying ophthalmoscope light. Table 9-1 lists common alterations of the body surface that can be categorized by fine needle aspiration. Figure 9-2 illustrates the diagnostic schema for a variety of surface and subsurface lesions.

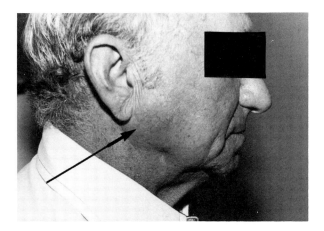

FIGURE 9-1: This patient was seen for an unrelated disorder, and was noted to have a shallow parotid bulge (*arrow*). On palpation it was firm. It yielded mucoepidermoid carcinoma on fine needle aspiration.

TABLE 9-1: Surface Targets for Fine Needle Aspiration

Benign	Malignant
Sebaceous cyst	Metastatic nodules
Lipoma	Sarcomas
Granular cell tumors	Leukemic infiltrates
Neural tumors	Lymphoma cutis
Neurilemoma	Mycosis fungoides
Neurofibroma	Kaposi's sarcoma
Nodular fasciitis[2]	Primary melanomas[5,15]
Fibromatosis	Primary squamous carcinoma
Calcifying epithelioma of Malherbe[8]	Basal cell carcinoma[8,10]
Lymphoid nodules	Small cell (Merkel cell)
Ganglia	carcinoma[12]
Inflammatory skin infiltrates	Implantation malignant nodules

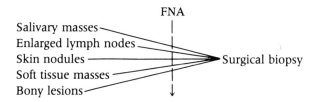

Comment: Surgical biopsy should always be preceded by FNA to guide the surgical approach and more often to forestall it. Sialograms can usually be eliminated.

FIGURE 9-2: Diagnostic schema for surface and subsurface lesions.

In no other anatomic region reviewed in this book is the diagnostic process so basic as in evaluation of the body surface. Technology, including imaging techniques and laboratory tests, contributes little to the lesional diagnosis. Of course, a large hilar mass demonstrated on x-ray film is compelling data in a patient with multiple subcutaneous skin nodules. However, before that point is reached, nodules must be discovered, and physical diagnosis, which leans heavily on inspection and palpation, is mandatory. Findings on inspection are evident in Case 9-1.

Case 9-1

Figure 9-3 illustrates the classical appearance of metastatic nodules. The patient was a 72-year-old retired urologist who had a level III melanoma removed from his left arm 1 year previously. He also had a left axillary dissection. He had noted the development of skin nod-

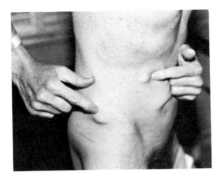

FIGURE 9-3: Subcutaneous nodules (metastatic melanoma) are indicated by the physician–patient. The skin can be moved over the nodules.

ules and presented himself for evaluation. He assumed the nodules were from the melanoma, but wanted confirmation.

There was no evident visceral disease. The nodules were in the subcutaneous compartment and the skin could be moved over them. On examination, several other smaller, unnoticed nodules were found. Fine needle aspiration was definitive. The disease generalized shortly thereafter.

COMMENT In this patient the history essentially made the diagnosis, but it is evident that such nodules are generic "tumors" (see Chap. 1) until specifically identified.

Inspection and palpation may be lost arts in medicine. Experience with resident training suggests that candidates in internal medicine may spend more time studying electrocardiograms and chest films than examining the patient. And within the discipline of physical examination, auscultation of the heart receives considerable emphasis compared to the techniques of inspection and palpation.

Inspection

The Scalp

The bald scalp can and should be inspected. Keratotic and pearly lesions of all types may be present, including actinic keratoses, squamous and basal cell carcinomas, and sweat gland tumors (see Chap. 2). The most commonplace bulge is a sebaceous or epidermoid cyst, but definitive diagnosis will require aspiration, because subcutaneous metastatic nodules can simulate benign cysts. The scalp is not a preferential site for cutaneous and subcutaneous metastases. Hematogenous metastases will colonize the scalp, presumably in the same proportion as other areas of the integument. Isolated ulcerative invasion of the scalp without contiguity to regional breast metastases has been recorded,[8] and Case 9-2 illustrates another example.

Case 9-2

This patient developed a crusted infiltration of the hair-covered scalp (Fig. 9-4). It was treated initially by a dermatologist, and failed to respond. Because of the history of mastectomy 3 years before, fine needle aspiration of the scalp lesion was done with a 25-gauge needle tangentially. Carcinoma cells were obtained that were typical of breast carcinoma. Regression took place with hormonal therapy. No other metastatic sites were detected at the time.

Direct lymphatic spread to the scalp with contiguity is also unusual. In our experience, it has occurred only during the *en cuirrasse* dissemination of breast carcinoma. An exception was illustrated in a 64-year-old patient who had metastatic breast carcinoma that had extended by a hematogenous route to the parotid nodes, and then by lymphatic spread to the neck and scalp (see Case 2-4).

In our experience, the common sources of hematogenous metastasis to the skin and therefore the scalp are melanoma and carcinomas of the lung, breast, kidney, pancreas, and gastrointestinal tract. However, no primary can be excluded. Scalp metastases from follicular thyroid carcinoma have been reported.[8]

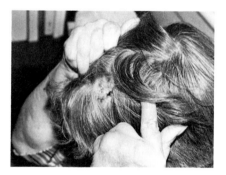

FIGURE 9-4: This patient has advanced rheumatoid arthritis (note hands), history of mastectomy, and a crusted nodular lesion of the scalp. Diagnosis of metastasis was made by fine needle aspiration.

Pigmented lesions must be noted, and should be considered suspicious if there is any nodular component (see below).

The Ears

Inspection of the ears must include the retroauricular region and the external ears. The common ear lesions noted on inspection are basal cell carcinomas along the edges of the pinna, and melanomas. Infiltration of the ear because of lymphoma is not rare and is illustrated in Case 9-3.

Case 9-3

This patient was a 72-year-old diabetic man (Fig. 9-5). He was partially deaf, and he wore a somewhat obsolete type of hearing aid. He was referred for evaluation of an abnormal blood count. On inspection, the lobe of his left ear was noted to be thickened and purplish. He had attributed it to irritation from the hearing aid. Further examination revealed that he had chronic lymphocytic leukemia. The ear was infiltrated with lymphoid cells that were demonstrated clearly on fine needle aspiration. A similar case with infiltration of the pinna has been recorded.[8]

The Eyes

Confrontational inspection of the face often will reveal an absence of symmetry of the eyes. Alterations of facial contour are often dismissed or simply do not register as an abnormal finding (see below). The elevation of per-

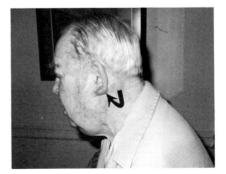

FIGURE 9-5: This patient with chronic lymphocytic leukemia presented with an infiltrated violaceous lesion (*arrow*) of his earlobe. Fine needle aspiration yielded sheets of mature lymphocytes.

iorbital skin, particularly under the eyebrows, should not be ignored. It may be the first evidence of a non-Hodgkin's lymphoma, as illustrated in the following case.

Case 9-4

The patient was a 77-year-old man with arteriosclerotic heart disease and moderate compensated congestive heart failure. He denied anorexia, weight loss, fever, or any systemic symptoms suggesting a pervasive disorder. On a routine examination, while checking the patient's blood pressure and state of cardiac compensation, his internist noted some swelling above the right eye and referred the patient for oncologic evaluation (Fig. 9-6).

On inspection, infiltrations also were noted in both anterior axillary folds and above the left breast (Fig. 9-7). Several skin nodules were evident on inspection of his torso. Fine needle aspiration at several sites, including the orbit, yielded lymphoid smears composed of poorly differentiated cells. Histologic examination of a surgical biopsy specimen confirmed a non-Hodgkin's lymphoma characterized as diffuse and poorly differentiated.

COMMENT In this case, fine needle aspiration served the purpose of immediately identifying the orbital lesion and demonstrating widespread cutaneous involvement, resulting in prompt treatment with chemotherapy.

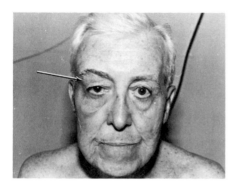

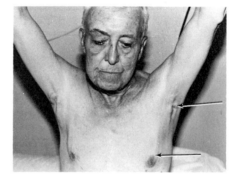

FIGURE 9-6: The swelling (*arrow*) above the right eye consisted of firm rubbery tissue over which the skin could be moved. Fine needle aspiration yielded lymphoid smears.

FIGURE 9-7: Infiltrations were palpable in both axillae and both breasts (*arrows*). These sites yielded similar lymphoid smears.

Proptosis of one eye in a patient with known primary cancer, particularly of the lung or breast, should raise immediate suspicion of retroorbital metastases. Figure 2-7 illustrates proptosis of the eye in a patient with metastatic chemodectoma arising in the parotid gland (see Case 2-6).

Metastases also occur in the orbit, and rarely to the anterior structures of the eye, including iris and lids. Such lesions are evident on careful inspection. An orbital lesion led to an unexpected diagnosis in Case A-5.

Enlargement of the lacrimal gland may be noted on inspection. In children, metastatic neuroblastoma may produce proptosis and periorbital ecchymoses, a cardinal sign.

Basal cell carcinoma of the eyelid or inner canthus should be evident on careful inspection.

The Face

On careful examination of a basal cell carcinoma at the root of the nose to plan radiation, an experienced radiotherapist failed to make note of a small but clearly evident nodular melanoma on the cheek, which was classified level III on excision. This failure is not particularly remarkable. It is related to the concept of focus. We tend to see what interests us, and this is no more evident than in reviewing the clinical practice of a variety of subspecialists who miss obvious pathology outside of their range of interest (see Case 10-1). An example is the occasional failure of a dentist to note an oral carcinoma immediately adjacent to a tooth he is treating.

Confrontational inspection of the face can reveal a variety of asymmetries in addition to those noted about the orbits and ears. These include

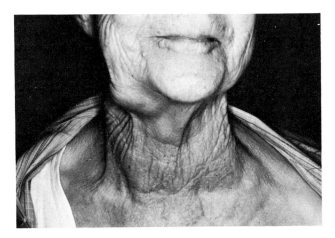

FIGURE 9-8: A firm parotid mass in this 66-year-old man yielded cytologic smears diagnostic of malignant mixed tumor.

bulging of a cheek because of tumor of a maxillary sinus, enlargement of a nasal ala or a lip (Fig. A-1), and parotid or submental swelling (Fig. 9-8; contrast with Fig. 9-1). Many of these are considered in Chapter 2, The Head and Neck Region, but Case 9-5 illustrates aspects of inspection and focus.

Case 9-5

A 61-year-old woman was referred by a plastic surgeon for fine needle aspiration of a parotid mass. This patient has been employed by the surgeon as a secretary for 6 years, but most recently had been employed by a dermatologist for 4 years. The surgeon had met her on the street and noted a fairly obvious parotid bulge. He was surprised to find that it had been present for more than 10 years. During her employment with him, she had worn her hair long to cover it. During her employment with the dermatologist, she had short hair, but he either had not noticed it or had not mentioned it.

COMMENT This case, of course, illustrates the limitations of casual inspection and the focus of the dermatologist, who ignored an obvious tumor.

Basal cell carcinoma often will escape notice on casual examination. Early lesions are bland, and may blend with the surrounding skin or may be considered part of a somewhat gnarled, wrinkled, or worn physiognomy, particularly in older men (Fig. 9-9). The small, pearly lesion with depressed

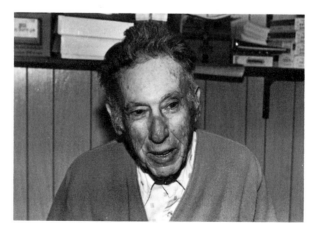

FIGURE 9-9: This elderly man had multiple facial lesions, not all of which were clinically diagnosable. (See Fig. 9-11.)

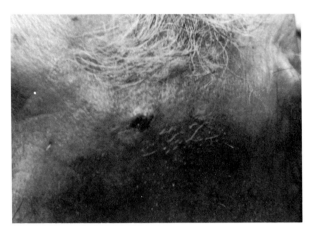

FIGURE 9-10: This lesion has elevated rounded edges with a depressed center. Clinically it is a typical basal cell carcinoma.

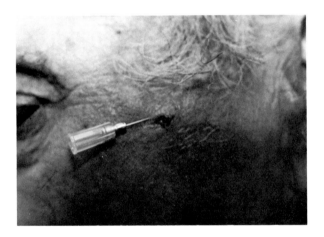

FIGURE 9-11: Fine needle aspiration yielded chronic inflammatory smears. The lesion regressed with local treatment.

center and rounded edges, however, is fairly characteristic. Differential diagnosis will become a consideration only if a lesion is noted by simple inspection in the first instance. Figures 9-10 and 9-11 illustrate that a "typical" basal cell carcinoma can turn out to be an inflammatory lesion.

The Neck

Abnormalities detected on inspection of the neck occur in organs considered in other chapters (thyroid, salivary glands, carotid body tumors, lymph nodes) and are a byproduct of a scanning examination for surface lesions and nodules. Figures 2-9A, 2-12 to 2-14, 3-5, and 3-8 illustrate types of lesions.

Apart from cutaneous lesions noted above, including primary melanomas, basal carcinomas, and squamous carcinomas, the major surface lesions occur after irradiation and surgery for a variety of head and neck tumors. Inspection of the incision or radiation site may detect the earliest evidence of recurrence crucial to salvage therapy. The curious recurrence of cancer precisely and exclusively within radiation portals has been noted in the literature,[3] and is seen more often in oncologic practice than is reported. Any skin thickening should be aspirated promptly.

PALPATION OF THE HEAD AND NECK

The hair-covered scalp requires palpation to disclose any lesions, and should be a routine part of an oncologic examination (Fig. 9-12). Searching palpation of the suboccipital region, angles of the jaw, submental areas, and triangles of the neck may disclose nodules and swellings not evident on inspection. Subcutaneous nodules may be found with greater regularity on stroking palpation than with selective patting of the tissues. Postirradiation and operative sites should be stroked for subtle early infiltrations.

Unlike the scalp, the more likely route of neck nodes and nodules is the lymphatic system. Dermal nodules arising by lymphatic permeation from contiguous recurrent breast carcinoma are most characteristic.

The Torso

The axillae, of course, can be inspected only on abduction of the arms. This is done routinely in breast examination in women (see Chap. 4), but Figure

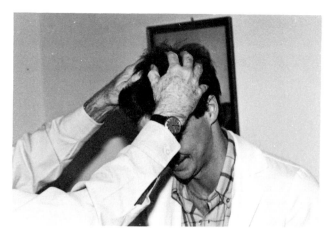

FIGURE 9-12: Palpation of the scalp should extend to the suboccipital region.

9-7 illustrates lesions in a man. Lack of symmetry of the breast, in men and in women, and bulges in the thoracic wall detected on simple inspection are sometimes the initial evidence of deep-seated disease unnoticed by the patient.

Surface lesions again appear in the post-treatment setting. After mastectomy, both the incisional scar, contiguous skin, and the radiation portal should be inspected carefully.

Lymphatic implants may appear as innocuous, sometimes slightly red, and discrete elevations several centimeters from the scar (Fig. 4-15). Fine needle aspiration with a 25-gauge needle will harvest a surprise yield of cancer cells. Post-thoracotomy incisions are occasional sites of implantation nodules (see below).

Other subcutaneous nodules resulting from hematogenous spread may be visible on inspection (see Case 9-1, Fig 9-3).

The Abdomen

Alterations in abdominal contour that are evident on inspection result from visceral abnormalities including hepatomegaly, splenomegaly, pelvic masses, metastatic masses, and ascites (see Chap. 6).

Apart from hematogenous tumor nodules, the umbilicus and periumbilical region are major points of inspection. Nodular infiltrations here are often of lymphatic origin. Paracentesis in patients with ascitic tumors may result in a tumor implant at the site of puncture. Figure 9-13A illustrates an obvious mass recurrent in the incision after laparotomy was done originally for stage III ovarian carcinoma. Aspiration of the mass is done simply, confirming the diagnosis (Fig. 9-13B).

PALPATION OF THE THORAX AND ABDOMEN

The oncologic examination of the thorax and abdomen should include fingertip palpation of all surgical scars to detect the earliest infiltration not evident on inspection. Stroking palpation of the body wall in search of metastases is important in the patient with known prior tumor. Skin nodules are usually asymptomatic, but not always as illustrated in the following case.

Case 9-6

A 46-year-old man presented 1 year after treatment of a bronchogenic carcinoma. The tumor had involved a right upper lobe bronchus without an evident pulmonary lesion on chest film but with widening of the superior mediastinum and early superior vena caval syndrome. Large cell undifferentiated carcinoma cells were found on bronchial wash. He was treated with radiation. There was complete disappearance of all radiographic evidence of tumor. He then received six cycles of chemotherapy with cisplatin and vinblastine sul-

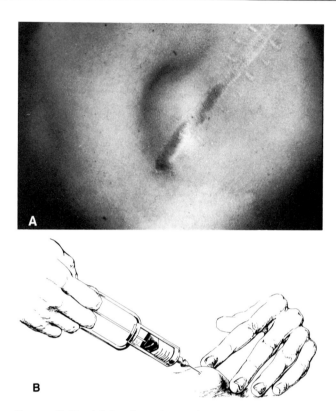

FIGURE 9-13: (*A*) Implantation nodule is seen in a patient with stage III ovarian carcinoma with malignant ascites. (*B*) This drawing illustrates aspiration of a nodule using a one-hand syringe.

fate (Velban). Follow-up chest films, bone scan, and chemistry profiles appeared to confirm his clinical complete remission at 1 year.

He returned complaining of a small, tender nodule under the skin of his right posterior hemithorax. It was firm, moved with the trapezius muscle, and measured 4 mm. On fine needle aspiration, a smear with abundant, poorly differentiated carcinoma cells was obtained. The remainder of the examination was entirely negative.

COMMENT The nodule could not be seen on inspection. Careful palpation might have detected it. Early attention was called to it by the tenderness.

Pelvis, Perineum, and Genitalia

Examination of the pelvis, perineum, and genitalia has been discussed in Chapter 7. Skin nodules of hematogenous origin may appear as they do in other areas. A lack of symmetry, particularly of the buttocks, may indicate a major, deep-seated tumor. Examination of the anal crease and perianal and anal tissue done at the time of digital rectal examination is important, since it is possible to pass an examining finger past a potentially lethal skin or mucocutaneous lesion, such as melanoma (discussed below) or squamous carcinoma. After abdominoperineal resection, recurrence of tumor may be heralded by surface nodules, which are easily visible and palpable. The patient may be unaware of them, or may have dismissed them as part of the scar.

Anal and genital warts usually can be recognized clinically, and do not become targets for fine needle aspiration.

Vulvar nodules secondary to metastatic hypernephroma were palpated and identified by fine needle aspiration.[9] Nodular alterations and infiltrations of the penis may occur, usually secondary to prostate carcinoma,[14] and may be identified easily by fine needle aspiration. Nodular alterations also occur with Peyronie's disease, which should not be confused. We have not observed secondary deposits in the scrotum.

Surface Changes

Pigmented Lesions

From the standpoint of inspection, pigmented lesions are the most evident surface changes. Clinicians repeatedly are being called upon to pass judgment on a variety of these lesions. It is certainly not uncommon for a patient visiting a cardiologist, gastroenterologist, or any variety of specialist or generalist to enlist an opinion about some newly observed pigmented spot or elevation. Because the vast majority are benign freckles, nevi, hemangiomas, or keratoses, they usually are dismissed. The alternatives are referral to a dermatologist or surgeon, a return visit to the referring general physician, or local excision by the examining physician if the spirit moves him.

What role, if any, does fine needle aspiration offer in management of primary pigmented lesions?

1. Clinical concern about any pigmented surface lesion varies from absolute certainty of its banal nature to high suspicion that it is a malignant melanoma. Many lesions that appear to be clinically benign may not warrant formal referral to a dermatologist, who may be inaccessible, or to a surgeon. Fine needle aspiration using a 25-gauge needle and a tangential technique (see Figs. 9-11, 9-22) will easily extract malignant melanoma cells, if they are present, from lesions several millimeters in diameter. Depending on the lesion, this is preferable to observation and postponement.

2. There are numerous sites in which incisional or excisional biopsy for diagnostic purposes is less desirable than having a preoperative diagnosis to plan definitive therapy (see Case A-1).

    a. Large facial freckles known as Hutchinson's freckle, particularly in elderly patients, not rarely show evidence of malignant melanoma. Prophylactic removal may require a major plastic surgical procedure, and is rarely undertaken. Careful observation for alteration in color or early nodular thickening followed by fine needle aspiration is a useful alternative.

    b. Pigmented lesions of the pinna of the ear, nasal frenum, or nasal alae, and vermillion lip border may be suitable targets for fine needle aspiration when the clinical status results in mild physician anxiety.

    c. Pigmented lesions of the anus, vulva, penis, and scrotum that are not clinically melanoma also may become targets for fine needle aspiration. It is more desirable to sample such a lesion than to postpone a decision.

    3.   Physicians sometimes are called upon to examine a patient with multiple lesions of the torso, particularly the back. Many of these lesions may be pigmented, and most are seborrheic keratoses. Scattered among them may be nodular pigmented lesions, raising mild suspicion of melanoma. Fine needle aspiration is a clinically useful technique in this context.

    4.   Finally, in experienced hands, particularly in the practice of clinical oncology, suspicious pigmented lesions in any site realistically may be targets for fine needle aspiration. It is important to remember that the color of a melanotic lesion may vary from black to tan to pink, to absence of pigment.

    Concern about dissemination of melanoma cells has been discounted because even incisional biopsy of pigmented lesions is acceptable to dermatologists.[6]

    Case 9-7 illustrates further use of fine needle aspiration in observing a clinical problem.

Case 9-7

The patient was a 78-year-old man who had a level IV melanoma widely excised from his right lateral chest wall with an accompanying axillary dissection. Recurrence infiltrated the scar and surrounding skin, producing an exophytic mass (Fig. 9-14). Fine needle aspiration yielded sheets of poorly differentiated, nonpigmented melanoma cells (Fig. 9-15). Treatment in the form of DTIC given intravenously for 5 days resulted in marked regression of the tumor mass, and suggested a marked cytolytic effect (Fig. 9-16). However, repeat fine needle aspiration of the tumor infiltrating the scar produced luxuriant tumor cells with no evidence of cytolytic effect. The tumor rapidly spread, leading to the death of the patient. It was presumed that the exophytic mass regressed because of poor vascular supply.

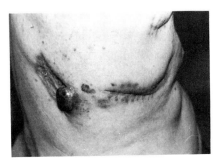

FIGURE 9-14: The incision and regional skin are infiltrated, producing an exophytic mass.

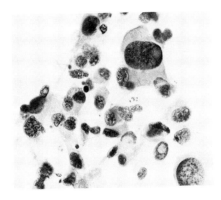

FIGURE 9-15: This smear is composed of polymorphous, dispersed, bizarre cells with nucleoli and intranuclear inclusions, characteristic of melanoma.

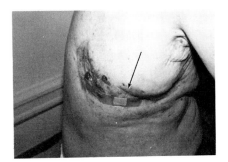

FIGURE 9-16: There was marked regression of the exophytic mass, but aspiration of the infiltrated scar (*arrow*) yielded florid melanoma.

The following two contrasting cases illustrate clinical problems that are resolved rapidly by fine needle aspiration.

Case 9-8

The patient was a 43-year-old woman referred by a general surgeon for evaluation of multiple, elevated, dark papules on her right thigh. Two years earlier, a level II melanoma had been widely excised from her knee. An inguinal node dissection had been done at the same time. Postoperatively, she developed an ileofemoral phlebitis. The surgeon interpreted the lesions as varicosities in a limb with compromised venous and lymphatic circulation.

Fine needle aspiration demonstrated melanoma cells. Individual lesions then were treated with intralesional bacille Calmette–Guérin

(BCG) with regression. The method allowed repeated sampling of the dermal lesions to judge regression.

Case 9-9

This patient was a 77-year-old woman referred by a neurologist for evaluation of disseminated dark papules on her right arm. He interpreted them as melanoma (Fig. 9-17). She had been referred to him for peripheral neuropathy involving that arm and had been to several physicians. The arm had been the site of an extensive congenital hemangioma, but its appearance had changed in the past 6 months. As many patients are, she was weary of visiting physicians and traveling to remote specialists.

Fine needle aspiration of several lesions yielded blood and a few endothelial cells, confirming the hemangiomatous nature of the lesions. There was no evidence of malignancy. The peripheral neuropathy remained unexplained but was attributed to possible effects of the vascular lesion. She was content with the diagnosis, and the clinical syndrome remained stable for a year.

COMMENT The clinical impressions of skilled physicians were supplemented usefully by examination of cytologic smears. The "shuttle syndrome," in which patients travel between doctors and cities, often can be interrupted by direct intervention with this simple technique.

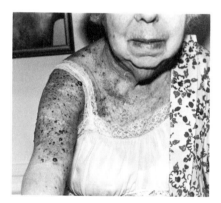

FIGURE 9-17: This patient had multiple dark papules that clinically resembled melanoma. The distinction was made easily with fine needle aspiration.

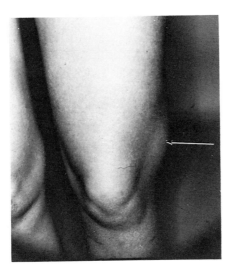

FIGURE 9-18: A lateral bulge (*arrow*) was known to the patient for 3 months. There was further delay by the physician for 2 months. Fine needle aspiration yielded a pleomorphic sarcoma.

Sarcoma: The Innocuous Swelling

When is a muscle bulge, a nodular cutaneous elevation, or an apparent lipoma a sarcoma? The late diagnosis of sarcoma is traditional. The evolution may be slow. The lesion is painless and unobtrusive. The characteristic patient evaluation is that "If it doesn't hurt, then it doesn't bother me." The characteristic physician response, depending on its size and rapidity of growth, is to postpone and check it again in a month, during which the patient may drift. There is a hesitancy to refer immediately for surgical biopsy because of the banal asymptomatic nature of the lesion (Fig. 9-18).

The usual swelling is in the extremities. This is illustrated in the following case.

Case 9-10

The patient was a 60-year-old man with a nodular goiter, for which he had studiously rejected surgical intervention. He finally consented to fine needle aspiration, which demonstrated degenerated colloid nodules. One year after this, he called his physician's attention to a bulge in the external surface of his upper left arm. He stated that it had been present and unchanged for 1 year. On inspection, it appeared to be an extra bulge in a muscular arm, not at all evident without special attention. On palpation, it was smooth, poorly defined, and measured approximately 2.5 cm by 1.5 cm. Again, he declined surgery but he agreed to fine needle aspiration. The material obtained was moderately cellular and consisted of oval cells with little cytoplasm. Nuclei were bland with no nucleoli. The impression was that of a benign lesion, but because a specific diagnosis could not be rendered, surgery was recommended. An ovoid lesion lying between muscle layers was found and extirpated.

The initial pathology report was that of a malignant spindle cell sarcoma, and further therapy was recommended. The Armed Forces Institute of Pathology thought it was a low grade hemangiopericytoma with limited malignant potential. The patient was referred to a large cancer center, where a tumor pathologist diagnosed (unequivocally, in his opinion) a benign schwannoma. No recurrence was evident at 1 year.

Several points emerge from study of this case:
1. Unobtrusive swellings may escape detection on routine examination. It is helpful to ask the patient if he has noticed any "lumps or bumps."
2. The length of time a lesion exists and its lack of symptoms are not decisive in recommending biopsy.
3. Benign but indefinable cytology mandates follow up with surgery.
4. Failure of cytology to conform to histology suggests that the lesion needs detailed study, as in Case 9-10 (three pathologists).

Where the swelling appears to be purely cutaneous, consideration should be given to dermatofibrosarcoma protuberans and to leiomyosarcoma of the skin.

Delay in Diagnosis

It is quite evident from the above discussion that small lesions may be highly malignant and potentially lethal tumors. At the same time, they may be unobtrusive, painless, and easily ignored. A systematic study of the problem has demonstrated that the patient and the physician are equally responsible for delay in diagnosis and that delay worsens the prognosis.[11]

Patient delay can be corrected by education. This has been demonstrated in the salutary effects resulting from self-examination of the breast (see Chap. 4).

Physician delay is a more complex problem. Failure to examine adequately and failure to recognize obvious pathology are deficiencies that can be corrected only by training. Postponing diagnosis of an apparently innocuous although visible or palpable lesion, however, can be circumvented by direct sampling of the lesion. Often the physician does not ignore the lesion, but simply postpones diagnosis because he believes surgical biopsy is unwarranted for an ''obviously'' benign disease. Many patients do not receive follow-up examinations.

The incorporation of the fine needle method into the daily practice habits or thinking of the physician will aid considerably in reducing delay.

Miscellaneous Surface Targets for Fine Needle Aspiration

There is a series of palpable surface lesions that are encountered infrequently, but that nevertheless must remain under clinical consideration.

NODULAR FASCIITIS

Nodular fasciitis may present as an enlarging subcutaneous mass, which may be tender. It is seen in young adults, most commonly in the neck, upper extremities, and torso. It varies in size up to 5 cm or 6 cm in diameter, and may be alarming. The cytologic picture is fairly characteristic, and fine needle aspiration offers the possibility of prompt preoperative diagnosis to relieve anxiety and the option of no surgery because it may spontaneously regress. The cellular yield may be quite abundant, and has been described.[2,13]

FIBROMATOSES

Fibromatoses have fairly characteristic clinical pictures and are unlikely targets for fine needle aspiration. Dupuytren's contracture is an example. Nevertheless, fibromatous nodules both in children and adults may be clinically puzzling. In this context, particularly in children, fine needle aspiration is useful. It can be anticipated that the yield may be meager in a collagenized lesion, but there is usually sufficient cellularity to provide clues to the diagnosis. More important, the absence of rich cellularity tends to exclude sarcoma. Surgery may or may not follow.

NEUROFIBROMA

Neurofibroma usually is recognized clinically because of the presence of multiple lesions and a clinical syndrome of von Recklinghausen's disease. Fine needle aspiration is not indicated in diagnosis of one of the pedunculated, molluscum-like lesions. However, a solitary neurofibroma may occur that is indistinguishable from other subcutaneous masses and sometimes is confused with an enlarged node. Fine needle aspiration is useful in suggesting a neural tumor.[13]

NEURILEMOMA (SCHWANNOMA)

Neurilemoma may present as an isolated, unidentified, subcutaneous mass, arising on a peripheral nerve. Usual sites are the extremities, head and neck, and thorax (intercostal nerves). Needle aspiration may produce excruciating pain, a unique reaction. The following case illustrates an interesting result of this observation.

Case 9-11

The patient was a 58-year-old woman with a history of right mastectomy at age 56. She was referred for evaluation and aspiration of a partially fixed right supraclavicular mass. On examination, no other nodes or masses were detected. The operative site was free of nodules. Fine needle aspiration produced severe pain. The clinical impression was that the needle had penetrated to the brachial plexus.

However, the cytology was that of a neural tumor. No evidence of metastases was present. Case A-9 also illustrates the importance of fine needle aspiration diagnosis of this neural tumor.

GRANULAR CELL TUMOR

Cytology of granular cell tumor of the skin is identified rather easily by an experienced observer. As in the breast,[8] it is a benign lesion.

CALCIFYING EPITHELIOMA OF MALHERBE

This lesion is a benign adnexal tumor of the skin that arises out of the hair matrix. Because of its more common location in the head and neck, it may be considered suspicious of a metastatic node. Fine needle aspiration yields a fairly characteristic picture.[8] Its identification is another example of the importance of sampling a mass of unknown origin before embarking on a major diagnostic search for a primary or carrying out surgical excision.

Two common lesions that ordinarily are not confused with any of the above, but that should be considered, are ganglia and lipomas.

GANGLIA

Ganglia, particularly of the wrist, are readily identified clinically. Where such a swelling is in question, needle aspiration will extract a thick, gelatinous material. A large-bore needle may be necessary, but extraction can be accomplished with a 22-gauge needle. In spite of rather easy clinical identification, fine needle aspiration serves the purposes of relieving patient anxiety and therapeutically reducing a tense swelling, even though temporarily.

GIANT CELL TUMOR OF TENDON SHEATH

Giant cell tumor of the tendon sheath, which is an unusual tumor, provides a unique target for fine needle aspiration. Its cytology is readily identifiable in the appropriate context. It is illustrated in the following case.

Case 9-12

The patient was a 66-year-old woman who visited a physician with a history of arthritis involving primarily the index and third fingers of her left hand (Fig. 9-19). The third finger in particular was enlarged and stiff, but was not painful. She had been treated intermittently for

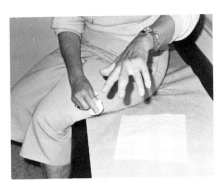

FIGURE 9-19: There is a fusiform
swelling of the third finger and a
lesser deformity of the index finger.
On palpation the third finger "mass"
had a rubbery texture.

2 years with antiarthritic medications and local heat treatments, with
no particular change. Sedimentation rate was 28 mm/h (Wintrobe)
and uric acid was 6.7 mg/dL.

On examination, the middle finger was enlarged. On palpation
there was a rubbery texture to the mass at the second interphalan-
geal joint. The index finger had minimal changes and the other fingers were uninvolved.

A fine needle aspiration was done (Fig. 9-20), yielding abundantly cellular smears. The report was as follows: "Fine needle aspiration yields numerous dispersed histiocytic 'cells' with occasional
multinucleated giant cells. *Diagnosis:* Consistent with giant cell tumor
of tendon sheath."

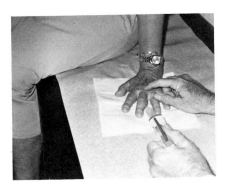

FIGURE 9-20: Fine needle aspiration
of the middle finger yielded a mixture
of fusiform and multinucleated giant
cells characteristic of giant cell tumor
of tendon sheath.

With a cytologic diagnosis of giant cell tumor of tendon sheath, the patient underwent hand surgery. The pathology report was as follows: "Microscopic sections of this soft tissue mass revealed proliferation of synovial lining cells and sub-synovial connective tissue. The component cells are spindle shaped, polyhedral, having round to oval nuclei. They are interspersed by dense, fibrous stroma. There is mild round cell infiltrate, several multinucleated giant cells, and aggregates of pigment-filled macrophages. The fibro–fatty tissue is seen partially surrounding it. *Diagnosis:* Giant cell tumor of tendon sheath."

COMMENT The surgery was successful, with complete recovery of mobility. The diagnosis was based on clinical, as well as cytologic, findings.

LIPOMAS

Lipomas are perhaps the most common surface lesion encountered in daily practice. They are fairly characteristic clinically and infrequently require aspiration. Their presence in atypical sites, such as the axilla or the breast, may prompt aspiration. They are often multiple, which confirms the clinical impression. Patients often express anxiety, and fine needle aspiration of a solitary lipoma or one from a multiple lipoma syndrome will alleviate anxiety. In general, the diagnosis can be made by simply observing the translucent material smeared on a slide. The cytology is characteristic.[13]

The Anxiety Factor

Rapid diagnosis of surface lesions, in contrast with postponement and return visit, clearly pays dividends in early discovery of metastatic nodules, sarcomas, and a variety of primary skin lesions (see above). Less evident but quite important is the sharp reduction in anxiety, which sometimes may be of morbid proportions, resulting from rapid diagnosis. Anxiety experienced by a physician is depicted graphically in an essay entitled *Lessons.*[4] The patient's surface "lump" was diagnosed as lipoma after considerable delay and unnecessary utilization of supplies and facilities (nursing, anesthesia, operating room, and surgeon).

Leukemia, Lymphoma, Mycosis Fungoides, and Kaposi's Sarcoma

A diffuse papular eruption occurs in acute monocytic leukemia. The patient may visit his general physician with vague symptoms and with such a rash. A preliminary diagnosis of a dermatologic disorder of unknown origin may be made. Dermatologic consultation may be inaccessible. A serology test and blood count usually are ordered. An abnormal blood smear should suggest the diagnosis. Aspiration of a papule with a fine gauge (25-gauge) needle will yield many dispersed blast cells. This is not only of great interest to the physician from a clinical pathologic standpoint, but it rules out a secondary dermatologic disorder engrafted on the leukemia.

Lymphoma cutis may take numerous forms. Characteristic is an elevated, smooth, violaceous, nontender lesion (Fig. 9-21). There may be multiple lesions. Figure 9-8 illustrates cutaneous infiltration that thickens the skin without producing a nodular elevation.

The most common site is the head and neck region.[1] Prompt fine needle aspiration and careful smears will answer the following questions immediately: (1) Is the material lymphoid? (2) Are the lymphoid cells small, well-differentiated lymphocytes or one of the varieties of large cell lymphomas (histiocytic; large cell, poorly differentiated lymphocytic; cleaved cell)? In one study, 44% were histiocytic types.[1] Nonmalignant lymphocytic infiltration may occur in the form of a benign lymphocytoma or in several dermatologic disorders. Although most lymphoid cutaneous lesions will come to surgical biopsy, particularly to distinguish nodular and diffuse non-Hodgkin's lymphoma, finding immature lymphoid cells will prompt an immediate staging workup. For the consulting oncologist, this is valuable because it will guide him in carrying out a bone marrow examination and selected blood studies in the same sitting.

The patient with mycosis fungoides may provide a longitudinal history beginning with dermatologic problems, including erythematous eczema. The lesions become targets for fine needle aspiration in the plaque stage. Characteristic cells with convoluted nuclei that are appreciated readily in cytologic preparations may be extracted.

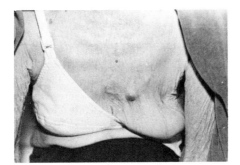

FIGURE 9-21: This patient had diffuse, poorly differentiated non-Hodgkins lymphoma involving abdominal nodes. The breast lesion was a cutaneous lymphoma deposit.

The early lesion of Kaposi's sarcoma may be an elevated pink or red papule. Although not diagnostically definitive, the extraction of slender fibrocytic cells rather than dispersed immature lymphoid cells will distinguish Kaposi's sarcoma from lymphoma cutis.

The Character of Metastatic and Recurrent Lesions

The physical characteristics of metastatic involvement of the skin depend to some extent on the mode of transmission of the tumor cells. Hematogenous tumor emboli ordinarily will produce a firm to hard subcutaneous mass over which the skin will slide. It may be fixed to underlying fascia. It can be controlled easily with one hand to allow puncture. The needle is usually introduced at an angle (Fig. 9-22).

Lymphatic tumor spread through dermal lymphatics will produce dermal nodules that move with the intact skin. Typical nodules are found in the skin of the chest wall during follow up after mastectomy. Satellite melanoma nodules are dermal and are spread by lymphatics (see above) in contrast with metastatic hematogenous melanotic nodules (see Fig. 9-3). A shower of black satellite nodules was interpreted as a curious development of varicosities by an experienced surgeon (see Case 9-8). Tangential aspiration with a 25-gauge needle easily yielded typical pigmented melanoma cells. If pigmented, metastatic subcutaneous hematogenous melanotic nodules may be seen through the skin.

Dermal nodules may appear initially as solitary lesions, then extend to form showers of nodules, and ultimately spread by contiguity in all directions from the original point of appearance.[14]

Implantation nodules may be found on careful follow-up examinations after numerous operative procedures. Two- or three-millimeter nodules may be palpated within the scar. Large subcutaneous nodules and masses may appear beneath or adjacent to the scar (see Fig. 9-14). In the early

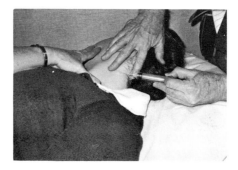

FIGURE 9-22: Aspiration of a superficial lesion using a plastic syringe without a handle.

weeks after tumor surgery, however, it is not unusual to feel fairly alarming nodularity beneath the scar, which on fine needle aspiration may yield some granulomatous or mild chronic inflammation.

Case 9-13 illustrates the unusual findings that a rather banal subcutaneous swelling may yield.

Case 9-13

The patient was a 54-year-old woman who noticed a painless swelling overlying the xiphoid process between her breasts (Fig. 9-23). General physical examination failed to reveal any gross disease, mass, or tumor. A chest x-ray and mammogram were negative. A fine needle aspiration yielded smears diagnostic of an epithelial tumor with many psammoma bodies (Fig. 9-24). This directed the examination to the ovaries, and the patient was referred for gynecological examination.

The patient had no gynecologic complaints. She was postmenopausal. Both adnexae appeared thickened. The cytologist insisted on exploratory surgery. At laparotomy, both ovaries were enlarged irregularly, and a total hysterectomy and bilateral oophorectomy were done. The diagnosis was psammomatous papillary carcinoma of the ovaries (Fig. 9-25). Following surgery, chemotherapy was administered. Fine needle aspiration of the residual subcutaneous mass re-

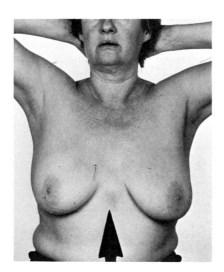

FIGURE 9-23: The subcutaneous mass (*arrow*) was surprisingly due to metastasis from a previously unknown ovarian primary.

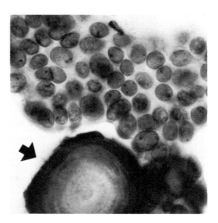

FIGURE 9-24: In this smear, psammoma bodies (*arrow*) are demonstrated clearly.

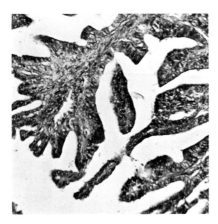

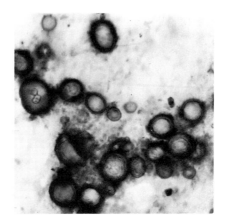

FIGURE 9-25: Tissue section, papillary carcinoma of the ovary.

FIGURE 9-26: Aspiration cytology smear. Psammomatous bodies remained after a metastatic mass was treated with chemotherapy.

vealed disappearance of the epithelial component, leaving many psammoma bodies behind (Fig. 9-26).

Summary

No other area challenges the clinician's powers of observation as does the body surface.[7] A large variety of lesions is readily available for examination and diagnosis. Most metastatic lesions are accompanied by a history of prior or concurrent primary tumor (as in Case 9-1). Careful inspection becomes, then, a crucial part of the oncologic follow-up examination.

The application of the principles of fine needle aspiration will enhance diagnostic sensitivity as well as rapidly establish a definitive diagnosis in most cases.

REFERENCES

1. Burke JS, Hoppe RT, Cibull ML et al: Cutaneous malignant lymphoma: A pathologic study of 50 cases with clinical analysis of 37. Cancer 47:300, 1981
2. Dahl I, Åkerman M: Nodular fasciitis: A correlative cytologic and histologic study of 13 cases. Acta Cytol 25:215, 1981
3. Diehl LF, Hurwitz MA, Johnson SA et al: Skin metastases confined to a field of previous irradiation. Cancer 53:1864, 1984
4. Frank SE: Lessons. JAMA 252:2014, 1984
5. Kline TS, Kannan V: Aspiration biopsy cytology and melanoma. Am J Clin Pathol 77:597, 1982

6. Knutson CO, Hori JM, Spatt JS Jr: Melanoma. In Current Problems in Surgery, pp 1–55. Chicago, Year Book Medical Publishers, 1971

7. Koop CE: Visible and Palpable Lesions in Children. New York, Grune & Stratton, 1976

8. Linsk JA, Franzen S: Clinical Aspiration Cytology. Philadelphia, JB Lippincott, 1983

9. Linsk JA, Franzen S: Aspiration cytology of metastatic hypernephroma. Acta Cytol 28:250, 1984

10. Malberger E, Tillinger R, Lichting C: Diagnosis of basal cell carcinoma with aspiration cytology. Acta Cytol 28:301, 1984

11. Robinson E, Mohilever J, Zidan J et al: Delay in diagnosis of cancer: Possible effect on the stage of disease and survival. Cancer 54:1454, 1984

12. Szpak C, Bossen EH, Linder J et al: Cytomorphology of primary small-cell (Merkel-cell) carcinoma of the skin in fine needle aspirates. Acta Cytol 28:290, 1984

13. Willems J-S: Aspiration biopsy cytology of soft-tissue tumors. In Linsk JA, Franzen S (eds): Clinical Aspiration Cytology, pp 319–347. Philadelphia, JB Lippincott, 1983

14. Willis RA: The Spread of Tumours in the Human Body. London, Butterworths, 1973

15. Woyke S, Domagala W, Czerniak B et al: Fine-needle aspiration cytology of malignant melanoma of the skin. Acta Cytol 24:529, 1980

10   The Skeleton

In clinical practice, patients with skeletal pains often are managed as arthritic or discogenic patients initially. Seasoned physicians will not rush to establish lethal diagnoses because they want to spare a patient unnecessary anxiety, and because primary and metastatic bone tumors are statistically uncommon and often incurable.

On the other hand, persisting in a diagnosis of arthritis or sprained back when neoplastic disease is the etiology of pain results in unnecessary morbidity. Diagnostic delay results from self-medication, suggestions by pharmacists, chiropractic manipulation, and routine films revealing ubiquitous degenerative joint disease. In one report, metastatic renal cell carcinoma presented as shoulder arthritis.[14]

Separating skeletal disorders from the total clinical picture may result in absurd decisions by the subspecialists. This is illustrated by the following case.

Case 10-1

The patient was a 62-year-old domestic worker diagnosed and treated in the oncology clinic for leiomyosarcoma metastatic to the lung. Diagnosis was established by a prior total abdominal hysterectomy for leiomyosarcoma of the uterus and fine needle aspiration of a pulmonary mass (see Chap. 5). The disease had progressed in spite of chemotherapy. The patient sustained a pathologic fracture of the femur and was admitted to the orthopedic service, where a procedure using cement was done satisfactorily (Fig. 10-1). She was seen subsequently in the oncology clinic quite depressed because her disability payments had been cut off retroactively, and she was suffering economically. She presented a copy of a letter from the orthopedist stating that she had recovered from the fracture and was ready to return to work. It was necessary to submit a letter indicating that the patient had advanced untreatable metastatic disease with a life expectancy of 3 months for her to continue to receive payments.

This is an example of the disorder known as "tubular vision." It highlights the importance of a clinical rather than a lesional approach to disease.

The rarity of primary bone lesions dictates that skeletal symptoms, particularly with identifiable alterations, must be viewed in the context of remote or systemic disease. Skeletal and "arthritic" and discogenic symp-

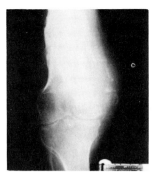

Figure 10-1: A pathologic fracture of the femur is immobilized by cement.

toms that are atypical, unconfirmed by appropriate ancillary studies, or fail to respond to treatment must be evaluated immediately for metastatic and infectious disorders. Fine needle aspiration has a well-defined role in this process (see Case A-15 in the Appendix).

Skeletal lesions become targets for fine needle aspiration following identification on x-ray films or scans. Such procedures are ordered routinely because of current skeletal symptoms or because of a current or prior neoplasm. Silent bone lesions often are detected during the perusal of films taken to investigate visceral symptoms. For example, it is not uncommon to identify blastic pelvic lesions in the film of an IVP taken to investigate a bladder outlet problem that turns out to originate in a prostate cancer.

The usual current symptoms and signs that mandate an x-ray study are pain, tenderness, and swelling overlying a bone. A painful lesion is illustrated in Case 10-4. Routine follow up of prior neoplasms to detect metastases in asymptomatic patients at times includes a total skeletal scan. Breast carcinoma is by far the most appropriate neoplasm to pursue by this technique. Routine skeletal scanning of asymptomatic patients with prior gastric, colonic, and renal carcinomas is inappropriate because the yield is low and because there is no currently effective treatment if a lesion is found. The asymptomatic prostate cancer patient will give a higher yield on scan, but whether any treatment is warranted on discovery of an asymptomatic bone lesion is a matter of debate.

In staging a current neoplasm, such as prostate, breast, and broncho-genic carcinomas, bone scan is probably useful before primary ablative therapy is undertaken, but it is not uniformly done.

With the widespread and often indiscriminate use of scanning, the use of skeletal films, particularly skeletal surveys, has declined. Finding a hot spot or lesion on scan should be followed by films for better delineation and localization of the lesion. However, skeletal films are not infrequently normal in the presence of a positive scan.

The Puncture

The fine needle, 22 gauge or smaller, is not designed for puncture of the intact bony cortex. The smallest gauge bone marrow needle used for sternal or posterior iliac puncture is 18 gauge. However, in our experience, the 22-gauge or 20-gauge needle can puncture the sternum, and it may be useful to puncture ribs (see Chap. 5). When inserted with a firm twisting motion, this needle can penetrate the thin cortex. Therefore, it is useful, particularly for rib aspiration in which careful control must be maintained to avoid skirting the rib and puncturing the lung.

The fine needle has its greatest utility in puncturing lytic bone lesions. Bone lysis can result in thinning of the cortex, disappearance of one cortical table, or total replacement of the bone by lesional tissue. This is illustrated in the following cases.

Case 10-2

The patient was a 63-year-old woman who attended the rheumatology clinic complaining of pain and swelling in her left knee with inability to bear weight. There was diffuse swelling of her leg above the knee, with loss of landmarks. Fluid within the knee could not be delineated. The tissues appeared moderately warm.

The patient was admitted, and a film revealed a diffuse lytic process (Fig. 10-2). There was no history of surgery. The patient did not smoke. General physical examination was not revealing, although her abdomen was somewhat obese and difficult to palpate.

The oncologist was asked to see the patient at the same time that the following studies and consultations were ordered by the resident: complete blood count; urinalysis; chemistry profile; Bence Jones protein in the urine; serum protein electrophoresis; urine im-

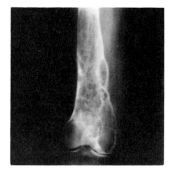

FIGURE 10-2: Diffuse lytic changes are seen in the distal femur.

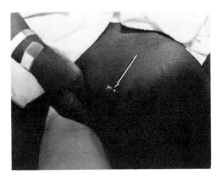

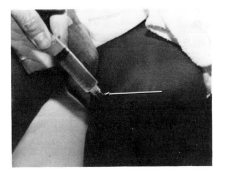

FIGURE 10-3: A fine needle with stylet in place (*arrow*) is inserted easily through the skin into the femur.

FIGURE 10-4: Aspiration is done at the bedside with a plastic syringe immediately available (*arrow*). Such a procedure can be done on routine rounds.

munoelectrophoresis; skeletal survey; bone scan; chest x-ray; and orthopedic, gynecologic, and oncologic consultations.

Following review of the film, a 22-gauge needle was inserted without anesthesia directly through the thin cortex (Figs. 10-3 and 10-4). Puncture yielded cytologic smears diagnostic of hypernephroma.

Many of the above studies were cancelled and an intravenous pyelogram was obtained, confirming the presence of a mass lesion in the lower pole of the left kidney.

Case 10-3

The patient was a 68-year-old retired steamfitter who visited his physician's office with pain, swelling, and tenderness in the metatarsal region of his right foot. Clinically, it had the appearance of gout. The patient was referred for an x-ray film (Fig. 10-5). Without clinical information, the radiologist reported "surgical removal of the second metatarsal bone."

The patient was referred for fine needle aspiration, and poorly differentiated adenocarcinoma was extracted. At this point, a workup was initiated with a chest x-ray, which revealed a small infiltrate in the right lung. The primary diagnosis proved to be bronchogenic carcinoma.

Where the bone harbors a lytic lesion and a thick cortex, it has been our experience on numerous occasions that fine needle aspiration of periosteal tissue of an involved bone will yield diagnostic smears. The needle

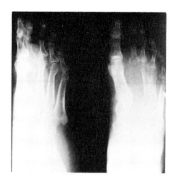

FIGURE 10-5: There is total lysis of the second metatarsal, which is interpreted radiologically as surgical removal of the bone.

tip is brought abruptly to the dense bony wall without attempting to penetrate it, and suction is applied with oscillation in the usual manner. The success of this maneuver is based on the likely fact that tumor cells situated in the marrow emerge through the marrow foramina to the periosteum without destroying the cortex. This was noted by von Recklinghausen,[18] but other mechanisms are not excluded.

Periosteal reaction because of unexpected acute leukemia has been aspirated with a fine needle, and the diagnosis has been established.[13]

The tumor may break out of the bone and form a soft tissue mass, which then becomes an easy target for fine needle aspiration, depending on accessibility.[17]

Finally, the bone may fracture because of pathologic changes, and puncture of the fracture site will yield diagnostic material.[17]

Where a lesion has been identified by an imaging procedure, it may be possible to perform a direct puncture using topographic landmarks or by simple palpation of a bony defect (see Case 2-6). Localized tenderness with or without swelling may guide an accurate office or bedside puncture. This is illustrated in the following case.

Case 10-4

The patient was a 71-year-old woman who was seen initially in September 1981 for a small mass in her left breast. A cytologic diagnosis of carcinoma was followed by a modified radical mastectomy. In 1983, a colonic polyp was resected endoscopically and a small focus of carcinoma was found in the tip. In September 1984, she complained of exquisite pain in her left rib cage with tenderness localized in the posterior sixth rib. A bone scan revealed a lesion in the area of tenderness as well as one in the fourth lumbar vertebra (Fig. 10-6).

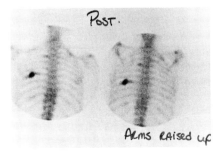

FIGURE 10-6: A distinct lesion in the left posterior sixth rib is noted on bone scan. Such a lesion can be punctured in the office or at the bedside if there is point tenderness.

The patient was referred for biopsy and opinion. The point of tenderness was so localized that a 22-gauge needle could be slipped easily into the rib at that point, yielding cells consistent with the original breast carcinoma. The patient was referred immediately for radiation therapy.

COMMENT Many lesions require fluoroscopic guidance, and may be reached provided they are evident on skeletal films. With negative films, positive lesions on scan are reached by careful evaluation of the target with the help of a radiologist and guided puncture. However, as in this patient, clinical findings may guide the puncture.

Skeletal Involvement

Primary Tumors

Radiographic differentiation of solitary primary tumors from solitary metastases is normally not difficult, but diagnosis may require coordination with morphology. Primary tumors arising from osseous tissue are seen rarely in a community hospital patient population, and even more rarely are referred for fine needle aspiration.

Major experience with the aspiration cytology of primary tumors of necessity has been gathered at major tumor institutions.[1,3,9,16,17] Needle biopsy with cytologic diagnosis of primary malignant bone tumors has been reported from Memorial Hospital for Cancer and Allied Diseases by Hajdu and Melamed.[9] Eighty-six aspiration specimens of osteogenic sarcoma, chondrosarcoma, malignant giant cell tumor, fibrosarcoma, chordoma, Ewing's sarcoma, plasmacytoma, and reticulum cell sarcoma gathered from

1960 to 1969 were studied. This paper concluded with the statement: "Properly used, needle aspiration cytology is a simple, rapid, and accurate diagnostic technique that can be applied to the study of bone tumors with minimal discomfort to the patient."

In a large aspiration cytology clinic (Karolinska), fewer than 10 patients with primary bone tumors out of a total of 10,000 patients are aspirated annually. This may be due in part to failure of the orthopedists to avail themselves of the service. However, the paucity of primary bone tumors is apparent. Therefore, attention must be directed to secondary tumors of the skeleton, which are common clinical problems.

Secondary Tumors

The skeleton becomes involved by tumor through several mechanisms. Invasion of bone by a contiguous neoplasm does occur, and may produce primary destruction of bone with lytic lesions identified on x-ray films. The primary tumor is usually available for puncture, and as a rule, this will explain the bone lesion.

A lytic lesion of the skull because of a meningioma is illustrated in Case A-4. They also have been noted in the literature.[5,8] Similarly, chordomas producing bone destruction are illustrated in Case A-2, and are cited by Willis.[18] In both of these tumors, the cause of the lytic lesion may be surmised, but cytologic or histologic studies are required for definitive diagnosis.

In destruction of facial bones by cancers of the sinuses, skin, nose, and mouth, the cause is self-evident. However, local bone destruction may occur without clear evidence of the local tumor producing the lysis. A common example is a rib destruction due to a peripheral bronchogenic carcinoma not specifically identifiable. This is illustrated in Figure 10-7 in which an anteroposterior (AP) view demonstrates absence of a rib section. Minimal pleural thickening was evident. Fine needle aspiration yielded poorly differentiated adenocarcinoma, and a primary tumor at the subpleural site was demonstrated subsequently. Fine needle aspiration may yield a specific diagnosis, but if the cytology is nonspecific, the question of local invasive tumor versus metastatic deposit remains unsettled.

Metastases of Hematogenous Origin

Metastases to bone are of hematogenous origin and are carried intially to the marrow.[18] Extracting metastatic deposits on routine sternal or iliac bone marrow aspirations when there is no gross, x-ray, or isotopic evidence of cancer is not at all uncommon, with oat cell carcinoma of the lung a leading source and example. Tumor grows expansively within the marrow cavity. Lytic tumors produce erosion, thinning, and cortical destruction, which allows penetration by a fine needle. The usual neoplasms are my-

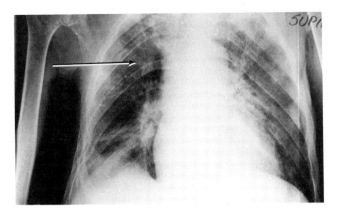

FIGURE 10-7: Absence of rib segment is noted (*arrow*). This yielded poorly differentiated adenocarcinoma on aspiration.

eloma, carcinoma of the breast and lung (which are common), hypernephroma (which is less common), and thyroid carcinoma (which is quite infrequent). All other neoplasms occasionally may invade the bone and produce lysis.

Even in the presence of known past or concurrent primary cancers, the etiology of bone lesions can only be surmised. This is illustrated in the following case.

Case 10-5

The patient was seen 1 year after treatment of a melanoma of the chest wall by wide excision and placement of a skin graft (Fig. 10-8). It was a nodular melanoma, level III. The patient had a history of arthritis and cervical and lumbar radiculopathy. He was followed up with routine examinations after removal of the melanoma, and was quite well until the abrupt onset of severe neck and lower back pain and pain in the extremities. He had not lost weight and was otherwise feeling well.

On physical examination, there was no evidence of local recurrence of the melanoma. His skin was clear of evidence of satellite skin lesions or remote skin nodules. There were no enlarged lymph nodes. His liver was not enlarged and no other masses were evident. His prostate was smooth, slightly enlarged, and firm.

Because of severe pain, he was admitted to the hospital where bone x-rays were carried out. The films demonstrated narrowing of disc spaces in the cervical and lumbar spine. In addition, a bone scan was done, and numerous areas of increased uptake were noted, diagnostic of disease metastatic to the skeleton. The radiologist was very

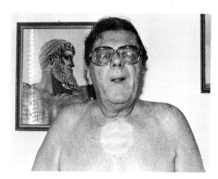

FIGURE 10-8: This patient had a cutaneous melanoma that was treated surgically with a graft. The sternum was
punctured on three successive occasions at the identical graft–skin margin
to demonstrate disappearance of metastatic melanoma cells with chemotherapy (DTIC).

skeptical that this could have arisen from the melanoma, and he fa-
vored prostate as a primary.

Before performing a fine needle aspiration of the prostate, a
nondirected sternal puncture was done with a 20-gauge needle.
Smears consisted of masses of pigmented melanoma cells.

Hematogenous metastases also are illustrated in Cases 10-2, 10-3, and
10-4 above.

FREQUENCY AND DISTRIBUTION OF METASTASES

The frequency of skeletal metastases can only be estimated, since an
accurate investigation would require longitudinal slicing and inspection of
long bones and the vertebral column, as well as multiple sampling of flat
bones at autopsy. Such procedures are impractical. However, skeletal metastases were discovered in 13.6% to 47.5% of carefully performed autop-
sies.[6,18]

Solitary skeletal metastasis is clinically a rare event if a longitudinal
history of the disease is kept in mind. Frequently, an initial solitary metastasis after mastectomy may be treated with irradiation, only to be followed
at varying intervals by the appearance of new skeletal lesions.

The distribution of skeletal metastases has been studied by several
observers.[2,4,10,18] The skull, ribs, vertebrae, pelvis, and proximal long bones
are affected most commonly. This may be related to the fact that these
bones harbor most of the red marrow. Within the vertebral column, the
lumbar spine is the preferential site, and within the vertebra, the body is
the usual site. However, disappearance of the lamina is a frequent x-ray

report, and lytic lesions of the spine, arch, and processes may become targets for fine needle aspiration. Not all destructive lesions are due to neoplasm. Case A-15 illustrates the sequence in such a case.

Lesions of the Skull

Targets for fine needle aspiration are identified easily by films of the skull (see Fig. 10-10; see also Fig. 2-8). The skull provides numerous targets, illustrated below. Osteoblastic lesions are not penetrated with a fine needle, but aspiration of the periosteum will often yield tumor cells (see above). Lytic lesions of the calvarium, on the other hand, are aspirated easily, although it must be emphasized that care must be exercised. A tangential approach is satisfactory. The site of puncture is identified by palpation (see Cases 2-6 and A-3), or puncture may be carried out under fluoroscopic control (see Case A-4).

Both Paget's disease and fibrous dysplasia may undergo sarcomatous degeneration.[12] The primary diseases usually are recognized by clinical and radiographic findings. Malignant alteration may produce swelling and tenderness. Malignant change should be recognized easily by cytologic smears.

Although the most common skull targets are of metastatic origin (see below), the following primary skull lesions should be kept in mind:

Paget's disease with sarcomatous degeneration
Fibrous dysplasia with sarcomatous degeneration
Cholesteatoma
Eosinophilic granuloma
Plasmacytoma

Solitary myeloma (plasmacytoma) may exist without evidence of systemic disease. When it is discovered, a general examination is done, including skeletal films, protein studies, and marrow aspiration. If results of studies are negative, primary plasmacytoma may be diagnosed and treated locally. Generalization of the disease will occur in most cases (see Case A-10).

Cholesteatoma is a benign lytic lesion with benign sclerosing edges which may occur in the calvarium. It is composed of squamous epithelium shedding keratin flakes (epidermoid cyst) and should be easy to identify by fine needle aspiration.

Eosinophilic granuloma is an inflammatory lesion that may present as a solitary lytic lesion of the calvarium. Cytologic diagnosis is rendered easily by an experienced cytopathologist. Clinical aspects are illustrated in the following case.

Case 10-6

The patient was a 24-year-old woman (Fig. 10-9) who reported to her physician complaining of a frontal headache. Analgesics produced temporary relief and the patient was referred for neurologic

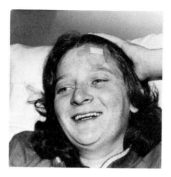

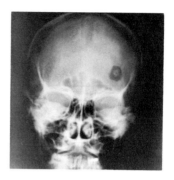

FIGURE 10-9: This patient had eosinophilic granuloma, left frontal skull. Transcutaneous puncture was done through a palpable defect. The puncture site is marked by a bandage.

FIGURE 10-10: Skull film with lytic lesion. The differential diagnosis was eosinophilic granuloma and osteomyelitis.

consultation. Skull films revealed a left frontal lytic lesion with a doughnut pattern. The differential diagnosis was eosinophilic granuloma and osteomyelitis (Fig. 10-10).

Using the skull film for guidance, the lesional defect could be palpated. Fine needle aspiration using a 22-gauge, 1-inch needle inserted tangentially yielded smears diagnostic of eosinophilic granuloma. A neurosurgeon planned surgery, proceeding with a covering plate.

The importance of diagnosing eosinophilic granuloma preoperatively is illustrated also in Case A-3.

The above lesions are mainly solitary. Metastatic lesions may be multiple. With a known primary such as breast or bronchogenic carcinoma, there is no reason to sample metastatic lesions. However, the ease of aspiration makes it important to sample solitary lesions, even with a known primary. The procedure may confirm that a stage I disease is, in fact, stage IV. On the other hand, an apparent stage IV disease may be redefined by the cytologic findings. This is illustrated in Case A-4.

The common primary tumors are breast, bronchogenic, and renal cell carcinomas and multicentric myelomas. However, any neoplasm may be a source. An unusual tumor is illustrated in Case 10-7.

Case 10-7

The patient was a 74-year-old man who visited his family doctor with a complaint of hemorrhoids. Examination revealed a bulge at

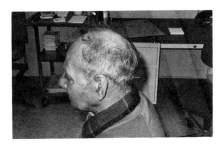

FIGURE 10-11: The contour of this patient's head was normal on visual inspection. A soft defect could be palpated.

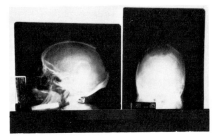

FIGURE 10-12: On these views of the patient's skull, a massive defect is illustrated dramatically.

the anal verge. Bleeding occurred easily on digital examination, and he was referred to a proctologist. A diagnosis of basaloid carcinoma of the anal canal was made. The patient was treated with radiation at his request with apparent clearing of the lesion.

One year later, he was seen by a neurologist because of persistent headaches. Results of physical examinations were negative, but his scalp was not palpated. The contour of his head was normal (Fig. 10-11). He was referred for a skull x-ray (Fig. 10-12). The massive defect was interpreted as a lytic metastatic lesion, and he was referred for fine needle aspiration.

Aspiration yielded smears consistent with small cell carcinoma. He was treated with radiation.

Although lesions commonly appear in the cranial vault, the occiput and mastoid regions must not be neglected. Lytic lesions of the skull base may be approached through the nose, cheek, and under the occipital ridge.[7] These punctures require fluoroscopic control. An example of puncturing through the cheek is illustrated in Case A-2. As shown in Figure 3-10, the needle may be passed through the nasal vestibule and enter the pituitary fossa. Cytologic diagnoses obtained include pituitary adenoma and craniopharyngioma (see Case 3-5).

The Cervical Spine

The bodies of the upper cervical vertebrae are punctured easily transpharyngially through the mouth (see Case A-10, Fig. A-35).

The lower cervical vertebrae are entered by a lateral approach with the patient supine. The needle remains posterior to the posterior margin of the sternocleidomastoid muscle and should be observed fluoroscopically entering the lesions. The anterior approach is illustrated in Figure 10-13.

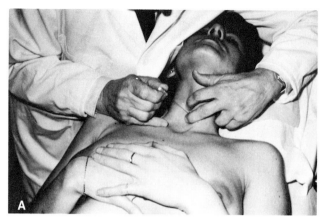

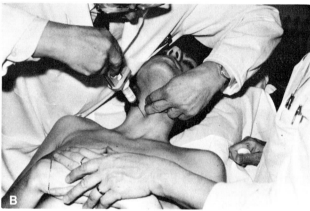

FIGURE 10-13: (*A*) A lytic defect in a cervical vertebra is punctured anteriorly by deflecting the larynx and manually inserting a needle. (*B*) Aspiration is then carried out.

Long Bones, Sternum, and Ribs

All long bones, the sternum, and the ribs are easily accessible. There may be exquisite localized tenderness, particularly in the sternum. In the presence of x-ray evidence of lytic lesions, direct puncture may be carried out. (The ribs are considered in greater detail in Chap. 5.)

Thoracic and Lumbar Vertebrae

The approach to lytic lesions and pathologic compression fractures of the vertebrae have been reviewed by Salzman.[15] A tangential approach under fluoroscopic control allows entrance of a fine needle into a vertebral body. The point of entrance is 6.5 cm from the lumbar spinous process and 4 cm from the thoracic spinous process, to avoid puncturing the lung.[15] A lead marker is placed with the patient in prone position. Where possible, a right-sided approach is preferable to avoid the aorta. In the thoracic region, the needle enters above the rib caudal to the involved vertebra.

The Pelvis

The bony pelvis is an ideal target for fine needle aspiration. The iliac wings, pubic, and ischial bones are reached easily. Using films and topographical landmarks, most lytic lesions can be aspirated. Less accessible targets may require fluororoscopy or CT scanning.

Case 10-8 illustrates problems in diagnosis and surprise findings.

Case 10-8

The patient was a 56-year-old electrician who developed a mild pain in his left hip region 3 months before he was seen in consultation. He attributed the symptoms to the maintenance of a cramped position during a recent construction job. The pain gradually increased, and he was seen and treated symptomatically by his family physician on three occasions with no relief. He then visited a chiropractor who x-rayed the area and told him he had no serious problem. With continuous pain, he was referred for consultation.

History revealed that he had smoked 50 pack years. His appetite and weight were stable and he had no gastrointestinal symptoms. On physical examination, there was evident clubbing of his fingers. Lungs were clear. No nodes or masses were palpated. The liver was not enlarged. Digital rectal and prostate examination were negative.

The film was reviewed and was deemed unsatisfactory (Fig. 10-14). Computed tomography of the area was requested, and it demonstrated a destructive lesion in the wing of the ilium (Fig. 10-15).

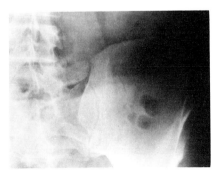

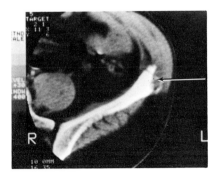

FIGURE 10-14: This is a film of left ilium with a poorly visualized lytic defect.

FIGURE 10-15: The lytic lesion is evident on CT scan. Fine needle aspiration yielded mucinous carcinoma.

Precisely at that point, there was point tenderness. A fine needle was passed through the thin cortex of the left iliac wing, and abundant cellular material diagnostic of mucinous adenocarcinoma was obtained. A chest film (Fig. 10-16) revealed a mass in the right lower lobe.

The final diagnosis was bronchogenic carcinoma with metastasis to the left ilium. The patient was referred for palliative radiation therapy to the ilial lesion. Hospitalization was not required. The patient was placed on protocol chemotherapy with partial regression of the lung tumor.

The sacrum may be approached from its posterior aspect or anteriorly by transrectal aspiration.

The most common pelvic bony lesion is prostatic metastasis, almost always osteoblastic and unsuitable for fine needle aspiration. The usual lytic lesions are metastatic, bronchogenic, breast, and renal carcinomas, and multiple myeloma.

Primary bone tumors occur. A chondrosarcoma indistinguishable radiographically from metastatic carcinoma has been described.[11]

Summary

The application of fine needle aspiration to the diagnosis of bone lesions is considerably simplified by the ease of visualization both on x-ray films and scans (Fig. 10-17). Palpation of defects and points of tenderness is an additional useful guide. It has been demonstrated repeatedly that diagnostic smears may be prepared from periosteal aspiration and that many bones can be punctured with needles as small as 20 gauge. The sternum and ribs, for example, are suitable targets at times. Frankly lytic lesions are entered and aspirated easily with even finer needles.

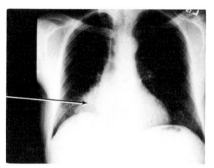

FIGURE 10-16: A mass (*arrow*) in the right lower lobe is evident. It was the source of the mucinous carcinoma.

X-ray alteration with or without pain, tenderness, swelling

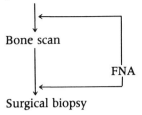

Bone scan

FNA

Surgical biopsy

Comment: Open bone biopsies are rarely necessary if FNA can be carried out. X-ray control may not be necessary if there is point tenderness, swelling, or palpable defect.

FIGURE 10-17: Diagnostic schema for bone lesions.

The importance of sampling solitary lesions has been demonstrated. It has been proven to change previous staging unexpectedly.

Cooperation among the primary physician, the radiologist, and the cytopathologist is essential.

REFERENCES

1. Agarwal PK, Wahal KM: Cytopathologic study of primary tumors of bones and joints. Acta Cytol 27:23, 1983
2. Aufses AH: Skeletal metastases from carcinoma of rectum, report of 8 cases. Arch Surg 21:916, 1930
3. Bhatia A: Letter: Problems in the interpretation of bone tumors with fine needle aspiration. Acta Cytol 28:91, 1984
4. Copeland MM: Skeletal metastases arising from carcinoma and from sarcoma. Arch Surg 23:581, 1931
5. Cushing H: Cranial hyperostoses produced by meningeal endotheliomas. Arch Neurol Psychiatr 8:139, 1922
6. Drury RAB, Palmer PH, Higman WJ: Carcinomatous metastases to the vertebral bodies. J Clin Pathol 17:448, 1964
7. Franzen S: Needle biopsy in skull base tumors. In Disorders of the Skull Base Region, pp 285–287. Stockholm, Proceedings of the Tenth Nobel Symposium, 1968
8. Grant FC: Cranial endothelioma. In Trans Phila Acad Surg. Ann Surg 81:1036, 1925
9. Hajdu SI, Melamed MR: Needle biopsy of primary malignant bone tumors. Surg Gynecol Obstet 133:829, 1971
10. Lenz M, Fried JR: Metastases to skeleton, brain, and spinal cord from cancer of breast and effect of radiotherapy. Ann Surg 93:278, 1931
11. Linsk JA, Franzen S: Clinical Aspiration Cytology. Philadelphia, JB Lippincott, 1983
12. Mirra J: Bone Tumors: Diagnosis and Treatment. Philadelphia, JB Lippincott, 1980

13. Phillips J, Goodman BN, Harding-Smith J et al: Fine needle aspiration cytology of an unusual presentation of leukemia. Acta Cytol 27:334, 1983
14. Ritch PS, Hansen RM, Collier BD: Metastatic renal cell carcinoma presenting as shoulder arthritis. Cancer 51:968, 1983
15. Salzman AJ: Imaging techniques in aspiration biopsy. In Linsk JA, Franzen S (eds): Clinical Aspiration Cytology, pp 25–40. Philadelphia, JB Lippincott, 1983
16. Stormby N, Åkerman M: Cytodiagnosis of bone lesions by means of fine needle aspiration biopsy. Acta Cytol 17:166, 1973
17. Willems J-S: Aspiration biopsy cytology of tumors and tumor-suspect lesions of bone. In Linsk JA, Franzen S (eds): Clinical Aspiration Cytology, pp 349–359. Philadelphia, JB Lippincott, 1983
18. Willis RA: The Spread of Tumours in the Human Body. London, Butterworths, 1973

Central Nervous System Lesions

11

Discrete lesions of the central nervous system will become targets for fine needle aspiration with greater frequency in the coming years. Although needle aspiration diagnosis is not new,[10,11] it has not reached general acceptance in the past because of the limited experience in microscopic interpretation. Techniques for reaching the lesion do not pose serious problems in the modern surgical and radiologic arena.[9,15,16] Puncture of the central nervous system is in fact a fertile field for the development of both simple and complex methods with varying instrumentation.

Familiarity with the potential for rapid diagnosis will be important to practicing clinicians, and appropriate dialogue with neurosurgical and radiology services is strongly indicated.

The frequency of interventional diagnosis and therapy for metastatic and primary brain tumors will vary from one institution to another. In one series, 101 patients underwent craniotomy for removal of metastatic lesions and during the same period 111 primary brain tumors were operated upon.[6] Where diagnosis by FNA (see below) is available, craniotomy for metastatic disease is unusual in our experience.

The Clinical Pattern

Lesions potentially suitable for fine needle aspiration are suggested by clinical examination but must be confirmed by radiographic studies. Computed tomographic (CT) scanning has simplified identification and localization. Before considering an invasive procedure, the full clinical picture must be reviewed, including history and physical examination. Prior and current neoplasms must be assessed carefully.

Solitary intracranial masses identified in patients with known past or current carcinomas of the lung, breast, gastrointestinal tract, and kidney, as well as melanomas, must be reviewed carefully before proceeding with intervention. The major primary tumor to consider is bronchogenic carcinoma. Brain metastases occurred in 26% to 41% of cases in five series reported by Willis.[17] In contrast, only 14 of 126 cases of prostatic carcinoma metastasized to the brain, and all were far advanced tumors.[14] The classic tumor in which brain radiation is instituted without further diagnostic intervention is oat cell carcinoma of the lung. It will colonize the brain in a sufficiently high percentage of cases to warrant prophylactic brain irradiation by some clinicians.

Elderly patients (age 80 years to 100 years) with past or current carcinoma (see above) probably will receive brain radiation for a solitary mass without diagnostic intervention.

Younger patients with liver or other metastases probably will receive brain radiation for solitary masses as well. On the other hand, younger patients without other evidence of metastases probably will be subjected to neurosurgical evaluation, including fine needle aspiration.

The number of variables is unlimited, but the clinical judgment of the primary physician is critical.

Where there is no known primary tumor, the patient should have a focused diagnostic workup, including chest x-ray, mammography, careful surveillance for cutaneous and ocular melanoma, and possibly intravenous pyelography.

Some primary brain tumors may be diagnosed on purely clinical findings, including angiography. Radiation may proceed without biopsy confirmation.

Multiple intracranial masses are almost invariably of metastatic orgin, although rare cases of multiple primary meningiomas or gliomas do occur.[1] Forty-four percent of 81 cases of primary lymphoma of the central nervous system were multifocal.[4]

Therefore, the final decision concerning the need for biopsy should rest on a collaborative approach that includes input from the primary physician, the neurologist or neurosurgeon, and the radiologist. It is important that the primary physician does not abdicate his role in the effort, since his knowledge of the patient's history and psychological profile is crucial to the decision process. In particular, he is responsible for a thorough patient evaluation including breast, pelvic, and rectal examinations that normally are not the province of the neurosurgeon or neurologist. Proceeding immediately from radiologic identification to neurosurgical intervention will not always be in the patient's best interest. Finally, fine needle aspiration carried out by the neurosurgeon is an excellent technique for resolving ambiguities.

It is in the interest of the clinician and the patient, when confronted with an intracranial mass, to try to resolve the problem at the regional or community hospital level rather than to shuttle the patient immediately to a referral center. Therefore, the clinician first must discuss with the pathologist his expertise in interpreting cytologic smears from aspirated brain and spinal cord lesions. Where experience is limited, smears can be referred to appropriate cytopathologists for primary diagnosis. This is entirely in keeping with the current practice of sending blood and urine specimens thousands of miles for special chemistry procedures. Expertise in securing appropriate cytologic specimens of intracranial and intraspinal lesions is the province of the neurosurgeon in cooperation with the radiologist.

Securing a Specimen by Fine Needle Aspiration

Access to a mass encased in bone (calvarium or spinal column) should be accomplished by the simplest method. Although reports of collections of brain tumors emanate from major referral centers, clinical problems arise repeatedly in community and regional hospitals. Such problems can be dealt with at the local level, where computed tomography (CT) is now readily available.

A simple technique involves localizing the mass with CT and placing a marker on the prepared scalp. When the marker on the scalp and the lesion on the scan are clearly visualized and related, the patient is taken to the operating suite. There, under local anesthesia, a twist drill produces a 1-mm hole down to the dura. A 22-gauge needle is passed through the hole down to the previously determined depth and the material is extracted. Aspiration is carried out at several depths to assure extraction of lesional material. A small hole allows direct puncture without deviation or angulation of the needle.

For deep-seated and in particular for small lesions, stereotactic techniques are emphasized. (These are illustrated in Case A-7 of the Appendix.) Such techniques are usually available only at referral centers where sufficient cases are collected to promote expertise and justify the technology.[8,9,15]

Aspiration during a craniotomy is useful for deep-seated lesions. Where cytopathologic expertise is available, rapid diagnosis analogous to frozen section can be offered. Failure to examine the specimen prior to closure may leave the patient with sutures in situ and no diagnosis. It is useful to encourage fine needle aspiration of all lesions at craniotomy even if surgical excision is contemplated. This will provide the pathologist with material for correlative study.[9] In addition, anticipated tumor resection cannot always be accomplished, and securing cytologic smears as an initial procedure is a good clinical habit.

Aspiration through a lytic lesion of the skull is accomplished fairly easily (as illustrated in Case A-4).

Optimally, smears should be prepared in the operating room and fixed in 90% ethyl alcohol. Air-dried smears also should be prepared, if possible, particularly if metastatic tumor is suspected. Time invested in learning and practicing the smear method will eliminate many of the problems in diagnosis that initially occur. None of this is feasible unless the surgeon and the pathologist have a commitment to this type of diagnostic approach.

Preoperative fine needle aspiration is an important adjuvant method. It is not necessary when radiographic evidence is pathognomonic of a tumor that can be treated with radiation (see above). If the symptoms mandate immediate surgery, as in some posterior fossa tumors, preoperative cytologic studies are not obtained. However, specimens taken at the time of surgery are useful, as noted above. Tumors that appear clearly to be operable meningiomas do not require preoperative identification. However, in elderly patients or in patients with other medical disability, diagnosis of an intracranial lesion by fine needle aspiration is preferable to hazardous exploratory surgery.

Finally, infarction of the brain may produce neuroradiologic changes difficult to distinguish from tumor. Fine needle aspiration will yield smears with a "dirty" appearance. There is necrosis intermixed with scattered remnants of gray matter containing degenerated astrocytes. Some areas may be fairly cellular. In other parts, there are foamy histiocytes and crystal formation.

Approach to Spinal Lesions

The approach to spinal lesions is based on the same principles as intracranial lesions. Access to the tumor may be accomplished through a guide needle or at the time of laminectomy. This is illustrated in the following case.

Case 11-1

A 24-year-old man was admitted to the hospital with increasing weakness in both legs. A mass was detected in the spinal canal. With the help of a guide needle introduced to the tumor site, a fine needle aspiration was done (Fig. 11-1). A large amount of mucoid material was obtained. The smears contained many cells gathered into rosettes characteristic of ependymoma (Fig. 11-2). The patient was treated with radiation.

Description of a lesion at T-10 is given in Case 11-2.

Case 11-2

The patient was a 46-year-old black laborer seen in 1976. His history was that of progressive difficulty in walking over 1 year's duration. During the 3 months preceding his visit to the office, the patient had been unable to work and had shown increasing clumsiness.

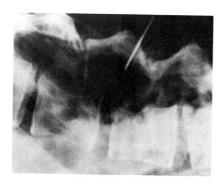

FIGURE 11-1: Fine needle aspiration of spinal cord tumor. Gelatinous material was extracted from ependymoma.

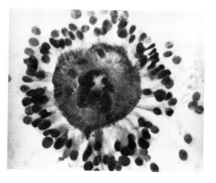

FIGURE 11-2: Aspiration cytology of ependymoma. Typical rosette.

Neurological examination revealed the presence of a spastic paraparesis. The right leg appeared to be weaker than the left leg. Ankle and knee clonus were present on the right. The patient's sensory deficit was patchy. There was a loss of vibratory sense about the left ankle compared to the right. There was diminution of position sense bilaterally.

Myelography was performed, and revealed the presence of an intramedullary defect at the T-10 level. At surgery, a cystic intramedullary tumor was recognized. The tumor was fusiform in shape. The cyst yielded brownish fluid on fine needle aspiration. The cyst was marsupialized by a small myelotomy. The patient tolerated the procedure well.

Cytologically, the smears were diagnostic of ependymoma.

The patient received postoperative radiation therapy. Reportedly, he was seen 6 months later riding a bicycle.

The Lymphomas

Discrete involvement of the central nervous system by non-Hodgkin's lymphoma is statistically an uncommon event.[5,7] Intracerebral involvement in Hodgkin's disease is considered even more uncommon. Cuttner and co-workers added 6 cases to a total of 28 collected from the literature up to 1979.[3] However, cord compression because of extension of both Hodgkin's and non-Hodgkin's lymphoma is an event seen frequently by clinical oncologists and radiotherapists. Such cases appearing sporadically in many community and regional hospitals will be reported infrequently.

Because lymphomatous involvement of the CNS may be successfully treated by radiation or chemotherapy, it is important that the clinician maintain an alert and expectant attitude regardless of the reported statistics.

The following questions should be reviewed and answered:

1. Is there a past or current diagnosis of lymphoma?
2. Did the screening examination in search of a primary include consideration of an undiscovered lymphoma?
3. Is the known non-Hodgkin's lymphoma a nodular or diffuse histiocytic type?

These questions are all raised in the following case.

Case 11-3

The patient was a 43-year-old woman admitted to the hospital with a suspected brain tumor. Thirteen years previously, a biopsy was done of a femoral lymph node, yielding a diagnosis of non-Hodgkin's lymphoma.

Clinical staging at that time revealed no other site of disease. The femoral region was irradiated. The patient was symptom free for 13 years. Three months prior to admission, the patient experienced headache, anxiety, and somnolence. Her physician could find no organic basis, and referred her for psychiatric opinion and finally for a neurological evaluation. At this point, her symptoms had progressed, and the neurologist made a clinical diagnosis of a large parietal mass.

General physical examination, apart from the neurological examination, was essentially negative although a node estimated at 1 cm in diameter was palpated high in the axilla. Breast examination including mammography was negative. Pelvic examination, chest x-ray, and intravenous pyelogram were all negative.

At this point, attention was directed to the history of lymphoma and slides were retrieved. Histologically, it was a nodular, poorly differentiated non-Hodgkin's lymphoma with one portion of the node exhibiting diffuse involvement.

The patient began to experience bilateral leg weakness and neurologically appeared to have a cord lesion in addition to the brain lesion. However, there was no block on myelogram.

At this point, following the identification of a large parietal mass on CT scan (Fig. 11-3), a fine needle aspiration was carried out using the twist drill method. Smears diagnostic of poorly differentiated non-Hodgkin's lymphoma were obtained.

In spite of radiation, the disease rapidly progressed and the patient died. At autopsy, histologic studies showed that the tumor was diffuse histiocytic non-Hodgkin's lymphoma. There was an intramedullary cord lesion that had produced transverse myelitis.

COMMENT The history of lymphoma was unusually remote in time and was not immediately brought to the attention of the clinicians. A

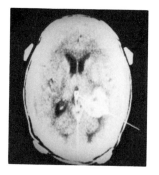

FIGURE 11-3: CT scan of head. Fine needle aspiration of intracranial mass (*arrow*) yielded smears diagnostic of non-Hodgkin's lymphoma.

solitary axillary node suggesting a possible breast primary could have been aspirated and at least could have excluded carcinoma. The diagnosis of lymphoma, particularly if poorly differentiated, also would have been possible from such a node. Review of the original pathology revealed a nodular lymphoma. The vast majority of brain lymphomas are diffuse histiocytic types. In this case, the metastases were diffuse in type.

Primary brain lymphoma, which is rare, is illustrated in the following case.

Case 11-4

The patient was a 71-year-old man admitted to the hospital in 1977 after having headache and increasing weakness of the left side of his body for 1 week. In 1966, a cerebrovascular accident had left him with mild left hemiparesis.

General physical examination apart from the neurological examination was not revealing. A chest x-ray and intravenous pyelogram were negative.

On brain scan, a large abnormal focus of activity was noted in the right hemisphere deep in the posterior right parietal lobe. It had the appearance of a tumor mass, probably glioblastoma multiforme. On angiography, the mass was partially vascular and was consistent with a glioma.

At craniotomy, a small amount of tissue was obtained. Several smears were prepared from deeply aspirated sites.

The tissue diagnosis was astrocytoma. The slides were submitted to the Armed Forces Institute of Pathology (AFIP) for confirmation.

The cytologic diagnosis was poorly differentiated lymphoma. The AFIP confirmed a diagnosis of lymphoma. The patient was treated with radiation therapy, and responded well.

Cytologic Potential

Depending on the level of cytologic expertise, the following brain lesions can be identified by fine needle aspiration.[9,15,16]

Metastatic tumors
Meningiomas
Astrocytomas
Oligodendrogliomas
Ependymomas

Medulloblastomas
Germinomas
Pinealomas

Skull base lesions are considered in Chapter 10.

Conclusion

Fine needle aspiration of the central nervous system has to this time received the least attention in the published literature.[12] Experience with exfoliative cytology is useful, but as pointed out by Rosenthal,[12] it cannot be used as a basis for diagnostic expertise in aspirated material. Where a commitment has been made to this method, correlative study of tissue and cytology by the pathologist is the best way to acquire cytologic expertise.[9,15] Where pre-extirpative aspiration has not been done, touch preparations will provide excellent cytologic detail.[2,11,13]

More important is the recognition by practicing clinicians that this is a feasible approach to the solution of clinical problems involving the brain and spinal cord. Many of these problems are part of an overall systemic disorder, such as metastatic carcinoma or lymphoma, in which major surgery will introduce an unwarranted degree of morbidity.

The clinician's interest will stimulate neurosurgical and pathology colleagues to undertake these diagnostic investigations. Reference to works by Rosenthal,[12] Willems,[15,16] and Liwnicz[9] is recommended.

REFERENCES

1. Bhangui GR, Roy S, Tandon PN: Multiple primary tumors of the brain including a medulloblastoma in the cerebellum. Cancer 39:293, 1977
2. Cardozo PL: Atlas of Clinical Cytology. Targa bv's-Hertogenbosch, 1975
3. Cuttner J, Meyer R, Huang YP: Intracerebral involvement in Hodgkin's disease. Cancer 43:1497, 1979
4. Henry JM, Heffner RR, Dillard SH et al: Primary malignant lymphomas of the central nervous system. Cancer 34:1293, 1974
5. Herman TS, Hammond N, Jones SE et al: Involvement of the central nervous system by non-Hodgkin's lymphoma. Cancer 43:390, 1979
6. Kishi K, Normura K, Miki Y et al: Metastatic brain tumor: A clinical and pathological analysis of 101 cases with biopsy. Arch Pathol Lab Med 106:133, 1982
7. Levitt LJ, Dawson S, Rosenthal DS et al: CNS involvement in the non-Hodgkin's lymphoma. Cancer 45:545, 1980
8. Lewander R, Bergström M, Boethius J et al: Stereotactic computer tomography for biopsy of glioma. Acta Radiol [Diagn] 19:Fasc 6, 1978
9. Liwnicz BH, Henderson KS, Masakuwa T et al: Needle aspiration cytology of intracranial lesions. A review of 84 cases. Acta Cytol 26:779, 1982
10. Marshall LF, Bryan J, Langfitt T: Needle biopsy for the diagnosis of malignant glioma. JAMA 228:1917, 1974

11. McMenemy WH: An appraisal of smears: Diagnosis in neurosurgery. Am J Clin Pathol 33:471, 1960

12. Rosenthal DL: Cytology of the central nervous system. Basel, S Karger, 1984

13. Russell DS, Krayenbühl H, Cairns H: The wet film technique in the histological diagnosis of intracranial tumors: A rapid method. J Path Bart 45:501, 1937

14. Taylor HG, Lefkowitz M, Skoog SJ et al: Intracranial metastasis in prostatic carcinoma. Cancer 53:2728, 1984

15. Willems J-S: Aspiration biopsy of tumors of the central nervous system and the base of the skull. In Linsk JA, Franzen S (eds): Clinical Aspiration Cytology, pp 361–370. Philadelphia, JB Lippincott, 1983

16. Willems J-S, Alva-Willems JM: Accuracy of cytologic diagnosis of central nervous system neoplasms in stereotactic biopsies. Acta Cytol 28:243, 1984

17. Willis R: Spread of Tumours in the Human Body. London, Butterworths, 1973

Appendix:
Case Panorama

Case A-1

A young child (Fig. A-1) was noted to have a slight enlargement of the nasal ala. The skin and mucosa were intact and the alteration was barely noticeable. The tissue was firm on bimanual palpation. Fine needle aspiration (Fig. A-2) yielded smears highly suggestive of embryonal rhabdomyosarcoma (Fig. A-3). The cytologic diagnosis was confirmed by electron microscopy using aspirated material (Fig. A-4). The tumor was removed, and the diagnosis was confirmed histologically (Fig. A-5).

COMMENT This is an example of lesions that appear in sensitive areas such as the nose, lips, ears, labia, anus, and penis. Such lesions can be sampled rather painlessly with a fine needle. Fine needle aspiration often will spare the patient an incisional biopsy.

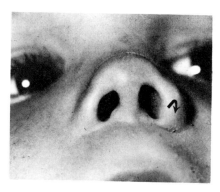

FIGURE A-1: Close-up of thickened nasal ala (*arrow*) in a 2-year-old child.

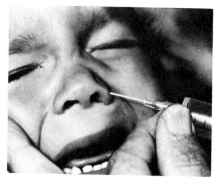

FIGURE A-2: Fine needle aspiration of the nasal ala.

Case A-2

The patient was a 78-year-old woman with vague head symptoms that prompted a skull film. A solitary destructive lesion was seen at the skull base.

There was no history of surgery. Complete physical examination

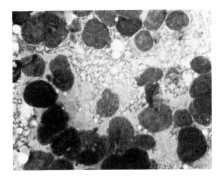

FIGURE A-3: Aspiration cytology. Poorly differentiated blastlike cells led to cytologic diagnosis of embryonal rhabdomyosarcoma in the clinical context.

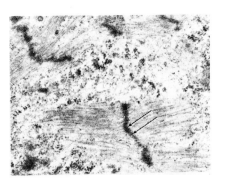

FIGURE A-4: Electron microscopy of aspirated cells. Z-lines (*arrows*) with attached microfilaments (actin filaments) are diagnostic.

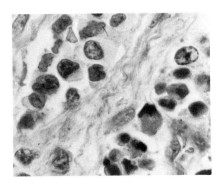

FIGURE A-5: Tissue section, biopsy of nasal ala. Diagnosis of embryonal rhabdomyosarcoma was confirmed.

failed to detect any primary lesion. A study for myeloma, including sternal puncture, was negative. Consideration was given to a primary lesion and the differential diagnosis included primary plasmacytoma and chordoma.

Under biplanar fluoroscopic control with the patient sitting up, awake, and cooperating (Fig. A-6), a guide needle was passed through the cheek toward the lesion (Fig. A-7). A fine needle was then introduced into the lesion and abundant mucoid cellular material was extracted. The cytologic diagnosis was chordoma (Fig. A-8).

COMMENT An attempt should be made to diagnose all basal skull lesions by fine needle aspiration. The cytology of pituitary adenomas, chordomas, craniopharyngiomas, and metastatic carcinoma is quite distinctive and these lesions are distinguished easily.

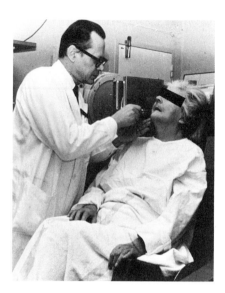

FIGURE A-6: A guide needle is passed through the cheek to the base of the skull under fluoroscopic control.

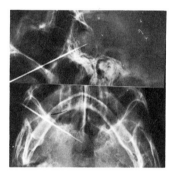

FIGURE A-7: Films of the destructive lesion of the skull base with guide needle in place. A fine needle has been passed through the guide and enters the target.

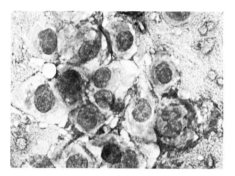

FIGURE A-8: Aspiration cytology. Round cells in dense mucinous stroma are characteristic of chordoma.

Case A-3

A 17-year-old girl (Fig. A-9), a former athlete, was seen in the aspiration clinic with palpable scalp lesions overlying lytic skull defects that were demonstrated on a skull film (Fig. A-10). Aspiration was done without fluoroscopy. It yielded typical smears of eosinophilic granuloma (Fig. A-11). This diagnosis was no surprise because it had already been established by an open biopsy of the fifth lumbar vertebra, which had required a laminectomy that resulted in the orthopedic defect seen in Figure A-12. The histologic diagnosis at that time was eosinophilic granuloma.

COMMENT The surgeon presumably was unaware that such a diagnosis could have been made by needle aspiration of the vertebra under radiographic control. Aspiration diagnosis could have been followed by radiation therapy. Although the patient felt well, her athletic career was curtailed. This case highlights the importance of awareness of the utility of fine needle aspiration for all clinical specialties.

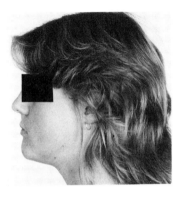

FIGURE A-9: This patient, a 17-year-old girl, had scalp masses palpable under her hair.

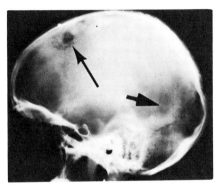

FIGURE A-10: Skull film. There are lytic lesions (*arrows*) underlying the scalp masses.

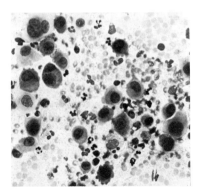

FIGURE A-11: Aspiration cytology. Atypical histiocytes, eosinophils, and polymorphonuclear leucocytes are characteristic of eosinophilic granuloma.

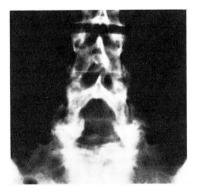

FIGURE A-12: Lumbar spine film. The spinal arch has been removed at L4.

Case A-4

In 1974, this patient, a 60-year-old woman (Fig. A-13), had back pain, diffuse osteoporosis, and elevated sedimentation rate. A gamma spike was seen on serum protein electrophoresis. In spite of this compelling picture, careful bone marrow studies and other confirmatory tests failed to demonstrate myeloma. Symptoms were intermittent for several years.

In 1981, the patient complained persistently of headache. A skull film was taken initially to evaluate this complaint. It revealed a solitary destructive lesion, and appeared to confirm a diagnosis of myeloma. However, sternal marrow was still normal, and therefore, an aspiration of the skull lesion was done with a 22-gauge needle under fluoroscopic control. The smear did not contain plasma cells,

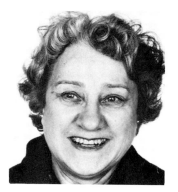

FIGURE A-13: Patient (aged 60 years) after recovery from surgery.

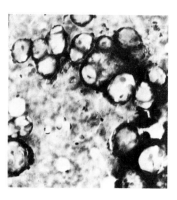

FIGURE A-14: Aspiration cytology. Whorled clusters of cells are characteristic of meningioma.

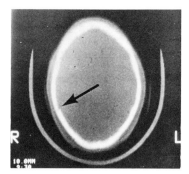

FIGURE A-15: CT view of skull. The *arrow* indicates a small erosive defect.

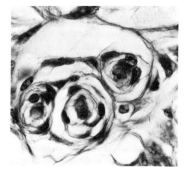

FIGURE A-16: Tissue section. Meningioma.

but did contain cell clusters typical of meningioma (Fig. A-14). In spite of this finding, a CT scan failed to show a mass lesion (Fig. A-15). However, at surgery a small meningioma was found. It was confirmed histologically (Fig. A-16). Lysis had been produced by erosion from within. The final diagnosis was benign monoclonal gammopathy and meningioma. The possibility of further evolution of the disorder to full-blown myeloma remained under consideration.

Case A-5

The patient was an 80-year-old woman complaining of pain in her left eye (Fig. A-17). Ophthalmologic examination by an eye specialist revealed a tumor at the inner corner. It was evident on CT scan (Fig. A-18). On careful palpation, the edge of this tumor could be detected. The eye specialist requested an immediate aspiration.

Smears were obtained and were examined promptly. They revealed a carcinoma composed of fairly small cells, some of which had purple intracytoplasmic inclusions (Fig. A-19). This was highly characteristic of breast carcinoma.

At this point, the patient was asked to disrobe for examination (Fig. A-20). A radical mastectomy had been done 15 years previously. The histology of the original tumor corresponded to the cytology of the aspiration.

COMMENT In this case, the cytologist was asked to see the patient during the course of the eye examination. For that reason, the puncture was done before history was obtained and physical examination was performed. It is evident that the discovery of a prior mastectomy

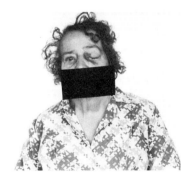

FIGURE A-17: This 80-year-old woman had pain in her left eye. She also had ptosis, medial ecchymosis, and a palpable mass.

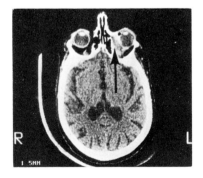

FIGURE A-18: CT view of the skull. A tumor (*arrow*) is pressing the left eye laterally.

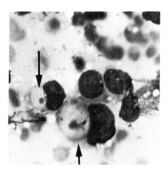

FIGURE A-19: Aspiration cytology. The cytoplasmic inclusions are characteristic of breast carcinoma.

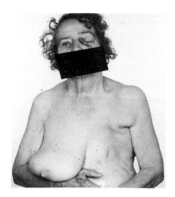

FIGURE A-20: Patient discloses mastectomy done 15 years previously.

would have raised the question of metastasis to the eye. The clinical picture would have guided the cytologic diagnosis, just as in this case the cytologic diagnosis directed the clinical examination.

Case A-6

A 76-year-old woman visited the clinic as a self-referred patient because of a soft swelling in the midline of her neck (Fig. A-21). It had been present for several years, but her family recently had encouraged her to have it investigated. There was no family history of thyroid disease. On examination, the mass was soft to firm and clinically appeared to be a cyst. However, during palpation a second, smaller, firm to hard nodule, of which she was unaware, was palpated in the right lobe of the thyroid. During the palpation, her face became flushed.

A scintigram was ordered. It revealed cold areas at the site of the cyst and at the second nodule (Fig. A-22).

At this point, aspiration of the cyst yielded typical tan cyst fluid containing pigmented histiocytes. Aspiration of the nodule yielded a typical cytologic picture of medullary carcinoma (Fig. A-23). Calcitonin level was elevated markedly.

Total thyroidectomy was done. The specimen is seen in Figure A-24.

COMMENT Clinically, this patient appeared to have a thyroid cyst, but careful examination revealed further disease of unknown character until the cyst was sampled. Pressing on the nodule produced a facial flush suggesting the release of vasoactive substances from the mass

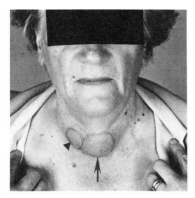

FIGURE A-21: Complex thyroid enlargement in a 76-year-old woman. A cystic mass (*barbed arrow*) and a solid tumor (*triangular arrow*) are delineated.

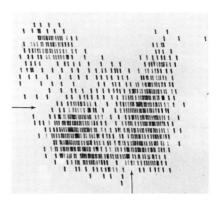

FIGURE A-22: Scintigram. Defects in pattern (*arrows*) are sites of cyst and tumor.

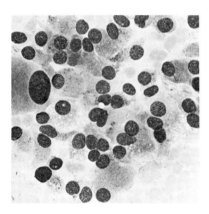

FIGURE A-23: Aspiration cytology. Fine reddish cytoplasmic granulation is characteristic with Romanowsky's stain.

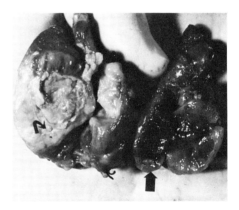

FIGURE A-24: Gross surgical specimen, thyroid. Hemorrhagic cyst (*thick arrow*) and pale fleshy medullary tumor (*curved arrow*) are evident.

into the bloodstream. This observation should suggest the diagnosis of medullary carcinoma to the clinician. Here, the scan displayed two cold nodules, one caused by a malignant tumor and the other by a benign cyst. Finding the medullary carcinoma and the elevated calcitonin level should prompt a study of family members.

Case A-7

A 23-year-old medical student had headaches for 6 months that were attributed to the pressure of his studies and depression. He fi-

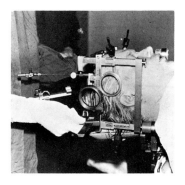

FIGURE A-25: Fine needle aspiration of deep brain lesion using stereotactic apparatus and a long fine needle (*white dot*).

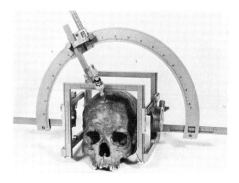

FIGURE A-26: Stereotactic apparatus.

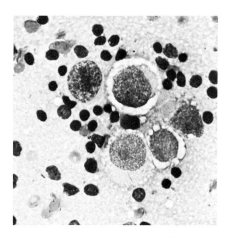

FIGURE A-27: Aspiration cytology. Large tumor cells intermixed with lymphocytes characteristic of seminoma are evident.

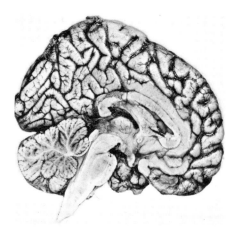

FIGURE A-28: Gross coronal section of brain. There is no evidence of a midline tumor.

nally was evaluated neurologically. CT scan revealed a midline tumor. The radiographic diagnosis was pinealoma.

Stereotactic biopsy was done, utilizing a fine needle (Fig. A-25). The stereotactic apparatus is shown in Figure A-26.

The smear contained a mixture of lymphocytes and large, dispersed malignant cells (Fig. A-27). Results of reexamination of the testes were negative, and a diagnosis of seminoma or midline germinal tumor was rendered.

The patient was treated with 3500 rads. His symptoms disappeared. However, he sustained a post-therapy depression, and committed suicide. At postmortem examination, there was no evidence of tumor (Fig. A-28).

COMMENT This technique allows presurgical diagnosis of almost all deeper brain lesions. Superficial lesions can be reached without stereotactic methods (see Chap. 11).

Case A-8

This patient, a 27-year-old man, came to the clinic with a left supraclavicular nodal enlargement that he had discovered (Fig. A-29). Fine needle aspiration yielded smears diagnostic of embryonal carcinoma (Fig. A-30).

This patient denied any abnormality of the testes. On examination a small (4 mm) mass was detected in the superior pole of his left testis. Fine needle aspiration yielded the same cytologic material.

COMMENT With present chemotherapy, this is a curable case.

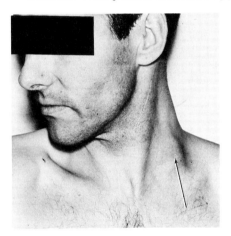

FIGURE A-29: A man (aged 27) with left supraclavicular mass (*arrow*).

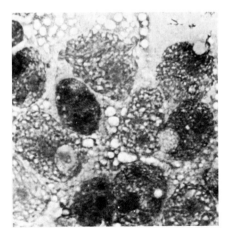

FIGURE A-30: Aspiration cytology. Vacuolated primitive cells are characteristic of embryonal carcinoma.

Case A-9

The patient was a 74-year-old woman who complained of difficulties in swallowing for about 4 months. She had lost considerable weight.

On examination, she appeared chronically ill. Examination of the head and neck revealed a hard lymph node palpable on the left side of the neck. An otolaryngologist visualized a papillary tumor rising from below into the hypopharynx. Barium swallow demonstrated a tumor in the upper third of the esophagus (Fig. A-31). Histopathologic diagnosis of an excised biopsy specimen was poorly differentiated squamous carcinoma.

Because of her age, poor nutrition, and apparent neck node metastases, the decision was made not to attempt therapy. However, aspiration of the node yielded not squamous cancer but a schwannoma (Fig. A-32). Therefore, the tumor appeared to be stage I, and the patient was treated with nutrition through a nasogastric tube, chemotherapy using the Price–Hill formulation, and radiation therapy, using only 2000 rads.

The tumor had disappeared on follow-up x-ray examination. Four years after therapy, the patient was remarkably fit (Fig. A-33).

COMMENT This case is cited not to illustrate an unusually favorable response to therapy, but rather to emphasize that palpation alone is not diagnostic of neck metastases. In this case, failure to identify the neck mass would have led to the patient's prompt demise.

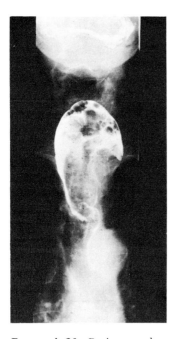

FIGURE A-31: Barium swallow. There is an exophytic tumor in the upper third of the esophagus.

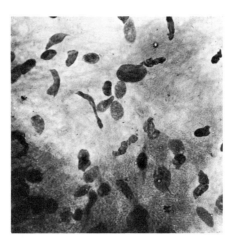

FIGURE A-32: Aspiration cytology, schwannoma. The smear was extracted from a cervical node. Squamous carcinoma was anticipated.

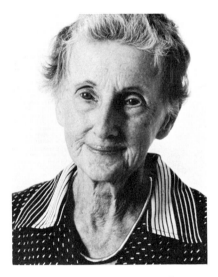

FIGURE A-33: The patient is shown 4 years after therapy.

Case A-10

A 70-year-old man complained of neck pains. An x-ray film of the cervical spine revealed destruction of the right half of the C-2 vertebra (Fig. A-34). The radiographic differential diagnosis was metastatic carcinoma or myeloma.

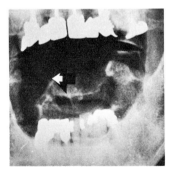

FIGURE A-34: Transoral film of cervical vertebrae. The right half of C-2 is not evident.

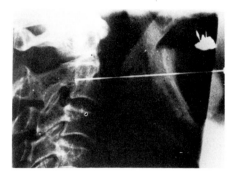

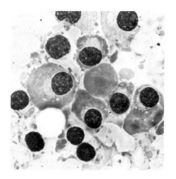

FIGURE A-35: Transpharyngeal puncture of C-2 vertebra using a long fine needle with x-ray control.

FIGURE A-36: Aspiration cytology. The smear illustrates typical plasma cell myeloma.

There was no history of a primary tumor. He was afebrile and otherwise asymptomatic. On physical examination, there was no adenopathy and no evidence of tumor in the head and neck region, abdomen, or rectum. The prostate was slightly enlarged and smooth.

Laboratory studies including blood count, urinalysis, chemistry profile, and serum protein electrophoresis were not revealing. A chest x-ray was normal. Results of sternal marrow aspiration were negative for myeloma and metastatic carcinoma.

Finally, under fluoroscopic control, the vertebra was punctured transpharyngeally (Fig. A-35). Smears obtained were crowded with plasma cells (Fig. A-36).

The patient responded to radiation therapy. On follow up several years later, the sternal marrow became infiltrated with myeloma cells, indicating dissemination.

Case A-11

The patient was a 68-year-old woman with a history of multiple primary cancers. Endometrial carcinoma was diagnosed in 1960, colon and ureteral carcinoma in 1980, and bronchogenic carcinoma in 1983. All four cancers were treated surgically with apparent success.

She was admitted by a pulmonary physician because of asthma. In the admitting physical examination, an enlarged liver was detected. Several defects were noted on liver scan, and an oncologist was consulted to consider which primary was responsible.

Fine needle aspiration of the liver yielded smears composed of carcinoma cells interpreted as breast cancer. At this point, the breasts were reexamined, and an ill-defined area of induration was palpated in the medial aspect of the right breast (Fig. A-37). Fine needle aspiration yielded smears identical to the liver aspiration.

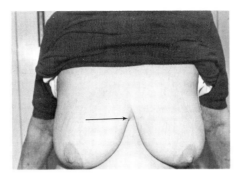

FIGURE A-37: Tumor of right breast. A barely perceptible alteration is evident (*arrow*). There was a hard nodule on palpation. It yielded carcinoma on fine needle aspiration. This patient had five primary cancers in all.

Further dissemination occurred, including right axillary nodal metastases.

COMMENT The importance of careful cytologic review is illustrated in this case. In problem cases, the clinician should discuss differential diagnosis and request tumor subclassification, if possible, from the cytopathologist.

Case A-12

This patient was a 53-year-old man. He had right supraclavicular nodal enlargement when he first was seen in 1982. Fine needle aspiration yielded smears suspicious for Hodgkin's disease, and surgical biopsy followed. The diagnosis was Hodgkin's disease, mixed cellularity. Clinical workup, including laparotomy, splenectomy, and liver biopsy, resulted in a diagnosis of pathologic stage IV based on findings of liver infiltration with Hodgkin's disease.

He was treated with alternating MOPP and ABVD chemotherapy programs with apparent complete remission. He then was followed at regular intervals with examinations and laboratory studies until June 1984, when he was involved in an automobile accident. Ultimately, a chest x-ray was ordered on August 1, 1984. It revealed multiple bilateral pulmonary nodules, with a radiographic diagnosis of metastatic carcinoma (Fig. A-38). At this time, the patient was afebrile and had a dry cough, but looked and felt well (Fig. A-39). He had been losing weight by dieting but maintained a satisfactory appetite.

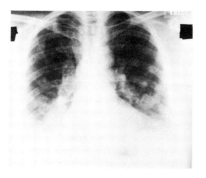

FIGURE A-38: Chest x-ray. There are multiple bilateral nodules on the lower lobes.

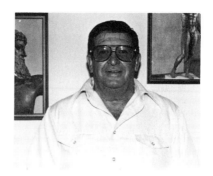

FIGURE A-39: Patient, aged 53, looked robust when the abnormal x-ray was obtained.

There was a long-term history of smoking cigarettes. The clinical differential diagnosis was metastatic carcinoma versus extranodal Hodgkin's disease. Fine needle aspiration of a pulmonary mass under fluoroscopic control was done as an outpatient procedure.

The cytologic smears were composed of necrosis intermixed with poorly differentiated carcinoma cells singly and in clusters.

Second malignancies after therapy for Hodgkin's disease are increasing in frequency.[1,2]

Case A-13

The patient was a robust, stocky, 52-year-old butcher who worked until the day he visited his physician, complaining of a tight abdomen. On examination, his abdomen was enlarged and firm. No organ enlargement was detected, and there was no fluid wave. On digital examination of the prostate, induration was noted. He was treated symptomatically, but returned in 2 weeks with right upper abdominal pain and vomiting. He was hospitalized and was started on intravenous fluids and suction.

Small bowel obstruction was relieved at laparotomy. Tissue submitted was inflammatory. The surgeon was unable to explore the abdomen thoroughly because the bowel was bound at numerous sites. Convalescence was delayed.

A CT scan failed to reveal a localized mass. A barium study demonstrated multiple areas of external compression (Fig. A-40). On palpation, an ill-defined elevated area was detected with the flat of the hand, and fine needle aspiration was done (Fig. A-41).

Smears consisted of dispersed, poorly differentiated carcinoma cells. At this point, fine needle aspiration of the prostate yielded poorly differentiated carcinoma, establishing the primary.

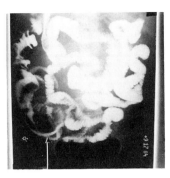

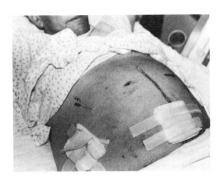

FIGURE A-40: Small bowel x-ray study. There are multiple loops of bowel with external compression (*arrow*).

FIGURE A-41: Direct bedside puncture of palpable, though ill-defined, mass yielded poorly differentiated carcinoma. Needle with stylus is *in situ.*

COMMENT Induration of the prostate, even though not typically malignant, warrants a fine needle biopsy, particularly in an obscure case. It is to be noted that tissue obtained at surgery failed to provide a positive diagnosis. This is not a rare event, and postoperative fine needle aspiration often will demonstrate malignant cells.

Case A-14

The patient was a 69-year-old retired violinist treated over a period of 3 years for multiple myeloma. He had sustained considerable loss of weight. He was studied as an outpatient for several weeks because of anorexia, malaise, and low-grade fever. Admission was prompted by an onset of abdominal pain. His liver was palpable at 4 cm, irregular, and slightly tender.

A liver scan (Fig. A-42) revealed a number of hepatic defects consistent with metastatic carcinoma. This was followed by an ultrasound study interpreted as showing an irregular defect (Fig. A-43). Following this, a CT scan revealed a major irregular defect in the right lobe (Fig. A-44). Finally, a gallium scan revealed a hot area in the right lobe consistent with abscess formation (Fig. A-45).

At this point, fine needle aspiration of the area yielded pus and a culture positive for anaerobic streptococcus. Treatment with antibiotics for 6 weeks resulted in resolution of the process. Total time spent in the hospital was 10 weeks. Time from admission to diagnosis was 4 weeks.

COMMENT It is evident that the profusion of studies could have been circumvented by the judicious application of fine needle aspiration early in the course.

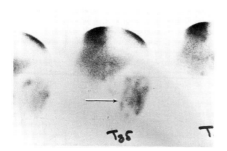

FIGURE A-42: Liver scan with multiple defects (*arrow*).

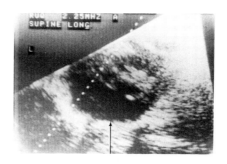

FIGURE A-43: Ultrasonogram with defect (*arrow*).

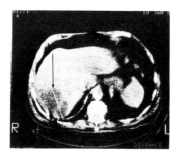

FIGURE A-44: CT scan with defect (*arrow*).

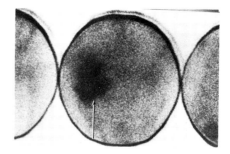

FIGURE A-45: Gallium scan with hot spot (*arrow*).

Case A-15

A 72-year-old man sought medical attention for severe backache. He had a slight fever and sedimentation rate of 100 mm/h (Westegren). On bone scan, pathologic changes were seen in the cervical and the lumbar vertebrae. X-ray films revealed a destructive lesion in the fourth lumbar vertebra, and metastasis from an undetected carcinoma was suspected.

Aspiration biopsy of the lumbar lesion was done under fluoroscopic control (Fig. A-46). The smears consisted of necrotic exudate with intact and necrotic granulocytes present (Fig. A-47). Diagnosis was osteomyelitis (spondylitis).

Following treatment with appropriate antibiotics, the destructive lesion healed.

COMMENT An important clinical point is made by this case. For example, this patient could have had a primary carcinoma at some time in the past. Now, with the presence of two hot spots on a scan

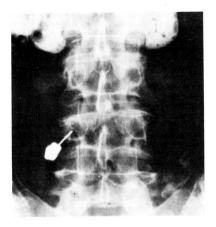

FIGURE A-46: X-ray film of lumbar spine with destructive lesion and needle *in situ.*

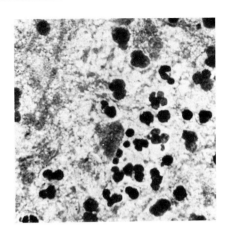

FIGURE A-47: Aspiration cytology. This is a partially necrotic inflammatory exudate.

and a lytic lesion, he might have become a candidate for therapy. The ease of fine needle aspiration of a lesion of this type should prevent any clinical misjudgments.

Case A-16

This patient was a 40-year-old man (Fig. A-48) who complained of pain when sitting. He was comfortable only with his feet up on his desk. He walked with a wide gait.

On initial review, results of a rectal examination were considered negative. A urologist believed the prostate was slightly indurated, and he did an aspiration, which yielded increased lymphocytes.

The patient was referred to the hematology service for a bone marrow study with presumptive diagnosis of lymphoma. The prostate was reexamined with deep palpation before the bone marrow puncture, and a mass was detected above the prostate. CT scan was ordered (Fig. A-49). It demonstrated a large pelvic mass.

Fine needle aspiration was carried out, and yielded smears diagnostic of schwannoma. The surgical specimen measured 10 cm in greatest dimension (Fig. A-50).

The patient was free of symptoms for 2 years.

COMMENT The clinical picture of a deep-seated lesion causing pressure was compelling. Deeper palpation identified the pathology, and fine needle aspiration allowed rational planning of a surgical procedure.

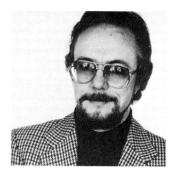

FIGURE A-48: Patient (aged 40) complained of pain on sitting, and had a wide gait.

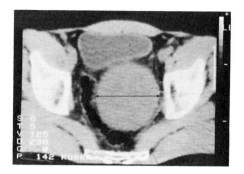

FIGURE A-49: CT scan of pelvis. This large mass (*arrow*) was detected on deep rectal palpation.

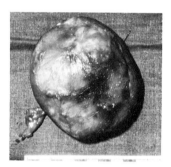

FIGURE A-50: Gross surgical specimen of a resected schwannoma.

Case A-17

The patient was a 56-year-old man who had a left upper quadrant mass with the contour of splenomegaly (Fig. A-51). General examination and bone marrow study were not revealing. His coagulation measurements were normal. A fine needle aspiration of the enlarged "organ" was done. It yielded dark reddish-brown fluid.

Contrast material was instilled into the cystic lesion, and a huge pancreatic cyst was revealed (Fig. A-52).

COMMENT The puncture of pancreatic and mesenteric cysts with a fine needle has not been accompanied by morbidity in our experience.

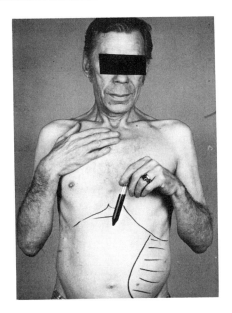

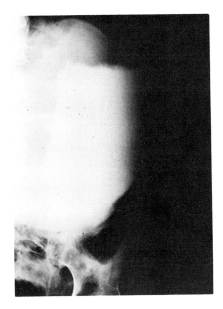

FIGURE A-51: The patient had a large palpable left upper quadrant mass (*horizontal lines*). Surprisingly, fine needle aspiration yielded fluid (*test tube*).

FIGURE A-52: X-ray film of abdomen. Contrast has been instilled, outlining a large pancreatic cyst.

Case A-18

This patient was a 32-year-old woman whose left thigh had been enlarged for several months (Fig. A-53). On palpation, a large tumor was evident in the medial aspect. Fine needle aspiration yielded smears diagnostic of a pleomorphic mesenchymal tumor (Fig. A-54).

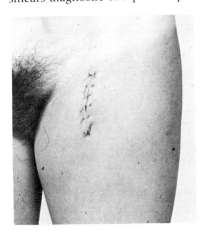

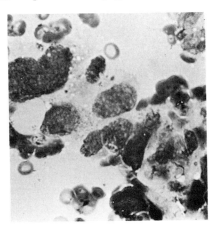

FIGURE A-53: Swollen left thigh with incisional biopsy site.

FIGURE A-54: Aspiration cytology. This is a pleomorphic sarcoma.

Local biopsy was done (see Fig. A-53), and the same diagnosis was rendered on histopathologic examination (Fig. A-55).

The patient was treated with radiation therapy, with considerable shrinkage of the mass. One month later, the entire mass was excised (Fig. A-56). Figure A-57 shows the postoperative appearance. The patient was symptom free at 5 years (Fig. A-58).

COMMENT Preoperative diagnosis allows presurgical radiation. In this case, surgical biopsy was done to confirm the cytology, but this is often not necessary.

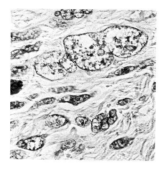

FIGURE A-55: Tissue section. Pleomorphic mesenchymal sarcoma.

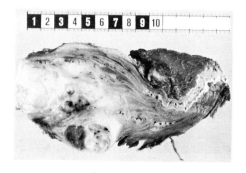

FIGURE A-56: Gross surgical specimen. The tumor exhibited marked effects of radiation.

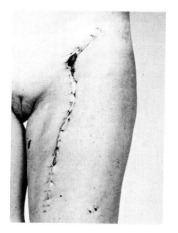

FIGURE A-57: Postoperative appearance of thigh.

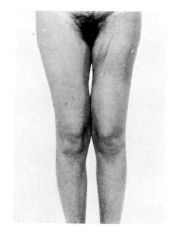

FIGURE A-58: Appearance of legs 5 years after treatment.

Case A-19

The patient had a palpable mass in his left bicep. Fine needle aspiration yielded 5 mL of thick brown fluid (Fig. A-59). Repeat aspiration of the indurated area yielded smears consistent with a poorly differentiated fibrosarcoma (Fig. A-60). The patient's arm is shown postoperatively in Figure A-61. He was operated on twice more, and then was treated with radiotherapy. He died 3 years after diagnosis of lung metastases.

COMMENT The patient's future often is determined by the first surgical intervention.

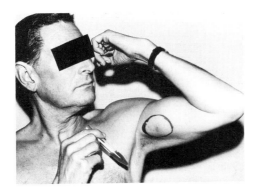

FIGURE A-59: Palpable mass (*circled*) of the left bicep. Removal of fluid (*test tube*) left residual induration.

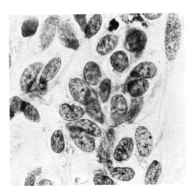

FIGURE A-60: Aspiration cytology. Spindle cell tumor.

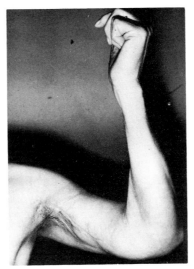

FIGURE A-61: Postoperative appearance of the arm.

Case A-20

A 52-year-old woman presented with a swelling at the metatarso-phalangeal joint of the right foot (Fig. A-62). Consultation with the rheumatology service, together with x-ray films of the foot, led to referral for fine needle aspiration.

The smear yielded a cytologic picture characteristic of synovioma (Fig. A-63).

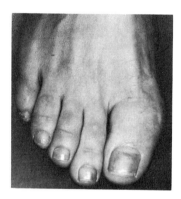

FIGURE A-62: Swelling at the first metatarsophalangeal joint simulated gout.

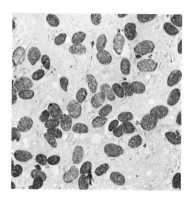

FIGURE A-63: Aspiration cytology. Oval cells are characteristic of synovioma.

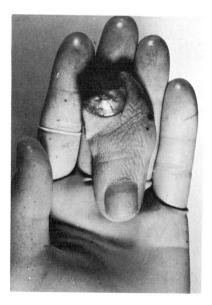

FIGURE A-64: Gross surgical specimen.

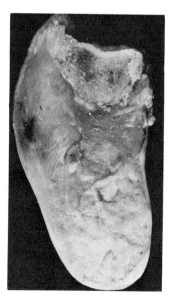

FIGURE A-65: Hemisection of specimen demonstrates tumor near the resection edge.

Aspiration was done, and the toe was amputated (Fig. A-64). Lengthwise section of the specimen demonstrates tumor at the resection edge (Fig. A-65). The disease disseminated, and the patient died of metastasis within 2 years.

COMMENT The presurgical diagnosis of synovioma should have permitted better planning and a more radical procedure.

Concluding Remarks

In these 20 cases, as in others throughout this book, we have sampled disease processes from head to toe. No region of the body is sequestered from access by the fine needle. In many cases, diagnosis was immediate. In others, the patient experienced an array of examinations, studies, and even surgical procedures before the diagnosis was documented.

Surprise findings that stimulate the thought processes and challenge the imagination appear regularly, to the delight of the thoughtful physician.

Once more, there is an opportunity for the practicing clinician to retain control of his patient without referral to many, often remote, specialists, or reliance on expensive technological procedures. Certainly this does not occur in all cases, but the potential exists.

Ordering a simple chest x-ray for diagnosis was hardly routine before 1950. The applications of radiology have proliferated during this period, because clinicians have become schooled in its marvelous ramifications and have employed it accordingly. In like fashion, fine needle aspiration should become an important tool in the clinician's armamentarium as the years pass. We hope this book will be a starting point for clinicians.

An old aphorism about patients and disease is worth remembering: More is missed in medicine by not looking than by not knowing!

REFERENCES
1. Brody RS, Schottenfeld D, Reid A: Multiple primary cancer risk after therapy for Hodgkin's disease. Cancer 40:1917, 1977
2. Schomberg PJ, Evans RG, Banks PM et al: Second malignant lesions after therapy for Hodgkin's disease. Mayo Clin Proc 59:493, 1984

Subject Index

The letter *f* following a page number indicates a figure; the letter *t* following a page number indicates a table.

Case History Index

The letter *f* following a page number indicates a figure.